Age and Anthropological Theory

Age and Anthropological Theory

Edited by DAVID I. KERTZER *and* JENNIE KEITH

with a Foreword by Matilda White Riley

Cornell University Press / Ithaca / London

First published 1984 by Cornell University Press.
Published in the United Kingdom by Cornell University Press Ltd., London.

International Standard Book Number (cloth) 0-8014-1567-5
International Standard Book Number (paper) 0-8014-9258-0
Library of Congress Catalog Card Number 83-21060
Printed in the United States of America

*Librarians: Library of Congress cataloging information
appears on the last page of the book.*

*The paper in this book is acid-free and meets the guidelines
for permanence and durability of the Committee on Production
Guidelines for Book Longevity of the Council on Library Resources.*

To MEYER FORTES, whose wisdom
and humanity remain a cherished memory

Foreword

A central challenge to social scientists today is how to deepen one's own discipline while at the same time broadening it through the pertinent new paradigms and knowledge developing in other disciplines. In much the same way that such important scientific specialties as biochemistry and neuroscience have crystallized at the junctures between disciplines, a multidisciplinary approach to age is now emerging. While anthropologists were among the first to recognize the social and cultural importance of age, the recent work in this area has been done largely in sociology and psychology. For anthropology to play its full part in these developments, a sharper conceptual framework is needed.

This volume speaks to this need. It examines the implications of a focus on age for theoretical development in the various realms of anthropology, in the belief that attention to age can act as a potent stimulus to the development of anthropological theory. Age impinges on social organization, for social roles are often linked to age. Aging is a universal process, experienced by every individual. Moreover, different people conceive of age in different ways. In all of these respects—in terms of social structure, the life course of individuals, and culture—age is clearly a major variable, but it has yet to receive the systematic attention it deserves. The essays in this volume address the question of how investigations of these manifold aspects of age can help to develop deeper insight into areas of traditional anthropological concern, such as domestic groups, kinship, political organization, and sociolinguistics.

This book is addressed primarily to the broad spectrum of anthropologists, whose perusal of the diverse and thought-provoking ideas presented here may stimulate them to consider the relevance of age for their own work, and thereby to contribute to the enrichment of anthropological theory. It is required reading as well for scholars in other disciplines who are concerned either with age as a feature of social organization or with aging over the life course from birth to death.

The initial impetus for the essays in this volume was a workshop organized by the Behavioral Sciences Research program of the National Institute on Aging (NIA) held in Bethesda, Maryland, on March 26–27, 1981. As preparation for the workshop, participants were exposed to a common set of background readings, now admirably synthesized in the section of the editors' introduction devoted to recent developments in the study of age in related disciplines. At the opening of the workshop, four principles from these background readings were enunciated:

- Aging can be understood only in dynamic terms. The aging process cannot be separated from the social, cultural, and historical changes that surround it. People do not grow up and grow old in laboratories. Therefore, we must learn how different cohorts age and how society itself is changed by these differences.
- Aging can be understood only from the perspective of its socioculturally patterned variability, both within a single society and across societies.
- Aging can be understood only within the framework of the total life course. People do not begin to age at any specific point in life. Rather, aging occurs from birth (or earlier) up until death. And within the total society, people of all ages are interdependent.
- Individual aging, wherever and whenever it occurs, consists of a complex interplay among biological aging, psychological aging, and interactions with the changing social and cultural environment.

It should be obvious from these basic principles that anthropologists have a great and as yet largely untapped contribution to make to the interdisciplinary study of age and aging. The necessity of studying human lives in their natural context, with emphasis on the complex interplay between cultural norms and social behavior, has long been a central anthropological tenet. Moreover, anthropologists, along with other social scientists, have become increasingly concerned in recent years with describing and explaining culture and behavior from a historical perspective.

The study of sociocultural variability, so important to research on age, is a central feature of anthropology, and anthropologists have made major contributions to scientific understanding of the myriad ways in which age is employed in various societies. Anthropologists have performed a valuable service, too, in cautioning against overgeneralizations from a limited range of societies regarding "universal" processes of age and aging. But though the study of aging from birth to death has deep roots in anthropology, the early work in ethnography and in culture and personality has led to few recent efforts in this direction. As the editors note in their introduction, despite the prominence of the concept of life stages in earlier anthropological work, this concept has so far been little developed beyond the descriptive level.

Finally, study of the interplay between biological and sociocultural forces in accounting for human behavior is one of the organizing principles of anthropology, particularly in the United States. American anthropology's traditional "four-field" approach to human study, with its requirement that both the biological and the cultural diversity of humankind be explored and interrelated, makes anthropology an especially fertile ground for research on the biological and cultural determinants of patterns of aging and age relationships. This book's chapters on primates and on human growth and development nicely sketch some of the important research that remains to be done in this area.

The authors' considered statements and those of the editors in their introduction identify a wide range of anthropological contributions, both actual and potential, to a fuller and more systematic understanding of age in such areas as norms, symbol and ritual, marriage and family, kinship, and power and conflict. One specific area of inquiry on marriage and family systems, for example, concerns the circumstances in which certain societies develop a large age differential between husband and wife. From a sociobiological perspective, the common pattern among higher nonhuman primates is for males to mate at older ages than females. The economic perspective points to the characteristic role of the human male in the productive process and his related need to acquire capital or expertise before he marries. Also involved are cultural norms and practices with regard to age at first marriage and to the remarriage of widows, for the greater the age differential between husband and wife, the greater the frequency of widowhood. Such differing perspectives illustrate how age and aging offer, in the words of the editors, "the nexus of biological, social, and cultural realities that anthropologists specialize in unraveling."

Prototypically anthropological, of course, is the cross-cultural approach, which can attack fundamental questions as to the sociocultural conditions that influence both the operation of age in the social structure and the variations in the aging process. Among such questions in the area of ritual and symbolism, for example, one focus for theory is on the circumstances in which age is most likely to be elaborated symbolically, with rituals marking age boundaries through which individuals pass. Perhaps, it is suggested, the rate of societal change may have a curvilinear relationship to intensification of age symbolism and ritual, as the hierarchical aspects of age may be ritually enforced in highly stable societies, while in highly fluid societies, as peers become significant sources of norm definition, conflict based on age may become more probable. A related focus of anthropological inquiry concerns the conditions in which age (as compared with class or ethnicity) becomes particularly salient as a basis for social interaction and social stratification. For example, does the development of strong kinship groupings, which are age heterogeneous, leave less room for age as a principle of social groupings? Are strong peer groups most often found in societies where kin are least well equipped to socialize their young? How is age involved in political power? Are older people, for example, more or less likely to enjoy positions of political influence in societies where they constitute only a small proportion of the population?

These are only a few of the directions in which anthropological theory may turn in a full-scale exploration of age and aging. Several emphases for such exploration are developed throughout this book: in cross-cultural terms, age and aging constitute an empirical domain about which little is known; they offer variables that promise to refine anthropological theory and offer a potential focus for theoretical development in their own right.

Such guidelines for future inquiry, coupled with the storehouse of existing facts and ideas, make this book a first of its kind in anthropology and an invaluable contribution to the emerging multidisciplinary study of age in society and aging over the life course.

MATILDA WHITE RILEY

National Institute on Aging
Bethesda, Maryland

Contents

Part Three   **Age and Culture**

Preface

This book admittedly aims to proselytize. We believe that the goals of anthropology can be significantly advanced if we pay more systematic attention to the role of age in human societies and cultural systems and to the variable nature of the life course. Of course, these subjects are hardly new to anthropologists. Quite the contrary; anthropologists have long been documenting the many ways in which age is employed in various societies and the rich diversity in the ways various cultures conceptualize and subdivide the life course. We believe, however, that not enough has been done to bring these ethnographic insights together in a more general theoretical framework, or frameworks, so that we can further advance our theoretical knowledge of the way social and cultural systems operate. Such work would not only benefit the development of anthropology as a discipline, it would also increase the impact of anthropology on the life-course research now flourishing in such neighboring disciplines as sociology, psychology, and social history.

The idea for this book originated in discussions between Matilda White Riley and David Kertzer in the late 1970s, shortly after Riley had become associate director for social and behavioral science research at the National Institute on Aging. Soon thereafter Jennie Keith joined in the early planning stages. In attempting to take stock of the importance of age and the life course to theoretical development in the mainstream of anthropology, we solicited the participation of anthropologists who had been en-

13

gaged in important theoretical work relevant to age, yet who had not previously focused their attention on age and the life course. We were eager to have these scholars consider how more systematic attention to the social use of age and cultural conceptions of the life course might profit their own subfields of interest. In other words, our intent was not to persuade people to abandon their own interests in anthropology, but rather to enrich them through systematic use of the age variable and the life-course perspective.

The book that grew out of these discussions is divided into three sections, each covering a broad area. In Part One the topic of age, evolution, and biology is addressed. The implications of age for research in biological anthropology are assessed, with one chapter on primate studies and another discussing age and life-course perspectives in human biological studies. Part Two considers how increased attention to age can further our understanding of social organization. Special emphasis is given to principles underlying kinship, domestic groups, economics, and power relations. Finally, in Part Three the multifarious links between age and culture are discussed. After an assessment of age as a variable in sociolinguistic research, the focus shifts to consideration of the way age is embedded in cultural systems and incorporated in symbolism and ritual. The authors relate their far-flung ethnographic examples—from India, China, Africa, Europe, South and North America—to a more abstract concern. Our goal is the full incorporation of age and the life course in the development of anthropological theory. This book begins to specify some benefits of that increased attention to age and the life course.

All but two of the chapters in this book are based on presentations to a workshop held at NIA headquarters; the exceptions are Rhoda Halperin's chapter on cultural economics and Ákos Östör's on symbolism and time. These chapters represent attempts to fill in important areas of anthropology not covered in the workshop. We would have liked to cover other areas, such as political anthropology, and we have tried to deal with some of those subfields at least briefly in our introduction. We hope our effort here may encourage scholars in some of those fields as well to turn their attention to the importance of age and aging.

The success of the workshop that generated this book was in good part the result of the outstanding work done by the NIA staff. Special mention should be made of Shirley Bagley's contribution in overseeing administrative arrangements and ensuring that the workshop went so smoothly and productively. Thanks are also due to Ron Abeles and other NIA staff members for their great help. We are also grateful to Pauline Federman and Helen Di Feliciantonio at Swarthmore College and to Julie Hodgkins and Jean Lee at Bowdoin College for preparation of the manuscript. Jennie Keith thanks Mary Etta Zwell of Project A.G.E. at Swarthmore for indispensable sleuthing and prodding. David Kertzer also thanks the Center for Advanced Study in the Behavioral Sciences, Stanford, where he was able to work on the final stages of the manuscript, supported in part by the John and Catherine MacArthur Foundation. A large role in the success of the workshop was played by Margaret Clark and Doris Mayer, who acted as discussants.

This whole endeavor has been made possible by the intellectual stimulation and prodigious organizational abilities of Matilda White Riley, one of the major figures in the development of the sociological study of age and a major influence in the interdisciplinary study of age and aging. To her we express our deep thanks and appreciation.

DAVID I. KERTZER

Stanford, California

JENNIE KEITH

Swarthmore, Pennsylvania

Age and Anthropological Theory

Introduction

Jennie Keith and David I. Kertzer

"What's in it for us?" That was the forthright question put to partici-pants in the workshop on age and anthropological theory which stimu-lated the papers in this volume.[1] The role of anthropologists in the recent expansion of social-scientific research on age and aging has been pri-marily altruistic: anthropology has given more than it has received to the life-course perspective emerging in sociology and psychology. An-thropologists, in their familiar role as purveyors of exotic data, have influenced life-course theorists in other disciplines, but as yet there has been little consideration of these neighboring developments by an-thropologists. Each author at the workshop was therefore asked to consid-er the implications of increased attention to the life course and age for a major anthropological subfield. All of the participants had done work with significance for cross-cultural study of the life course, but few had seen themselves as specialists on age or aging.

Our starting point was the idea that both individual aging and the use of age as a principle in social organization must be taken into account in attempts to discover patterns of human behavior. The emphasis is not on

1. We are grateful for the comments of Paul Baltes, Cynthia Beall, Glen Elder, James Fernandez, Renate Fernandez, Meyer Fortes, Christine L. Fry, Richard Lerner, and Sherry Ortner.

the product of the aging process but on the process itself and its relationships to social, cultural, and historical context. The following chapters point out significant aspects of aging and age: (1) in cross-cultural terms, age and the life course are *empirical* domains about which little is known; (2) age and aging offer *variables* whose inclusion will refine theory in many areas of anthropology; (3) age and the life course offer a potential focus for *theoretical development* in their own right.

There are certain universal biological principles of aging—all humans enter the world as dependent infants, gradually grow and acquire greater capacities, and ultimately die—with which all societies must cope if they are to survive and which all cultural systems manage in one way or another. In seeking a better understanding of age and the life course, we are interested not only in the direct relationship between these biological processes and their social implications but also in the very diverse ways in which peoples develop symbolic systems that conceptualize the life course and the process of time itself. While age can be conceived simply in terms of chronology, this perspective is satisfactory neither for the biological anthropologist, who notes a disjunction between chronological and biological time, nor for the social-cultural anthropologist, who sees the life course as culturally constructed. Indeed, in our study of different cultures the biological definition of the life course as beginning at birth (or conception) and ending at death may be too constraining. People's earthly lives may be seen as part of a continuum that extends beyond the material realm.

Two questions provide an appropriate introduction to the role of age in anthropology. First, why have anthropologists not paid more theoretical attention in recent years to general issues of the use of age in human societies and the varying cultural conceptions of the life course? Second, why should we pay more attention to these issues in our future efforts— what's in it for us? As structuralists point out, ambiguous category boundaries are often perceived as dangerous and are usually subjected to mythic elaboration. Age appears to have received this treatment from some anthropologists. As cultural specialists, sociocultural anthropologists are hypersensitive to the clarity of nature/culture boundaries; high priests rush to the rescue when these boundaries are threatened by too much stress on the biological aspects of human adaptations. Perhaps because of its continuous and dynamic biological basis, age has been even more eligible for assignment to the nature or biology side of the boundary than such characteristics as kinship and sex, whose biological foundations are more stable. A mythologized view of age has been presented in which age is a primitive element of society, always superseded as more complex principles, such as kinship, emerge (e.g., Needham 1974, Schurtz 1902). As Meyer Fortes points out, however, in human communities "nothing is nature." We might add: "but culture makes it so." Since all of human culture rests on a biological foundation, each community's definition of the nature/culture boundary is part of a cultural map, and a promising topic for anthropological investigation.

From another angle, as the physical anthropologists at the workshop observed, human aging may be seen as a product, or by-product, of culture. Phyllis Dolhinow's chapter makes clear, for example, that the social support required for longevity is not extended to other primates, who are permitted dependence only in infancy. It has been proposed that experienced elders offered adaptive advantages in human—and therefore cultural—populations (Katz 1978). The intricacy and subtlety of the biological/cultural interweave that makes age a difficult subject also offer a fitting topic for anthropological analysis. Such efforts will require that physical anthropologists extend their view of development beyond maturity, as Cynthia Beall's chapter argues, and that physical and sociocultural anthropologists work jointly to develop cross-cultural approaches to human aging. If, as David Maybury-Lewis states in his chapter, a theory of age is impossible except as part of a theory of society, then the converse is also true. Adequate theories of society must take account of aging and age.

Previous Anthropological Research on Age and the Life Course

The subject of age has appeared in the ethnographies and theoretical work of anthropologists, but those appearances have been limited in revealing ways (see Keith 1980a, Fry 1980, Fry n.d., Holmes 1976, Keith n.d. for reviews of anthropological research on age). First, most work on age as domain, variable, or theoretical focus has been done in those societies where physical aging is most firmly under cultural control through formal systems of age grades, groups, and sets. More recent analysis of the role of age in these societies has been broadened in several ways significant for the life-course perspective. Anthropologists are asking new questions about old systems, and also taking some old interests to new places. The relationship of age systems to other aspects of social organization is now a major question, which in turn raises more complex questions about geographic distribution of formal age systems. If age sets do not always provide warriors, if they are not always active politically, then under what conditions do they appear? And how is age related to other principles of social organization? (See Stewart 1977, Baxter and Almagor 1978, Foner and Kertzer 1978, Kertzer 1978 for recent reviews of formal age systems.) Maybury-Lewis' chapter on age and kinship in Central Brazil discusses the complementarity of these two principles in public and private, male and female spheres of social action.

The presence of a case from Central Brazil represents another way in which research on formal age systems has broadened its horizons: such studies have gotten away from an almost exclusively African focus. Identification of the social significance of age with a particular type of formal system found in East Africa has been an obstacle to thorough analysis of age in society. Extension of geographic range, even in the study of formal structures, is an important step toward consideration of wider variation, and is thus also a step toward consideration of different uses of age, including those that are less formal and explicit. Just as not all kinship systems have unilineal descent groups, age categories and prescribed social relationships based on age exist in the absence of elaborate age setting. Especially in those societies where age has its greatest salience in private and informal domains, greater attention to age will fill out the ethnographic record in the same ways as recent research on sex roles has helped to correct the previous bias toward public, formal (and predominantly male) culture.

Discrepancies between age-set norms and behavior have also introduced a wider life-course view in interpretation of formal age systems. Age sets have long evoked the image of egalitarian brotherhood. Agemates, however, do not always put these values into action. Fraternal ties among adolescents may weaken under the strain of power differentials in the middle years (Almagor 1978). Parallels between old people in many industrial societies and the young warrior age grades famous in ethnographic literature suggest that there may be a life-stage aspect to age-set egalitarianism. Residents in many types of retirement housing in the United States, France, and England create communities whose egalitarian norms are expressed in such frequently heard statements as "We're all old people here" (Keith 1980b, 1982a). Age equality appears most likely to be invoked by those who are equally excluded from major resources and arenas of decision making. In many communities, those in the age categories that precede and follow social maturity have less access to resources and influence than those in the middle years, although they are physically capable of full social participation. They are consequently most likely to appeal to age equality as a source of leverage for agemate solidarity and as a protective insulation from the consequences of a low rank on the status ladder outside the age group. The error of equating age sets and egalitarianism came from failure to place peer ties in a life-course context: ties to agemates have various meanings at various life stages, in various cultural contexts, at various historical moments (see Almagor 1978, Keith 1982b).

Ethnographers have also described the hierarchical aspect of age relations in reports of societies labeled gerontocracies. Here, too, static perspectives have produced distortion. As more recent analyses point out, many powerful elders, as among the Tiwi of Australia, achieved their positions through lifetimes spent shrewdly accumulating both material and social resources. Although seniority may have been a requisite for their achievements, it was not an ascriptive guarantee (Almagor 1978). Even in such societies as Samburu, where authority, often ritually based, is ascribed to the old, variation appears within their cohort in ability to command respect and obedience. The life-course perspective on gerontocracy produces a more accurate if less exotic picture, and in doing so makes comparison across societies more plausible. The ritual curses of elder age grades may be interpreted as the use of an ascriptive rationale in an attempt to maintain achieved position. Viewed in this more abstract manner, the gerontocratic strategy may well appear in modern societies where old people organize to protect financial gains now threatened by economic and political change (Keith 1982b:chap. 6). Formal age systems have also both waxed and waned in historical times, offering an opportunity for exploration of factors that promote cultural elaboration of age as well as a warning that even in the most rigidly defined age structures time seeps in to shape the experiences of members of different cohorts (Buxton 1958, Le Vine and Sangree 1962).

A second and by now classic way in which age has appeared in the anthropological literature has been in the "life-cycle" approach taken in ethnographic reports. Many ethnographies, particularly those written in earlier decades, contain a chapter headed "Life Cycle"; many have several chapters or subsections headed "Infancy," "Adulthood," "Old Age." These descriptions of age norms and sometimes age-related behavior, however, are seldom used in the other chapters as integral parts of the analysis of other aspects of social life. The life course itself is seldom seriously considered as a cultural unit—that is, as it is culturally defined as a whole—or subdivided into life stages (Fry and Keith 1982). S. F. Nadel's (1952) analysis of witchcraft in Sudan is an early exception, as he correlates the number of age grades and their consequent congruence to physical capability with patterns of intergenerational witchcraft accusation. Recent quantitative cross-cultural research reveals the relationship between recognition of two categories of old people, the "intact" and the "decrepit," and their differential treatment. Even in societies in which older people are prescribed an honored position, they may be abandoned or killed if they enter the "decrepit" category (Glascock and Feinman 1980). Ethnoscientific study of age categories has been carried out among Masai and in an American city (Kirk and Burton 1977, Fry 1976). Formal analysis of age terms revealed the following: key dimensions, such as responsibility, underlying cognitive organization of life-course categories; correlations between social characteristics, including life stage, of respondents and the number of age categories they identified; personality traits attributed to individuals and the age categories to which they were assigned. The meaning of an entire life also varies as a unit for planning and evaluation. The number, content, and interrelations of "careers," such as occupational, ritual, or reproductive careers, into which life may be divided are variable. Cultural prescriptions of a normative road map for life also vary in both content and strictness (Le Vine 1978, Fry and Keith 1982).

Although life history has long been an important anthropological technique, the resulting information has not often been used to interpret life-course processes themselves. Life histories have more often been employed as sources for "salvage ethnography" of vanishing groups and as evidence of child-rearing practices. Such anthropologists as Barbara Myerhoff and Gelya Frank are now using life histories as a means of understanding culturally shaped responses to old age as well (Langness and Frank 1981 review life history as a technique in anthropology).

Anthropologists have burned the life-course candle at both ends. Until recently the only life stages examined thoroughly in terms of human development, norms, and transitions were those at the youthful end (Mead 1928, J. Whiting and Child 1953, B. Whiting 1963). In the last fifteen years, anthropological research has also been focused on the latter end of the life course, but with some of the same restrictions that limited work on youth. An early and continuing theme in anthropological work on old age, for example, is that of status and treatment. Since Leo

Simmons' landmark review of the information on old age in the Human Relations Area Files, researchers relying primarily on quantitative comparative research methods have attempted to identify societal correlates of the position of old people (Simmons 1945; Press and McKool 1972; Maxwell and Silverman 1970; Glascock and Feinman 1980, 1981). Because in this research old people are usually seen via secondary analyses of data not collected with issues of aging in mind, old age is isolated from the dynamics of both cultural and life-course context. As a source of hypotheses about bases of status and treatment through life, however, these studies are a stimulating springboard for the firsthand ethnographies of age that anthropologists are beginning to do. Clearly, many themes of what is now labeled the life-span or life-course perspective have been present in anthropology throughout much of its history and are more visible now because of recent anthropological study of old age.

The Life-Span Perspective in Psychology and Sociology

The years since the late 1960s have witnessed a remarkable development of perspectives on age in psychology and sociology (Featherman 1981). These achievements are all the more noteworthy because they represent a convergence of the theoretical viewpoints of the two disciplines. Various terms have been given to this new orientation; we use Matilda White Riley's "life-course perspective" (Abeles and Riley 1977). Riley (1979a:4–5) has identified four "central premises" of this perspective:

1. Aging is a lifelong process. . . . It starts with birth (or with conception) and ends with death.
2. Aging consists of three sets of processes—biological, psychological, and social; and these three processes are all systematically interactive with one another over the life course.
3. The life-course pattern of any particular person (or cohort of persons all born at the same time) is affected by social and environmental change (or history).
4. New patterns of aging can cause social change. That is, social change not only molds the course of individual lives but, when many persons in the same cohort are affected in similar ways, the change in their collective lives can in turn also produce social change.

In this perspective, aging is seen as a continuous process of change involving individual-level processes interacting with a changing society. The rapid scholarly adoption of this approach is evident in, among other indicators, the publication of the annual series *Life-Span Development and Human Behavior*. Dedicated to interdisciplinary work, the series is edited by psychologist Paul Baltes and sociologist Orville Brim, Jr. To appreciate the significance of this perspective, whose principles may seem apparent enough at first sight, let us look briefly at what has happened since the late 1960s in psychology and sociology.

Life-Span Developmental Psychology

The psychological study of age and age-related phenomena has traditionally been compartmentalized into limited age categories. Infant specialists had little to do with specialists in adolescence, and neither had any scholarly contact with those who studied old age. This segregation was reflected in professional labels, with "developmental psychology" referring to the study of individuals up to the time of physical maturity and "aging" referring to psychological changes that occur after this point is reached (Birren and Renner 1977:3). Underlying these distinctions was the belief that the individual's various psychological functions mature during childhood and adolescence, reach a plateau at adulthood, and then begin to decline in old age (Baltes, Reese, and Lipsitt 1980:69–70). Thus one series of researchers studied the rise and one the decline, but there was little interest in the plateau.[2]

Although psychology has a long history of interest in the life span, particularly in Germany and Austria (Baltes 1979, Groffman 1970, Reinert 1979, Thomae 1979), the large-scale rejection of the traditional distinction between development and aging came about only in the late 1960s in the United States, under the influence of a group of scholars at the University of Chicago (Havighurst 1948, 1973; Neugarten 1968, 1969, 1977) and, most systematically, a group of developmental psychologists who initially coalesced at West Virginia University in the early 1970s (Goulet and Baltes, eds., 1970; Baltes and Schaie 1973a; Datan and Ginsberg, eds., 1975). Among the most active of these workers have

2. One forcefully stated rejection of this perspective is provided by Hans Thomae (1979:294), who states that the " 'mature' person who remains changeless and motionless in the face of different challenges, threats, and increasing opportunities of the adult years is a stereotype, having no psychological reality." It should also be noted that, coming from a different theoretical orientation in psychology, Erik Erikson (1963) stimulated interest in psychological development beyond childhood.

been Paul Baltes and Warner Schaie, who argue that psychological change takes place throughout the individual's life course, and that psychologists need to examine "life-span change in terms of antecedent conditions and their associated mechanisms" (1973b:369) without assuming that any one part of the life course is necessarily the most important (cf. Brim and Kagan 1980:1). With the burst of scholarly interest in this approach, it is suggested that "a kind of paradigm shift" is now taking place "in the way developmental psychology is conceptualized" (Baltes, Reese, and Lipsitt 1980:67).

When we take a long-term view of human development, the problem of social change becomes evident. Each cohort ages in different historical circumstances and thus individuals' environmental stimuli and opportunities vary with their historical location. Development, then, is not seen simply as the unfolding of a biologically rooted ontogeny in the context of a specified series of environmental variables, but as a complex interaction between biologically determined processes and an ever-changing society. As Baltes and Sherry Willis have suggested (1979:18–19): "traditional developmental psychology's benign neglect of these other change phenomena may have seriously limited the psychological study of ontogenetic change. That is, lack of concern for the biocultural context in which the individual develops may have resulted in an over-emphasis on age-segmented, normative, intraorganismic (personological) models of development."

Of particular interest to anthropologists is the prominence of the concept of the "life event" in recent work in life-span psychology. With chronological age per se being rejected as a meaningful variable, and with a focus on the antecedents of behavior through the life course, research has turned to the study of life events and their impact on individuals. David F. Hultsch and Judy K. Plemons (1979:17) broadly define a life event as a "noteworthy occurrence" in an individual's life. They divide these occurrences into those that are "experienced as a part of the usual life course," such as marriage and the death of a loved one, and "cultural events" that have an exogenous origin but affect individuals, such as warfare and natural catastrophe (1979:18–19). Orville G. Brim and Carol D. Ryff, who have further refined the life-event concept, have gone so far as to argue that "life events are as integral to life-span development theory as are atoms and other lesser particles to physical theory" (1980:368). In short, life events become the basic units for analysis, and the relationship in occurrence, timing, and sequencing of life events (e.g., marriage, death of parent, finishing education, birth of child) provides the data for the study of psychological changes that take place through the life course of the individual.

While life-span psychologists have generally recognized the importance of cultural change through time for an understanding of psychological processes at the individual level, few such studies have been conducted outside the industrialized nations of the West. Yet it is clear that the life-span goal of analytically distinguishing between biologically rooted developmental processes and those that are culturally and historically variable cannot be reached without such cross-cultural study. Indeed, Solomon Cytrynbaum and his colleagues (1980:471), in an article on midlife development for the American Psychological Association handbook on aging research, listed as the number one need for midlife development research in the 1980s the "extension of existing work with predominantly white middle- and upper-class males to women, blue-collar and cross-cultural samples." Among the most active researchers in this field has been David Gutmann, an anthropologically trained psychologist, who observes (1977:302):

> The comparative psychology of aging is a field that lacks concepts, methods, and investigators. Indeed, the useful literature is mainly produced by ethnographers and sociologists, by those with, at best, incidental interest in the psychology of aging.
>
>   . . . we find almost no comparative studies—those conducted by the same investigator(s) using the same tools and theoretical conceptions across cultures—of the sort required to either test or generate a developmental, "species" conception of aging psychology.

The one prominent exception to Gutmann's generalization is his own work, which has involved a comparative psychological study of middle-aged and older individuals in a variety of nonindustrialized societies, including the Mexican Maya, the Navajo, and the Israeli Druze. His goal has been to test his hypothesis that a personality shift is a universal aspect of aging. As women age, he claims, they become more autonomous, competitive, aggressive, and instrumental, while men become more passive, expressive, and dependent. In short, Gutmann sees a universal psychological cross-over effect, a process that could be verified only through the kind of cross-cultural research he has undertaken (Gutmann 1975). He sees his work as taking the framework most often applied to infancy and early childhood—that of biologically rooted ontogenetic development—and applying it to adulthood and old age (1977:303).

The Sociological Study of Age

At the same time as interest in aging throughout the life course has burgeoned in psychology, some sociologists have heralded the emergence of a sociology of age. As in anthropology, there has been sporadic interest in age as a principle of social organization among sociologists (e.g., Sorokin 1941, 1947; Parsons 1942; Eisenstadt 1956), yet only since the late 1960s have systematic attempts been made to construct a framework for the sociological analysis of age (Featherman 1981). Along with these theoretical developments, empirical applications have become increasingly common in such fields as social stratification (Blau and Duncan 1967, Featherman 1980), socialization (Brim 1966, Mortimer and Simmons 1978), and the family (Elder 1978; Hareven 1978/79, 1980; Rossi 1980; Vinovskis 1977).

Since the late 1960s two broad theoretical perspectives have emerged. The publication in 1968 of Bernice L. Neugarten's *Middle Age and Aging,* a product of the University of Chicago's human development program, marked the full emergence of a social-psychological and cultural perspective on age. The emphasis is on how "the individual organizes his life course and interprets his life experience" (Neugarten and Hagestad 1976:35) within a system of societal norms that specify age-appropriate behavior and expectations. The same year marked the publication of the first of three volumes on aging and society by Riley and her associates (1968), a work that culminated in *A Sociology of Age Stratification* (Riley, Johnson, and Foner 1972). With contributions from such scholars as Talcott Parsons, Robert K. Merton, John A. Clausen, and Norman B. Ryder, this volume reflects the development of an approach to the study of age in society which focuses on the societal as well as the individual level.

These two schools have continued to organize much of the theoretical and empirical sociological work on age. They have also proved to be of great relevance to anthropologists, though few anthropologists have heretofore been familiar with both of them. We thus think it useful to provide a summary of the main principles of each approach.

In Neugarten's *sociocultural* approach, people's lives are ordered by societal norms regarding age-appropriate behavior, roles, and status. At the societal level, this system can be viewed as one of social control, bolstered by negative sanctions employed against individuals deemed guilty of age-inappropriate behavior (Neugarten, Moore, and Lowe 1965:713). Each society has its own cultural timetable for an individual's appropriate social progress through the life course, and people's behavior corresponds closely to these norms. Social control is achieved not only through social sanction but also by people's internalization of these norms regarding culturally appropriate timing:

> Age norms and age expectations operate as prods and brakes upon behavior, in some instances hastening an event, in others delaying it. Men and women are aware not only of the social clocks that operate in various areas of their lives, but they are aware also of their own timing and readily describe themselves as "early," or "late," or "on time" with regard to family and occupational events. [Neugarten, Moore, and Lowe 1965:711].

This system of societal age norms is identified with "social time," a concept that Neugarten and Nancy Datan (1973:57) link to the earlier work by anthropologists on age-graded social systems. Each society is characterized by an "age-status system" (Neugarten and Hagestad 1976:35) which, in addition to ordering roles in society on the basis of age and sequence (e.g., jobholder before husband), affects individuals' cognitive maps. People come to have a "mental map of the life cycle" and therefore "anticipate that certain events will occur at certain times" (Neugarten and Hagestad 1976:35).

The affinities of this approach to anthropological paradigms are clear and derive from the involvement of anthropologists in the Chicago human development program. Incorporated, on the one hand, is the anthropological study of formally age-graded societies, which is expanded to handle all societies in the Neugarten formulation. On the other hand, the concern with culture, and especially with a cognitive approach, links this perspective to anthropological work and makes it a congenial approach for many anthropologists.

By contrast, the *age-stratification* approach has thus far been little known and little used by anthropologists.[3] There are both theoretical and practical reasons for this lack of attention. Theoretically, the age-stratification approach puts more emphasis on societal-level elements than on

---

3. For an exception, see A. Foner and Kertzer 1978, 1979.

individuals, and operates at a more abstract level than most anthropological work. Practically, the nucleus of scholars involved in the development of this perspective did not include anthropologists. Moreover, the kinds of historical documentation called for by the age-stratification approach are not often used by anthropologists (Le Vine and Sangree 1962, Legesse 1973, and Lamphear 1976 are outstanding exceptions), so that this approach was initially less appealing than the age-norms approach of Neugarten and her associates.

The age-stratification system consists of a series of age strata, each associated with a bundle of roles and statuses, and a series of cohorts passing through each stratum at different points in historical time. From the societal perspective, age serves as one mechanism (others are sex and social class) which structures roles and allocates individuals to these roles. Individuals must pass from one set of socially structured roles to another as they age, and in doing so they must learn "to adapt to new roles and relinquish old ones" (Riley 1976:191). These changes may constitute a source of strain for the individual, who must leave behind familiar roles (and sometimes the people who go with them) and take on new ones.

A key part of this model is cohort analysis, building on Ryder's (1965) seminal work. A cohort, for these purposes, consists of all individuals (in a specified population) who were born in a certain time period (i.e., a birth cohort). "Cohort" is almost always used in this "etic" sense, although a more "emic" usage has been recommended by Irving Rosow (1978) and employed by Corinne Nydegger (1977) and J. Kevin Eckert (1978). The various cohorts proceed through the age strata at different points in historical time, and thus each is affected in a unique way by historical events. The experiences of each cohort are products of both universal processes of aging and the historically and culturally specific processes that act on the cohort. One of the major aims of the age-stratification approach is to determine how sociohistorical changes are reflected in the way different cohorts age, and how the characteristics of different cohorts may bring about sociohistorical change. In this way, "cohort analysis opens the door to deeper understanding of the systematic interdependence between changes in the lives of individuals and changes in society, both past and future" (Riley 1979b:112).

The age strata through which the cohorts pass are themselves changing over time. These changes reflect economic changes, as when a depression forces children to leave school to supplement their families' income;

political changes, such as wars, which alter the age of marriage and the age of retirement; and demographic changes, such as epidemics, which require socially needed roles to be filled by individuals previously considered too young or too old (Riley, Johnson, and Foner 1972:17). What we see here are alterations over time in age-appropriate norms and practices of allocation of roles, that is, the "set of mechanisms for the continual assignment and reassignment of individuals of given ages to the appropriate roles" (Riley 1976:200). Of course, a society's roles themselves change over time as well.

Cohorts are differentially affected by historical events because of their different age-stratum locations at the time of the events. But cohorts can also be seen as forces for social change, as the characteristics of different cohorts interact with the age-stratification system of the society. As Ryder recognized years ago, an especially large or small cohort may have profound implications for the experience of the members of that cohort and for the society itself (1965:845). Unusually small cohorts may find plentiful opportunities, for the supply of desired roles is greater than the demand (Riley 1976:212). The size of one cohort also may have a great influence on the experience of another, as when the steep rise in the U.S. birth rate following World War II provided tremendous demand for teachers who were members of an earlier cohort (see Waring 1975). Yet the relationship between cohort flow (the succession of cohorts moving through the life course) and social change is, in fact, more complex than simple demographic aspects might indicate, as Riley, Johnson, and Foner (1972:522) point out:

> A particular cohort can be disruptive of existing arrangements if it differs from neighboring cohorts in size, characteristics, or manner of response to early socialization or to historical events. Pressures for change can also be exerted by imperfections in the articulating processes, as allocation and socialization may be out of phase with each other, as socialization may qualify people inadequately for the roles available, or as allocation may fail to assign the numbers and kinds of people appropriate to meet current demands. In such ways, the age-related processes, interacting with one another and with the given role structure, can threaten social stability over the life course of any particular cohort.

As roles in society change, in other words, problems may ensue in the allocation of people and the proper socialization of individuals for the new roles (1972:449).

Cohorts should not be assumed to be homogeneous entities, however. Cohort analysis involves not only intercohort comparisons but also examination of intracohort variation. Since members of the same cohort have different characteristics, they not only may show different life-course patterns but may also be differentially affected by the same historical events. Thus to understand how macro-level processes affect the life course of individuals and to understand better the mechanism by which social change takes place, cohorts must often be disaggregated into appropriate subgroupings on the basis of their characteristics (Elder 1981, Hogan 1981).

One of the ways an age-stratification system may change is as a result of its delegitimization in the eyes of certain cohorts in the society. In any stratification system some strata have more prestigious and rewarding roles than others; thus a familiar issue in the study of stratification arises: Why do people in the lower strata participate in a system in which they appear to be disadvantaged? Anthropologists have often raised this question in regard to reportedly gerontocratic societies that have high rates of polygyny. The answer must be found in the combined study of control of resources, socialization, and ideology.

Sociologists who adopt the age-stratification perspective are interested in the changing experiences of the cohort over time, in relationships at any one point in time among the various cohorts or strata, and in the relationships within an age stratum. The question of age solidarity has received considerable sociological attention since the writings of Karl Mannheim (1952) and S. N. Eisenstadt (1956). A central issue is the extent to which people conceive of themselves as sharing a common identity with others of approximately the same age, and the extent to which their behavior reflects such age solidarity. It is recognized that other social identities cross-cut age, and that these identities may prove to forge more important bonds of solidarity. Implied in age-stratification analysis, then, is the relationship between age as a principle of stratification and other principles of stratification, such as class and sex.

These cross-cutting bases of allegiance can also be seen as a means through which conflict between age strata is reduced. To the extent that people see their basic interests as lying in their lineage membership, for example, they are presumably less likely to form interlineage groupings on the basis of age commonality. This issue has received a great deal of attention in the anthropological literature on African age-group systems, and some scholars argue that a formalized age-group system is incompatible with a strong lineage system (Eisenstadt 1956, Baxter and Almagor 1978:19, Gulliver 1968).

Together with parallel developments in life-span developmental psychology, work in the sociology of age stratification has served to identify several analytical problems in the study of aging and social change. The age-stratification framework makes clear that if the significance of age and the nature of the aging process are to be understood, people must be viewed through time. This may appear to be obvious, yet hundreds of analysts have attempted to base statements about the aging process entirely on cross-sectional data. They have looked at the characteristics of individuals in different cohorts and concluded that the differences among them are due to the aging process in that society (or even to universal properties of aging). Yet such analysts are often guilty of what has been called the "life-course fallacy," that is, neglecting the possibility that differences between cohorts are due not to life-course changes but to the different characteristics and experiences of the cohorts themselves (Riley 1973). Taking the classic case, the fact that older cohorts in the United States were found to receive lower IQ scores than younger cohorts does not mean that intelligence decreases with age. IQ is related to amount of formal education, and older cohorts had received less schooling than younger cohorts.[4]

The related analytical pitfall, the cohort fallacy, is one in which the analyst attributes variation in characteristics between two cohorts to the different slices of history to which they have been exposed. In a familiar example, the fact that older people vote more conservatively than younger people in the United States has sometimes been explained as reflecting the different historical situations in which the cohorts grew up. Yet another possible interpretation is that these are life-course differences, that there is a tendency for people to vote more conservatively as they grow older (Bengtson and Cutler 1976).

As anthropologists we must be aware of this difficulty because so much of our work is based on nonlongitudinal data derived from fieldwork. The age-stratification approach, like the life-span developmental psychology approach, calls for greater emphasis on longitudinal data. While anthropologists often face considerable obstacles in acquiring such data, it is significant that there has been an increased movement toward historical

---

4. Similar fallacies afflict many studies of biological aging, including research on "secular trends" in age at menarche and age at achieving full adult size. See Tanner 1981.

study in anthropology since the early 1970s. Elizabeth Colson and Thayer Scudder's (1978) report on their thirty years of fieldwork among the Gwembe Tonga, for example, offers a superb view of the complex connections of historical change, cohort experience, intergenerational relations, and individual aging. Allocation schemes, for instance, initially weakened the position of older men, who lost valuable land. Eventually, however, the seniority principle was reasserted by another cohort of old men, who had obtained the desirable plots in the new land apportionment of their youth. Nancy Foner's chapter in this volume indicates the light that can be shed on the anthropological study of change through use of an age-stratification perspective.

The Future of Age and the Life Course in Anthropology

Human Development

The two routes to social-scientific study of age and the life course represented by the human development and age-stratification approaches offer useful guideposts for expanded anthropological explorations of age as empirical domain, variable, and focus for theory. In response to the human development emphasis on the individual life course, workshop participants stressed the need for research on the life course as a cultural unit: as Andrea Sankar's chapter shows, the American middle-aged and medicalized view of the life course as linear and declining is not universal. Very little empirical effort has been directed toward documentation of variation in the shape or subdivisions of the life course. As Ronald Cohen puts it, we have little information about various cultural "theories" of aging.

Empirical gaps in life-course data are most dramatic in physical anthropology and linguistics. As the chapters by Cynthia Beall and Penelope Eckert show, human development in these two areas has been arbitrarily ended at a very early age. Most sociolinguistic research concentrates efforts to explain variation in speech on speakers below 35; and in physical anthropology, human growth and development have been essentially *child* growth and development, human adaptability essentially child and adolescent adaptation. Although it is perhaps most striking that we do not yet have adequate cross-cultural understanding of the physical trajectories of aging, it is also significant for further research that we do not have adequate documentation of cultural definitions of the life course.

Life-span research in anthropology requires both the physical baseline and the "emics" of the life course in various cultural contexts.

As a variable in other areas of anthropological interest, cultural definitions of the life course have not been thoroughly explored, but scattered studies suggest they may have significant effects. In the study of Sudanese witchcraft mentioned earlier, Nadel (1952) used the number of age categories in the life course as a major variable: the more categories, the greater the congruity of social and physical age and the less the likelihood of conflict between younger and older men. At the workshop, Ronald Cohen suggested that the presence of prelife and postdeath stages reduces conflict over generational succession. Research on the status of old people in various societies also suggests that cultural definition of the entire life course as a unit for planning and evaluation of individual lives promotes support for the old, because their care is viewed as reciprocity for their earlier efforts, rather than unrequited support of dependents. The intact/decrepit distinction discussed earlier has consequences for the very survival of the elderly, as those in the decrepit category may be insulted, abandoned, or murdered even in communities that respect and treat well their more competent older members.

As an area of theoretical interest, the life course has been considered mainly in terms of its subcategorization. In research in the United States, Fry discovered that the number of age categories differentiated by the people she interviewed varied with their stage in the domestic cycle. Her hypothesis, similar to those derived from other ethnoscientific research, is that the number of age grades distinguished is related to the age heterogeneity of individuals' kin networks. In short, people make as many distinctions as they need (Fry 1976; cf. Frake 1962).

Fortes suggested during the workshop that measurements of age from one domain might invade another, with potential effects on expected and consequently actual patterns of human development, such as chronological schedules for sitting, talking, walking. This use of public time scales in the privacy of the family may have important effects on parent–child relations and on absorption of achievement values, as well as on development of the indicated behaviors.

Age Stratification

The age-stratification paradigm raises the issues of age and aging to a societal level. Workshop discussion on this more abstract level concentrated on the interrelationships among age and other principles of social organization. Although the stratification model, by definition, stresses the hierarchical aspect of age relations, ethnographic examples from Africa and central Brazil reveal the other face of age, the egalitarian and harmonious bonding of peers. Maybury-Lewis describes the complementarity of age and kinship in central Brazil, where in general the male world of the village center is opposed to a more private, informal domestic and female sphere at the periphery. In these societies, age as an element of formal dual organization is viewed as a principle of harmony, in contrast to the divisiveness perceived as inherent to kinship. The Masai-type organizations of East Africa have also been interpreted as counterbalances to the more conflictual relations of kin (Spencer 1976). Family and peer contacts of old people in age-homogeneous communities in modern industrial settings also suggest that more explicit age grouping and greater access to age peers promote harmonious family interaction (Keith 1980b, 1982a; Jonas 1979).

These parallels raise broad theoretical questions about the conditions and consequences of various uses of age as a principle of social organization. When is age likely to be the basis of what types and degrees of social differentiation, on cognitive, ideological, interactional, or corporate dimensions (Keith 1981, 1982b)? How are these degrees and types of boundary definition interrelated? And how are they related to differentiation based on other social characteristics, such as kinship and class? Complete ethnographies of age will be required to answer these questions, but some preliminary propositions have been made. Rhoda Halperin's chapter offers a framework for comparative analysis of age and the organization of ''cultural economics'' at various levels of societal complexity. Philip Gulliver (1968), among others, outlines a hydraulic model with some life-course implications: age bonds recede in significance as other bases of differentiation increase. The middle years consequently bring a decrease in salience of age ties in many societies, as other loyalties and identities take precedence. The subtle variation documented for other ascriptive identities, such as ethnicity, suggests, however, that research directed toward age links in a broader range of societies will reveal more complex patterns of age salience, which varies by, among other things, situation, type of issue in a conflict, and age characteristics of social participants.

Although most of the data available on age differentiation are from societies with highly formalized age organization, age, of course, plays a role in more informal and private domains. As Fortes points out in his chapter, the measurement of one's life-course position in the private domestic sphere is likely to be based on generation, while in the more public arenas outside the household, age may be indicated by chronology. Since age does have potential significance in both public and private spheres, it is a useful focus for theoretical questions about the interrelationship of those two fields of social action. Fortes proposes that chronological measurement is likely to invade the domestic domain when political organization reaches the state level. Eisenstadt (1956) long ago proposed, for example, a correlation between the degree of discontinuity between basic organizational principles of social life within the household and beyond it and the existence of age-homogeneous groups as "interlinking spheres." The interrelationship of public and private spheres also offers a hypothesis about the appearance of the frequently described "liberated" older women who are admitted to various male privileges after menopause: the sharper the distinction between domestic and public domains, the more likely that women will undergo dramatic role shift after menopause (see Brown 1982, Cool and McCabe 1983). To hazard an even broader speculation, conflict across age lines may be related to the private/public distinction in a curvilinear pattern. If the domestic sphere encompasses most social life, as in very small societies, personal knowledge and multiplex ties among individuals are likely to interfere with age-based conflicts. If the distinction between private and public domains is extreme, then age groups are likely to form and to mediate age-related conflict.

Norms

The acquisition and maintenance of norms by young people have been extensively examined. In such research the adult roles analyzed are those of guide and enforcer. A life-span perspective offers a more complex view. First, as an empirical domain, norms in connection with age have not been thoroughly reported. Human development researchers in the United States and in Japan, for example, have discovered the changing salience of norms of age-related behavior as individuals age (Neugarten, Moore, and Lowe 1965, Plath and Ikeda 1975). As people in these two societies grow older, age norms become more highly charged emotionally, and the individual's own normative position aligns more closely with his or her perception of the normative standards of others. Cross-cultural comparative research could document life-span patterns of norm salience and suggest explanations for variation. As noted earlier, we still do not have systematic observations of the factors that promote the appearance of the bawdy old women of ethnographic notoriety. Gutmann's proposed universal personality shift toward passivity for men and mastery for women may account for these patterns in some societies, but counterexamples have been presented (Werner 1981).

As a variable within the realm of normative theory, age would permit more subtle interpretation of the mechanisms by which norms are transmitted, enforced, and created. Criticism of the emphasis placed on traumatic initiation as essential to role change in youth is reinforced by accounts of rites of passage at later life stages which accomplish transitions across major role shifts without hazing (Legesse 1973, 1979). The conservative theme in discussions of rites of passage as means of moving individuals through established roles is also challenged by the creativity of old people in several modern societies, who have invented both transition rituals and the new roles into which they lead. As Myerhoff's chapter reveals, observations at this later stage offer insight into the creative potential of liminality. These same old people are often subjected to formal socialization attempts by younger members of society—institution administrators, family counselors, income-maintenance bureaucrats—so that the age roles of socializer and subject are reversed (Legesse 1979). This contradiction of previous status often produces resistance to formal socialization and development of informal alternatives, in a pattern similar to that described by Erving Goffman (1961) in connection with total institutions. Observation of socialization at later points in the life course also provides information about ''stripping'' of previous identities, usually considered only in the special settings of institutions or utopian communities (Kanter 1972).

Observations of old people who have created communities in several modern societies also show the tremendous force of peer sanctions at this life stage. The parallel to adolescence raises the question of whether there are certain life stages at which age norms are particularly salient and age peers particularly powerful reference groups. The commonalities between adolescence and early old age in modern societies offer a starting point for propositions: these are periods of transition, of powerlessness, and of identity confusion. Cross-cultural research could document variation in life stages that have those characteristics and thus facilitate evaluation of hypotheses about their relationship to salience and sanctioning of age norms.

Ethnographic research on norms, since it has focused on youth, has also emphasized transmission of existing standards. Recent studies of old-age communities, however, show the old people as creators of norms. Observations from this farther end of the life course consequently stimulate hypotheses about conditions under which norms are created. Propositions from gerontologists, which might be evaluated cross-culturally, point to development of a high level of community among agemates as the key prerequisite for creation of norms (Keith 1980b discusses factors that promote age communities).

As a focus for normative theory in its own right, age suggests several themes. Under what conditions does age become the subject of normative emphasis, for example? New and relatively undefined social situations may place an emphasis on ascriptive characteristics, as students of urban ethnicity have argued (Mitchell 1956; and see Hess 1972 on age). Rapid social change may highlight age differences and concentrate attention on the way members of different age categories ought to behave. The relationship of age norms to expectations in other domains is also a promising area. When is the egalitarian face of age dominant, as opposed to its hierarchical and more conflictual potential? The complementarity present in the available ethnographic evidence is a useful starting point. In other words, propositions about the two faces of age norms need to take account of differentiation of at least two social arenas, the domestic and the public. When the hierarchical aspect of age is accentuated within the domestic sphere—that is, in conflicts of authority, succession, and inheritance—the egalitarian theme may be most likely to appear in age groups outside the household. This reasoning suggests, for instance, that stress on egalitarianism should be more intense in patrilineal than matrilineal societies. As we mentioned earlier, egalitarianism is also likely to be emphasized among agemates if their age category is collectively out of power.

Symbol and Ritual

As a domain for empirical investigation on symbol and ritual, the life course itself has not yet been thoroughly documented. Not only the external and internal shape of the life course but also the symbolic markers or signals of each life-course identity have yet to be reported in the many types of society that do not have highly explicit age-grade systems. The symbolic marking of life-course boundaries is particularly interesting in contrast to those of other ascriptive identities, as the boundaries are typically maintained while individuals pass through them—a circumstance considered highly problematic in the study of ethnic boundaries, for example.

As a variable in the study of other social features, life stage offers new insight into rites of passage, as we have already proposed. In addition, the meaning of ritual in general appears to vary with stage in the life course. Myerhoff suggests, for instance, that ritual is particularly important to the old because of impending death. Fortes makes a more general argument that ritual is always a bridge across discontinuity. In this sense, ritual should be elaborated at points of greatest social discontinuity in the life course, and individuals should be most likely to participate in available rituals when they feel discontinuities most acutely. As Myerhoff's chapter proposes, immigrant and other elderly people with "disrupted histories" should be eager participants in and creators of ritual.

As a focus for theory, the symbolic and ritual aspects of age have been little considered. In what circumstances, for instance, is the life course likely to be most elaborated in symbolic and ritual terms? Rate of change may have a curvilinear relationship to intensification of life-course symbolism and ritual. In highly stable communities, the hierarchical aspects of age may be ritually enforced, and symbolic signals (clothing, hair styles) of age categories in a seniority ladder abundant. Highly fluid social systems may also emphasize age, as members of different cohorts react to change in different ways, traditional seniority systems are disrupted, peers become more significant sources of norm definition, and age conflict is more likely. As Victor Turner (1959) observed long ago, conflict is most likely to be shifted to a ritual plane when it involves opposing norms, which are in turn more likely to develop in circumstances of social change.

As the age stratification theorists frequently remind us, none of these patterns is static. Individuals, of course, move through different life-course categories; the structure of these categories may also change. As we pointed out earlier, formal age organization has intensified as well as waned in traditional societies in recent centuries. Observers of American politics also point out that increasing awareness of age differences, due in part to demographic changes that have increased the proportion of old people in the population, may increase the likelihood of age-based political action by those individuals who mature in this more age-conscious atmosphere (Cutler 1981). Dramatic changes in age demography are a type of social change particularly likely to increase the salience of age differentiation. If age differentiation becomes more formal and explicit in the United States, the greater salience of age, feared by many as a source of conflict, may eventually promote some of the mediating aspects of formal age organization observed in other societies (Keith 1981).

Marriage and the Family

Probably no area of anthropological research has made more use of a life-course framework than marriage and family studies. The "domestic cycle" (Goody 1958) has long been an organizing principle in ethnographies of family life, and as a result we have hundreds of ethnographies containing observations on age relations in the context of marriage and the family. Thus in this field we are in a more favorable position than we are in such areas as language use, for much of the empirical data on age and the life course are already available.

Analytical attention thus far, however, has focused on the kinship group or family as the unit of study, at the expense of a focus on the individual life course. Age as a variable, as distinct from position in the domestic group, has yet to be systematically analyzed. The chapters by Meyer Fortes and Eugene Hammel represent an important first step toward the needed synthesis, outlining several important issues and working toward a conceptual scheme for analyzing domestic age relations.

The wide variability found in age at marriage, especially the widespread custom of having a large age gap between husband and wife, raises intriguing questions regarding the relationship between age and social structure. What are the implications of an average age at first marriage of puberty for women and over 30 for men, as in some Australian and African societies? Hammel notes that in such cases the marital life-course experience of men is very different from that of women. At the beginning of marriage, the man occupies a dominant position, while as the man grows old the woman's power relative to his increases. Indeed, even when the husband's and wife's ages are more equal, the wife may become more independent of the husband during the course of their lives. Among the Gonja and Ashanti in West Africa, Goody reports (1976:123), "most wives returned to their natal kin after the menopause, abandoning the conjugal state to look after (and be looked after by) their brothers. . . . In this case a man's holding of wives decreased rapidly after middle age."

Sexual difference in age at marriage is also related to polygyny, for the basis of polygyny is almost universally higher age at marriage for men than for women. There is in fact a complex relationship between age and polygyny. Goody (1976:122) notes, for example, that polygyny is closely connected with bridewealth, and in many societies it is the elders that control the property suitable for bridewealth payment. Indeed, in some cases a man must decide whether to invest his wealth in another wife for himself or to provide a wife for one of his sons. Thus polygyny has implications for the age relations not only between men and women but between men and other men. Such ramifications may be seen, too, in societies that practice the levirate, where a man's widows are assigned in marriage to his surviving brother (Clignet 1970:90). In such societies, a man's relative age in the sibling group has implications for the number of women he ultimately marries.

Age relations among siblings are in turn affected by the practice of polygyny. As Fortes notes, the matrisibling group (children of the same mother) has a much narrower age range than the patrisibling group (children of the same father). A man with many wives may have children who are older than his junior wives. Age relations among siblings have attracted a certain amount of attention, particularly in terms of inheritance (e.g., primogeniture) and marriage priority. These are two of the areas where conflict among siblings is frequently manifest. Although its intensity and the norms for its management vary, as Fortes points out, such conflict may be a cultural universal.

It is not enough to look at the age of the man or woman and at their relative ages (in Hammel's terms, the spouses' ABSAGEs and RELAGEs) in order to examine the impact of age relations on their family lives. It is important also to determine how many children they have and the number of each sex, and also what their ages are. In contemporary Western society this is of course a commonly recognized issue, identified with the limitations imposed on parents (particularly mothers) of small children. But the matter is more complicated, for children are not only an economic burden; in many societies they also constitute an economic opportunity. Enid Schildkrout (1978) provides a nice illustration, showing the multifarious cultural ramifications of such age relations among the urban Hausa of Kano. The occupational history of the women cannot be understood apart from their relationship to their children and to foster or surrogate children over time. Because of the Islamic rule of purdah, women can become petty merchants only if they have children available to do their marketing. Changing norms of age-appropriate behavior for the children (e.g., going to school) thus have ramifications on characteristic age-linked patterns of economic activity for women.

To advance our theoretical understanding of the use of age in family and marriage systems we must pose some larger questions. We limit ourselves to just one of these questions here, by way of illustration. Under what circumstances do societies develop a large age differential between husband and wife? This question reveals the multiple perspectives that must be employed in the theoretical development of the role of age in family and marriage systems. Sociobiologists would certainly point to the common higher primate pattern in which males attain sexual maturity and adult body size later than females, and would want to address the biological bases of the age differential between mates. Most social anthropologists, stressing the variability in this pattern among societies, feel more comfortable with an economic explanation, based on the male's role in the productive process and his related need to acquire capital and/or expertise before marriage. Demographic factors also have to be considered, including the central role of age at marriage in the determination of total fertility and hence the rate of population growth. This consideration leads to the related issue of cultural norms and social practice with regard to the remarriage of widows, for the greater the age differential between husband and wife, the greater the likelihood of widowhood. Demographically, it is the woman's marital condition through her reproductive years, not the man's, that is of basic importance to societal levels of fertility. Thus any attempt to explain the husband–wife age differential on the basis of population control has to confront the related cultural issue of norms governing widow remarriage.

Kinship

The available ethnographic documentation on age in the context of kinship is less substantial than that found for age in the domestic sphere. Hammel's chapter, for example, takes up the issue of the extent of age homogeneity within a culturally defined generation. In many kinship systems equality among such kin-defined generation mates is assumed, but such solidarity is presumably undermined by the wide diversity of ages among generationally defined groupings (see also Legesse 1973; Needham 1974; Kertzer 1982, 1983). Little systematic ethnographic work, however, has yet been done on this issue. Similarly, while certain social relationships are implied by particular kinship relations in a society, the actual nature of individual dyadic relations is presumably heavily influenced by the relative ages of the individuals involved. Moreover, as people age, the nature of their relationship tends to change. The relationship between a man and his father-in-law may be hypothesized to depend on the age difference between them: the greater the age gap, the less the familiarity. Moreover, this relationship may be thought to change in response to the absolute ages of the two men. Contrast these observations with the traditional normative approach to kinship study, which tends to produce a much more static, simplistic, and hence erroneous description of kin relations.

The relationship between age and kinship systems involves a complex interaction between cultural norms and demographic characteristics within a context of individuals and groups striving to serve their own interests. While for Maybury-Lewis age and kinship operate equally in social organization, Hammel makes the provocative claim that the cultural norms that define a kinship system may be rooted at a more fundamental level in the age characteristics of a population: "We may profitably regard the systems of symbols and mutual expectations that are the culture of kinship as adaptive mechanisms to cope with the vagaries of demographic structures." This, of course, is an area in which Hammel (and Wachter 1977, Hammel et al. 1980) has been working for several years, but the demographic basis of kinship systems remains a largely unexplored field.

How do age structures and age relations constrain kinship systems? We must limit ourselves to two examples here. When a kinship system is based on rules governing prescriptive marriages between kinship units, an individual must have kin who actually fall into the prescribed category in order to marry appropriately. If such kin are too old, however, they are likely to be already married or in any case considered inappropriate in terms of cultural age norms (themselves linked to such factors as fertility, as in the case of the unmarried postmenopausal woman). Thus the age structure of the population, influenced by the kinship system (as reflected in marital age norms and hereditary longevity), limits the feasibility of certain kinship systems and may encourage the development of others.

Our second example is provided by one of the common features of kinship systems, the distinction made between generations. Indeed, Fortes argues that generation is more important than age in the family context, that age in the chronological sense is an imposition on the domestic sphere by the state. The long anthropological tradition of kinship terminology study, based on the link between principles of terminological grouping and principles of social grouping, has demonstrated the central role played by generational distinctions in kinship systems. Yet as we have noted, when people are grouped in the same generation by virtue of descent from a common ancestor, they are not necessarily of the same chronological age, and the farther back the common ancestor is traced, the greater is the age range in the generation of descendants. One may owe deference to another's senior generational standing, yet be chronologically older than that person. This tension may have two effects. In some cases efforts are made to reconcile the principles of generation and chronological age by altering the generational placement of an individual on the basis of age. This is not unlike the more frequently noted practice of altering an individual's kin relationship to accord better with social relationships. Yet it is also likely that such tension between generational principles and chronological age principles has through time constrained the development of the generational principle in kinship systems. The fact of age, in other words, sets limits on the kinds of cultural kinship norms that may be institutionalized and that prove viable.

In attempting to aid development of a theory of age and the life course, we can look at this question in a somewhat different way. Following the tradition of Eisenstadt (1956), we may ask whether there is an inverse relationship between the importance of kinship and that of age in a society. Under what conditions does age become particularly salient as a basis for social interaction and social stratification? Do highly developed kinship groupings leave less room for age as a principle of social grouping? A considerable amount of recent sociological attention has been devoted to the relationship between class and age as systems of stratification (A. Foner 1979), yet little work in the past quarter century has looked at age and kinship in these terms.

Power and Conflict

The relationship between age and political power has been noted in many ethnographies, and is familiar to those who study the United States and other Western societies as well. In anthropology the fullest development of this issue has come in analyses of gerontocracy, in societies where the elders (generally male) rule. Of course, political power is closely tied to economic power, and the political influence associated with various portions of the life course is generally correlated with the amount of property controlled. In many societies, power and property are embodied in the number of wives an individual has accumulated. Hence Paul Spencer (1965:299–300) proposes a "gerontocratic index" based on the concentration of polygyny among older men. The notable exception to this equation of political influence with economic resources concerns the importance of ritual knowledge and ritual practice among the elders in bolstering their political influence even in the absence of economic control (see, for example, Werner 1981). Yet we must be careful to distinguish between formal norms and formal behavior on the one hand and actual struggle for power on the other. Even in societies where political supremacy is the prerogative of the elders, there are ways in which younger men may gain the upper hand (La Fontaine 1978:14–15, Goody 1976:122–23). In many cases, too, gerontocracy is more achieved than ascribed, as advancing years give men an increasing advantage in accumulation of wives or property, but no guarantee of attaining them (Almagor 1978, Keith n.d.).

To what extent and under what circumstances do old and young form political pressure groups to further their separate interests?[5] Aside from analyses of the unusually formalized system found in societies that have named age sets, little cross-cultural work has been done by anthropologists on this topic, especially in comparison with the voluminous sociological literature on Western societies. Maybury-Lewis, writing of central Brazil, makes the point that age-based groupings are more fragile than kinship-based units. Similar observations have been made in regard to East Africa (e.g., Gulliver 1968:16). This finding is no doubt related to the strength of emotional ties within the family, but it is also linked to the advantage kinship groupings have as ongoing property-controlling units with a means of continuous replenishment that age-based groupings obviously lack. In this regard it is worth underlining Maybury-Lewis' point that age-based groupings are often perceived as socially integrative forces that tend to counteract the disruptive influence of kinship divisions, tying together people who belong to different kinship groups.

One of the most fundamental aspects of political leadership is that of succession. Indeed, this is also one of the major nodes of political struggle and intrigue. Succession is obviously linked to aging, and any society must have some mechanism whereby younger people replace older ones in positions of political power. As Hammel has noted, the very distribution of power may be partly a product of the population's age structure. The fact that in most human societies throughout history few people lived past age 50 (Washburn 1981; see also Dolhinow, chap. 1 in this volume) meant that the elderly constituted a tiny part of the community. Whether

5. For an interesting discussion of this issue, analyzing youth–elder conflict in terms of class struggle, see Terray 1975.

the elderly are more or less likely to enjoy positions of political influence where they constitute such a small segment of the community remains an open question.

With the evolution of chiefdoms and states, problems of succession took a different form (Goody 1966). Here again, though, questions of age relations remain central. In some cases, in some historical periods, fraternal succession was the rule, while in others succession was governed by the filial principle (see Southwold 1966:118). Notions of age-appropriateness appear to favor fraternal succession, for the sight of an infant king has always seemed odd. Yet filial succession may foster greater harmony between ruler and heir, giving it an advantage over the fraternal succession system. Under fraternal succession, the heir's interest in serving a long term himself has unsettling implications for the life expectancy of the ruler.[6]

The concepts of power and conflict are, of course, at the heart of any theory of age stratification. We are far from knowing the extent to which age serves as a basis of social stratification, or the conditions in which age is most highly developed as a basis of power differentiation. And turning from a societal level to an individual perspective, we need to determine the life-course power curve found in different societies, plotting age against political influence and economic position. By doing so we will be in a better position to explain the extent of societal variability in the use of age to stratify roles and statuses. While this kind of comparison has been attempted in gerontological studies (Cowgill and Holmes, eds., 1972), full life-course treatment, including developments through the middle years, has barely begun.[7]

Conclusion

If the reason to increase our attention to the life span is the same as the familiar reason to climb Mount Everest, because it's there, it is also true that this particular mountain is the kind that anthropologists are best suited to climb. As process and principle, the life course and age are present in every society, but strongly shaped by cultural context, the

6. That filial succession produces its own conflicts between ruler and heir is, of course, well known. We are concerned here, though, with the relative conflict (and resources to challenge authority) in filial and fraternal succession.

7. See N. Foner 1984 for an early attempt in this direction.

traditional formula for anthropological puzzles. Age and the life course also offer the nexus of interacting biological, social, and cultural realities that anthropologists specialize in unraveling.

As we suggested earlier, many themes of the life-course perspective have long been present in anthropology, and the availability of cross-cultural ethnographic data has encouraged this approach in other disciplines. Both human development processes and the structural significance of age in society have been explored by anthropologists, though such studies have been limited to certain life stages, regions, and domains of activity. We have done the preliminary exercises; it is time to begin full-scale exploration.

Though we have emphasized how increased attention to age and the life course can benefit anthropological theory, we do not believe that research in this area should be constrained by traditional disciplinary boundaries (cf. Super and Harkness 1981). Indeed, one of the most exciting aspects of the recent blossoming of life-course and age-stratification research is its interdisciplinary nature. Psychologists, for example, are not only pleading for increased attention to the impact of changing historical conditions on psychological processes; some are also proclaiming the need to understand human development, in evolutionary terms, as the product of the interaction of the changing organism and the environment that human culture has been continuously changing (Lerner and Busch-Rossnagel 1981). Similarly, social historians, many identified with the *Annales* school, have increasingly come to see the life course as culturally constituted (e.g., Ariès 1962). As anthropologists advance beyond traditional lines of anthropological inquiry, disciplinary boundaries should not serve to isolate communities of scholars and scholarship. Rather, some of our greatest achievements come about when problems traditionally posed in one discipline stimulate research in others, and when perspectives that originate in one discipline are used to place in new perspective problems traditionally faced in another.

Age should not be simply equated with old age, as is commonly done, for this approach will only create a new kind of "area study" similar to regional specializations that already tend to Balkanize theoretical development. The recent research reports on old age, like new data from a previously unexplored region, can of course be a stimulus to theory. But for that stimulus to take effect, data on old age must be integrated into broader questions about age and the life course; and those life-span issues must, in turn, be linked to theoretical effort in the mainstreams of anthropology.

REFERENCES

Abeles, Ronald P., and Matilda White Riley
　1977　A Life-Course Perspective on the Later Years of Life: Some Implications for Research. New York: Social Science Research Council.
Almagor, Uri
　1978　Equality among Dassanetch age-peers. *In* Age, Generation, and Time, ed. Paul T. W. Baxter and Uri Almagor. London: Hurst.
Amoss, Pamela
　1981　Religious participation as a route to prestige for the elderly. *In* Dimensions: Aging, Culture, and Health, ed. Christine L. Fry. New York: Praeger.
Amoss, Pamela, and Stevan Harrell, eds.
　1981　Other Ways of Growing Old. Stanford: Stanford University Press.
Ariès, Phillipe
　1962　Centuries of Childhood. New York: Knopf.
Baltes, Paul B.
　1979　Life-span developmental psychology: Some converging observations of history and theory. *In* Life-Span Development and Human Behavior, ed. Baltes and Orville G. Brim, Jr., vol. 2. New York: Academic Press.
Baltes, Paul B., Wayne W. Reese, and Lewis P. Lipsitt
　1980　Life-span developmental psychology. Annual Review of Psychology 31:65–110.
Baltes, Paul B., and K. Warner Schaie
　1973a　Life-Span Developmental Psychology: Personality and Socialization. New York: Academic Press.
　1973b　On life-span developmental research paradigms: Retrospects and prospects. *In* Life-Span Developmental Psychology: Personality and Socialization, ed. Paul B. Baltes and K. Warner Schaie, pp. 365–95. New York: Academic Press.
Baltes, Paul B., and Sherry L. Willis
　1979　Life-span developmental psychology, cognitive functioning, and social policy. *In* Aging from Birth to Death: Interdisciplinary Perspectives, ed. Matilda White Riley, pp. 15–46. Boulder: Westview Press.
Baxter, Paul T. W., and Uri Almagor
　1978　Introduction. *In* Age, Generation, and Time, ed. Baxter and Almagor, pp. 1–35. New York: St. Martin's Press.
Bengtson, Vern L., and Neal E. Cutler
　1976　Generations and intergenerational relations: Perspectives on age

groups and social change. *In* Handbook of Aging and the Social Sciences, ed. Robert H. Binstock and Ethel Shanas, pp. 130–59. New York: Van Nostrand.

Birren, James E., and V. Jayne Renner
1977   Research on the psychology of aging: Principles and experimentation. *In* Handbook of the Psychology of Aging, ed. Birren and K. Warner Schaie, pp. 1–38. New York: Van Nostrand.

Blau, Peter, and Otis D. Duncan
1967   The American Occupational Structure. New York: Wiley.

Brim, Orville G., Jr.
1966   Socialization through the life cycle. *In* Socialization after Childhood, ed. Orville G. Brim, Jr., and Stanton Wheeler, pp. 1–50. New York: Wiley.

Brim, Orville, G., Jr., and Jerome Kagan
1980   Constancy and change: A view of the issues. *In* Constancy and Change in Human Development, ed. Brim and Kagan, pp. 1–25. Cambridge: Harvard University Press.

Brim, Orville G., Jr., and Carol D. Ryff
1980   On the properties of life events. *In* Life-Span Development and Human Behavior, ed. Paul B. Baltes and Brim, 3:367–88. New York: Academic Press.

Brown, Judith K.
1981   Cross-cultural perspectives on the female life cycle. *In* Handbook of Cross-Cultural Human Development, ed. Ruth H. Munroe, Robert L. Munroe, and Beatrice B. Whiting. New York: Garland.
1982   Cross-cultural perspectives on middle-aged women. Current Anthropology 23(2):143–56.

Buxton, J. C.
1958   The Mandari of the southern Sudan. *In* Tribes without Rulers, ed. David Tait and John Middleton. London: Routledge & Kegan Paul.

Clark, Margaret
1972   Cultural values and dependency in later life. *In* Aging and Modernization, ed. Donald Cowgill and Lowell D. Holmes. New York: Appleton-Century-Crofts.

Clark, Margaret, and Barbara Anderson
1967   Culture and Aging: An Anthropological Study of Older Americans. Springfield, Ill.: Charles C. Thomas.

Clignet, Remi
1970   Many Wives, Many Powers. Evanston, Ill.: Northwestern University Press.

Colson, Elizabeth, and Thayer Scudder
1981   Old age in Gwembe District, Zambia. *In* Other Ways of Growing Old, ed. Pamela Amoss and Stevan Harrell. Stanford: Stanford University Press.

Cool, Linda, and Justine McCabe
1983   The "scheming hag" and the "dear old thing": The anthropology of aging women. *In* Growing Old in Different Cultures, ed. Jay Sokolovsky. Belmont, Calif.: Wadsworth.
Cowgill, Donald
1974   Aging and modernization: A revision of the theory. *In* Late Life: Communities and Environmental Policy. Springfield, Ill.: Charles C. Thomas.
Cowgill, Donald, and Lowell Holmes, eds.
1972   Aging and Modernization. New York: Appleton-Century-Crofts.
Cuellar, José
1978   El Senior Citizens Center. *In* Aging: Life's Career, ed. Barbara Myerhoff and Andrei Simic. Beverly Hills, Calif.: Sage.
Cutler, Neal
1981   Political characteristics of elderly cohorts in the twenty-first century. *In* Aging: Social Change, ed. Sara B. Kiesler. New York: Academic Press.
Cytrynbaum, Solomon, Lenore Blum, Robert Patrick, Jan Stein, David Wadner, and Carole Wilk
1980   Midlife development: A personality and social systems perspective. *In* Aging in the 1980s: Psychological Issues, ed. Leonard W. Poon, pp. 463–74. Washington, D.C.: American Psychological Association.
Datan, Nancy, and Leon H. Ginsberg, eds.
1975   Life-Span Developmental Psychology: Normative Life Crises. New York: Academic Press.
Eckert, J. Kevin
1978   Experimental cohorts among American men. Paper presented to the annual meeting of the Gerontological Society, Dallas.
1980   The Unseen Elderly. San Diego: Campanile Press.
Eisenstadt, S. N.
1956   From Generation to Generation. Glencoe: Free Press.
Elder, Glen H., Jr.
1975   Age differentiation and the life course. Annual Review of Sociology 1:165–90.
1978   Approaches to social change and the family. American Journal of Sociology 84:S1–S38.
1981   History and the life course. *In* Biography and Society, ed. Daniel Bertaux. Beverly Hills, Calif.: Sage.
Erikson, Erik
1963   Childhood and Society. 2d ed. New York: Norton.
Featherman, David L.
1980   Schooling and occupational careers: Constancy and change in worldly success. *In* Constancy and Change in Human Development, ed. Or-

ville G. Brim, Jr., and Jerome Kagan, pp. 675–738. Cambridge: Harvard University Press.

1981   The Life-Span Perspective in Social Science Research. New York: Social Science Research Council.

Fennell, Valerie
1981   Older women in voluntary organizations. *In* Dimensions: Aging, Culture, and Health, ed. Christine L. Fry. New York: Praeger.

Foner, Anne
1972   The polity. *In* Aging and Society, vol. 3: A Sociology of Age Stratification, ed. Matilda White Riley, Marilyn Johnson, and Anne Foner. New York: Russell Sage Foundation.

1979   Ascribed and achieved bases of stratification. Annual Review of Sociology 5:219–42.

Foner, Anne, and David I. Kertzer
1978   Transitions over the life course: Lessons from age-set societies. American Journal of Sociology 83(5):1081–1104.

1979   Intrinsic and extrinsic sources of change in life-course transitions. *In* Aging from Birth to Death: Interdisciplinary Perspectives, ed. Matilda White Riley, pp. 121–36. Boulder: Westview Press.

Foner, Nancy
1984   Ages in Conflict: A Cross-Cultural Perspective on Inequality between Old and Young. New York: Columbia University Press.

Frake, Charles
1962   The ethnographic study of cognitive systems. *In* Anthropology and Human Behavior, ed. T. Gladwin and W. C. Sturtevant. Washington, D.C.: Anthropological Society of Washington.

Fry, Christine L.
1976   The ages of adulthood: A question of numbers. Journal of Gerontology 31:170–77.

1980   Toward an anthropology of aging. *In* Aging in Culture and Society, ed. Fry. New York: Praeger.

n.d.   Culture, behavior, and aging in the comparative perspective. *In* Handbook of Aging and Psychology, ed. James Birren and K. Warner Schaie 2d ed. New York: Van Nostrand Reinhold, forthcoming.

Fry, Christine L., ed.
1981   Dimensions: Aging, Culture, and Health. New York: Praeger.

Fry, Christine L., and Jennie Keith
1982   The life course as a cultural unit. *In* Aging from Birth to Death: Sociotemporal perspectives, ed. Matilda W. Riley, Ronald Abeles, and Michael Teitelbaum. Boulder: Westview Press.

Glascock, Anthony, and Susan L. Feinman
1980   Toward a comparative framework: Propositions concerning the treatment of the aged in non-industrial societies. *In* New Methods for Old

Age Research, ed. Christine L. Fry and Jennie Keith. Chicago: Center for Urban Policy, Loyola University.

1981 Social asset or social burden: An analysis of the treatment for the aged in non-industrial societies. *In* Dimensions: Aging, Culture, and Health, ed. Christine L. Fry. New York: Praeger.

Goffman, Erving
1961 Asylums. Garden City, N.Y.: Doubleday.

Goody, Jack
1976 Aging in non-industrial societies. *In* Handbook of Aging and the Social Sciences, ed. Robert Binstock and Ethel Shanas. New York: Van Nostrand Reinhold.

Goody, Jack, ed.
1958 The Developmental Cycle in Domestic Groups. Cambridge: Cambridge University Press.

1966 Succession to High Office. Cambridge: Cambridge University Press.

Goulet, L. R., and Paul B. Baltes, eds.
1970 Life-Span Developmental Psychology: Research and Theory. New York: Academic Press.

Groffman, Karl J.
1970 Life-span developmental psychology in Europe: Past and present. *In* Life-Span Developmental Psychology: Research and Theory, ed. L. R. Goulet and Paul B. Baltes, pp. 53–68. New York: Academic Press.

Gulliver, Philip
1963 Social Control in an African Society. London: Routledge & Kegan Paul.

1968 Age differentiation. *In* International Encyclopedia of the Social Sciences 1:157–62. New York: Macmillan.

Gutmann, David
1975 Parenthood: A key to the comparative study of the life cycle. *In* Life-Span Developmental Psychology: Normative Life Crises, ed. Nancy Datan and Leon H. Ginsberg. New York: Academic Press.

1977 The cross-cultural perspective: Notes toward a comparative psychology of aging. *In* Handbook of the Psychology of Aging, ed. James E. Birren and K. Warner Schaie, pp. 302–26. New York: Van Nostrand.

Hammel, Eugene A., Chad K. McDaniel, and Kenneth W. Wachter
1980 Vice in the Villefranchian: A microsimulation analysis of the demographic effects of incest prohibitions. *In* Genealogical Demography, ed. Bennett Dyke and Warren T. Morrill, pp. 209–34. New York: Academic Press.

Hammel, Eugene A., and Kenneth W. Wachter
1977 Primonuptiality and ultimonuptiality: Their effects on stem-family-household frequencies. *In* Population Patterns in the Past, ed. Ronald D. Lee, pp. 113–34. New York: Academic Press.

Hareven, Tamara K.
1978/ Cycles, courses, and cohorts: Reflections on theoretical and meth-
79   odological approaches to historical study of family development. Jour-
        nal of Social History 12:97–109.
1980   The life course and aging in historical perspective. *In* Life Course:
        Integrative Theories and Exemplary Populations, ed. Kurt W. Back,
        pp. 9–25. Boulder: Westview Press.
Havighurst, Robert J.
1948   Developmental Tasks and Education. New York: David McKay.
1973   History of developmental psychology: Socialization and personality
        development throughout the life span. *In* Life-Span Developmental
        Psychology: Personality and Socialization, ed. Paul B. Baltes and K.
        Warner Schaie, pp. 3–24. New York: Academic Press.
Hess, Beth
1972   Friendship. *In* Aging and Society, vol. 3: A Sociology of Age Stratifi-
        cation, ed. Matilda White Riley, Marilyn Johnson, and Anne Foner.
        New York: Russell Sage Foundation.
Hogan, Dennis P.
1981   Transitions and Social Change. New York: Academic Press.
Holmes, Lowell
1976   From Simmons to the seventies: Trends in anthropological gerontol-
        ogy. International Journal of Aging and Human Development
        7:211–20.
Hultsch, David F., and Judy K. Plemons
1979   Life events and life-span development. *In* Life-Span Development and
        Human Behavior, ed. Paul B. Baltes and Orville G. Brim, Jr., 2:1–36.
        New York: Academic Press.
Jonas, Karen
1979   Factors in development of community in age-segregated housing. *In*
        The Ethnography of Old Age, ed. Jennie Keith. Special issue of An-
        thropological Quarterly 52(1):49–60.
Jones, G. I.
1962   Ibo age organizations, with special reference to the Cross River and
        North Eastern Ibo. Journal of the Royal Anthropological Institute
        92:191–210.
Kanter, Rosabeth Moss
1972   Commitment and Community: Communes and Utopias in Sociological
        Perspective. Cambridge: Harvard University Press.
Katz, Solomon
1978   Anthropological perspectives on aging. Annals of the American Acad-
        emy of Social and Political Science 438:1–20.
Keith, Jennie
1979   The Ethnography of Old Age. Special issue of Anthropological Quar-
        terly 52(1).

1980a "The best is yet to be": Toward an anthropology of age. Annual Review of Anthropology 9:339–64.

1980b Old age and community creation. *In* Aging, Culture, and Society, ed. Christine L. Fry. New York: Praeger.

1981 Old age and age differentiation: Anthropological speculations on age as a social border. *In* Aging: Social Change, ed. Sara B. Kiesler, James N. Morgan, and Valerie Kincade Oppenheimer. New York: Academic Press.

1982a Old People, New Lives: Community Creation in a Retirement Residence. Chicago: University of Chicago Press (2d paperback edition of Ross 1977).

1982b Old People as People: Social and Cultural Influences on Aging and Old Age. Boston: Little, Brown.

1984 Ask an anthropologist: A review of cross-cultural research on old age. *In* Handbook of Aging and The Social Sciences, ed. Robert Binstock and Ethel Shanas. New York: Van Nostrand Reinhold, forthcoming.

Kerns, Virginia

1980 Aging and mutual support relations among the Black Carib. *In* Aging in Culture and Society, ed. Christine L. Fry. New York: Praeger.

Kertzer, David I.

1978 Theoretical developments in the study of age-group systems. American Ethnologist 5:368–74.

1982 Generation and age in cross-cultural perspective. *In* Aging from birth to death: Sociotemporal Perspectives, ed. Matilda W. Riley, Ronald Abeles, and Michael Teitelbaum. Boulder: Westview Press.

1983 Generation as a sociological problem. Annual Review of Sociology 9:125–49.

Kirk, Lorraine, and Michael Burton

1977 Meaning and context: A study of contextual shifts in meaning of Massai personality descriptions. American Ethnologist 4:734–61.

Kleemeier, R. W., ed.

1961 Aging and Leisure. New York: Oxford University Press.

La Fontaine, J. S.

1978 Introduction. *In* Sex and Age as Principles of Social Differentiation, ed. La Fontaine, pp. 1–20. New York: Academic Press.

Lamphear, John

1976 The Traditional History of the Jie of Uganda. Oxford: Clarendon Press.

Langness, L. L., and Gelya Frank

1981 Lives: An Anthropological Approach to Biography. Novato, Calif.: Chandler & Sharp.

Legesse, Asmarom

1973 Gada. New York: Free Press.

1979 Age sets and retirement communities. *In* The Ethnography of Old Age, ed. Jennie Keith, pp. 66–69. Special issue of Anthropological Quarterly 52(1).

Lerner, Richard M., and Nancy A. Busch-Rossnagel
1981   Individuals as producers of their development: Conceptual and empirical bases. *In* Individuals as Producers of Their Development, ed. Lerner and Busch-Rossnagel. New York: Academic Press.

Le Vine, Robert
1978   Adulthood and aging in cross-cultural perspective. Items 31/32:1–5.

Le Vine, Robert, and Walter Sangree
1962   The diffusion of age-group organization in East Africa. Africa 30(2). Africa 30(2).

Mannheim, Karl
1952   The problem of generations. *In* Mannheim, Essays on the Sociology of Knowledge, pp. 276–320. New York: Oxford University Press.

Maxwell, Robert, and Philip Silverman
1970   Information and esteem. Aging and Human Development 1:361–92.

Mead, Margaret
1928   Coming of Age in Samoa. New York: Morrow.

Mitchell, J. Clyde
1956   The Kalela Dance: Aspects of Social Relationships among Urban Africans in Northern Rhodesia. Manchester: Rhodes-Livingston Paper no, 27,

Mortimer, Jeylan T., and Roberta Simmons
1978   Adult socialization. Annual Review of Sociology 4:421–54.

Myerhoff, Barbara
1978   Number Our Days. New York: Dutton.

Nadel, S. F.
1952   Witchcraft in four African societies. American Anthropologist 54:18–29.

Needham, Rodney
1974   Age, category, and descent. *In* Remarks and Inventions, ed. Needham. London: Tavistock.

Neugarten, Bernice L.
1968   Adult personality: Toward a psychology of the life cycle. *In* Middle Age and Aging, ed. Neugarten, pp. 137–47. Chicago: University of Chicago Press.
1969   Continuities and discontinuities of psychological issues into adult life. Human Development 12:121–30.
1977   Personality and aging. *In* Handbook of the Psychology of Aging, ed. James E. Birren and K. Warner Schaie, p. 626–49. New York: Van Nostrand.

Neugarten, Bernice L., ed.
1968   Middle Age and Aging: A Reader in Social Psychology. Chicago: University of Chicago Press.

Neugarten, Bernice L., and Nancy Datan
1973 Sociological perspectives on the life cycle. *In* Life-Span Developmental Psychology: Personality and Socialization, ed. Paul B. Baltes and Warner Schaie, pp. 53–69. New York: Academic Press.

Neugarten, Bernice L., and Gunhild O. Hagestad
1976 Age and the life course. *In* Handbook of Aging and the Social Sciences, ed. Robert H. Binstock and Ethel Shanas, pp. 35–55. New York: Van Nostrand.

Neugarten, Bernice, Joan W. Moore, and John Lowe
1965 Age norms, age constraints, and adult socialization. American Journal of Sociology 70:710–17.

Nydegger, Corinne
1977 Multiple cohort membership. Paper presented at the annual meeting of the Gerontological Society, San Francisco.
1980 Life course transitions. *In* New Methods for Old Age Research, ed. Christine L. Fry and Jennie Keith. Chicago: Center for Urban Policy, Loyola University.

Parsons, Talcott
1942 Age and sex in the social structure of the United States. American Sociological Review 7:604–16.

Plath, David, and Keiko Ikeda
1975 After coming of age: Adult awareness of age norms. *In* Socialization and Communication in Primary Groups, ed. Thomas R. Williams. The Hague: Mouton.

Press, Irwin, and Michael McKool
1972 Social structure and status of the aged. Aging and Human Development 3:297–306.

Reinert, Guenther
1979 Prolegomena to a history of life-span developmental psychology. *In* Life-Span Development and Human Behavior, ed. Paul B. Baltes and Orville G. Brim, Jr., 2:205–54. New York: Academic Press.

Riley, Matilda White
1973 Aging and cohort succession: Interpretations and misinterpretations. Public Opinion Quarterly 37:35–49.
1976 Age strata in social systems. *In* Handbook of Aging and the Social Sciences, ed. Robert H. Binstock and Ethel Shanas, pp. 189–217. New York: Van Nostrand.
1979a Introduction. *In* Aging from Birth to Death: Interdisciplinary Perspectives, ed. Riley, pp. 3–13. Boulder: Westview Press.
1979b Aging: Social change and social policy. *In* Aging from Birth to Death: Interdisciplinary Perspectives, ed. Riley, pp. 109–20. Boulder: Westview Press.

Riley, Matilda White, and Anne Foner
  1968   Aging and Society, vol. 1: An Inventory of Research Findings. New
          York: Russell Sage Foundation.
Riley, Matilda White, Marilyn Johnson, and Anne Foner
  1972   Aging and Society, vol. 3: A Sociology of Age Stratification. New
          York: Russell Sage Foundation.
Rosow, Irving
  1978   What is a cohort and why? Human Development 21:65–75.
Ross, Jennie-Keith (Keith, Jennie)
  1975   Social borders: Definitions of diversity. Current Anthropologist
          16:53–72.
  1977   Old People, New Lives: Community Creation in a Retirement Resi-
          dence. Chicago: University of Chicago Press. (See Keith 1982.)
Rossi, Alice S.
  1980   Aging and parenthood in the middle years. *In* Life-Span Development
          and Human Behavior, ed. Paul B. Baltes and Orville G. Brim, Jr., pp.
          37–205. New York: Academic Press.
Ryder, Norman B.
  1965   The cohort as a concept in the study of social change. American
          Sociological Review 30:843–61.
Schildkrout, Enid
  1978   Roles of children in urban Kano. *In* Sex and Age as Principles of
          Social Differentiation, ed. Jean S. LaFontaine. London: Academic
          Press.
Schurtz, Heinrich
  1902   Altersklassen und Männerbunde. Berlin: Reimer.
Simmons, Leo
  1945   The Role of the Aged in Primitive Society. New Haven: Yale Univer-
          sity Press.
Sokolovsky, Jay, and Carl Cohen
  1978   The cultural meaning of personal networks for the inner city elderly.
          Urban Anthropology 7:323–42.
  1981   Being old in the inner city: Support systems of the S.R.O. aged. *In*
          Dimensions: Aging, Culture, and Health, ed. Christine L. Fry. New
          York: Praeger.
Sorokin, Pitirim A.
  1941   Social and Cultural Dynamics: Basic Problems, Principles, and Meth-
          ods. Vol. 4. New York: American Book Company.
  1947   Society, Culture, and Personality. New York: Harper.
Southwold, Martin
  1966   Succession to the throne in Buganda. *In* Succession to High Office, ed.
          Jack Goody. Cambridge: Cambridge University Press.

Spencer, Paul
 1965 The Samburu: A Study of Gerontocracy in a Nomadic Tribe. London: Routledge & Kegan Paul.
 1976 Opposing streams and the gerontocratic ladder: Two models of age organization. Man 11:152–74.
Stewart, Frank
 1977 Fundamentals of Age-Group Systems. New York: Academic Press.
Super, Charles M., and Sara Harkness
 1981 Figure, ground, and gestalt: The cultural context of the active individual. *In* Individuals as Producers of Their Development, ed. Richard M. Lerner and Nancy A. Busch-Rossnagel. New York: Academic Press.
Tanner, J. M.
 1981 A History of the Study of Human Growth. Cambridge: Cambridge University Press.
Terray, Emmanuel
 1975 Classes and class consciousness in the Abron kingdom of Gyaman. *In* Marxist Analyses and Social Anthropology, ed. Maurice Bloch. New York: Wiley.
Thomae, Hans
 1979 The concept of development and life-span developmental psychology. *In* Life-Span Development and Human Behavior, ed. Paul B. Baltes and Orville G. Brim, Jr., 2:281–312. New York: Academic Press.
Turner, Victor
 1957 Schism and Continuity in African Society. Manchester: Manchester University Press.
Vinovskis, Maris
 1977 From household size to the life course. American Behavioral Scientist 21(2):263–87.
Waring, Joan M.
 1975 Social replenishment and social change: The problem of disordered cohort flow. American Behavioral Scientist 19(2):237–56.
Washburn, Sherwood L.
 1981 Longevity in primates. *In* Aging: Biology and Behavior, ed. James L. McGaugh and Sara B. Kiesler. New York: Academic Press.
Werner, Dennis
 1981 Gerontocracy among the Mekranoti of central Brazil. Anthropological Quarterly 54:15–27.
Whiting, Beatrice
 1963 Six Cultures. New York: Wiley.
Whiting, John M. W.
 1981 Aging and becoming an elder: A cross-cultural comparison. *In* Aging:

Stability and Change in the Family, ed. Robert W. Fogel et al. New York: Academic Press.
Whiting, John M. W., and Irvin Child
1953   Child Training and Personality. New Haven: Yale University Press.

Part One / Age, Evolution, and Biology

1

The Primates: Age, Behavior, and Evolution

Phyllis Dolhinow

All primates, human and nonhuman, male and female, experience an orderly, biologically based sequence of changes during their lifetimes. It is important to appreciate what is uniquely human, and we may identify these patterns both by comparing ourselves with living nonhuman primate relatives and by our best guesses as to behaviors that characterized early stages of our evolution. When the goal is to understand human behavior, the investigation should start with humans (Washburn 1978a, 1978b, in press; Washburn and Dolhinow n.d.); but because the other chapters in this volume focus on humans, I shall emphasize the life-course development of some nonhuman primates. The major functional stages of life described here are immaturity, adolescence, adulthood, and aged adulthood. Selection acts on each stage of development, and throughout a nonhuman primate's life its behavior is related directly to the biological events of maturation and aging. Because their biological timetables differ, males and females experience significant differences in social maturation. Age and correlated physiological events affect most systems of social behavior, such as reproduction, caregiving, and social rank. Although there are grave implications for a monkey's or ape's survival if the early maternal support system is damaged, a nonhuman primate never experiences anything comparable to the strong networks of social support that characterize a human's entire life. It is not just the old human that needs social support—humans at all ages require and get a great deal of support from their society.

Nonhuman Primate Stages of Life

Stages of development are usually identified as immaturity (infant and juvenile), adolescence (subadult), and adulthood (sometimes further subdivided into young, middle, and old adult). The definition of each stage is fairly consistent from one kind of primate to another, although the length of a specific stage may vary among genera because biological rates of development and length of life vary among phylogenetic groups. The following comments are very general and are intended to apply to both Old World monkeys and apes. Since the life span and the length of the various stages vary, emphasis will be on events rather than on specific lengths of time. It is necessary to study development longitudinally as well as in a cross section, since the behavior of cohorts at each age may vary when they have substantially different experiences.

Passage through the stages of development is biologically determined for the nonhuman primate. In contrast, a human can be moved from one stage to the next by social decree or ritual; the age at which an individual moves from immaturity to maturity, for example, varies from culture to culture. Variations in the human view of subadulthood or adolescence are well documented, and the history of the concept of childhood has been discussed (see, for example, Ariès 1965). In contrast, the nonhuman primate is totally unable to vary the normal progress of an individual through life stages.

The Infant

The first few days to weeks of life, designated as the neonatal period, are characterized by relative helplessness and dependency on the major caregiver. The degree of helplessness varies among genera, from the precocious African ververt monkey (Struhsaker 1967) to the slow-maturing African apes (Fossey 1979; Goodall 1967, 1968; Hamburg and McCown 1979; Kingsley 1977). Most primate infants need to be carried, nursed, protected, and looked after by the mother and/or other adults for a period varying from days to months after birth (Kaufman 1970; McKenna 1979a, 1979b).

The color of a monkey's natal coat often differs from that of the adult of the species (Napier and Napier 1967, Roonwal and Mohnot 1977), an adaptation that is not understood. The contrast may be marked, as in one dusky gray Southeast Asian langur, whose young infant is bright orange (S. H. Curtin 1976). Other natal coats offer a lesser contrast with adult pelage (Altmann 1980). Natal coat color generally lasts for the period of marked dependency and then gradually turns to the adult shade and pattern. Infancy, however, lasts longer than the natal color, and toward the end of this first period of life the young primate becomes increasingly independent of its major caregivers (see, for example, Altmann 1980; Jay 1962, 1965).

As infant coordination improves, the young animal strives to increase independence from restraining adults. It seeks to leave, to explore, and to play; and it is the caregiver that restrains and restricts during the early months of life (Dolhinow and Murphy 1982). By the time of weaning, which usually marks the end of the infant period, the immature monkey is able to live without major assistance from its mother. It can obtain its own food, recognize danger, and act appropriately in stress, and it is familiar enough with its social unit's routines and patterns of behavior so that it can follow daily life events on its own. Some infants may continue to maintain a great deal of contact with the mother after weaning, but this is not generally the case. Varying degrees of dependence may survive weaning; but the major focus of the mother's attention is directed toward care of her most recently born infant, and the just-weaned turns to its peers and elders. Weaning marks increasing independence for the great ape, but because it matures more slowly than a monkey, the young chimpanzee or gorilla may continue to have a very important, strong relationship with its mother.

The strongest tie of infancy for both monkey and ape is with the biological mother. This is a bond that may persist for some time, depending on the kind of primate (Dolhinow 1980). Never again in the nonhuman primate's life will it experience such physical or emotional dependency. The mother–infant relationship is an elegant and complex system of biologically motivated as well as socially acquired interactions. The net result is a female that is motivated to care for her infant and an infant that is biologically and emotionally equipped to elicit and receive this care. The mother or other important caregiver may still play a role in the juvenile's life, but her newest infant has taken the old infant or juvenile's place at her ventrum and in her attentions.

The Juvenile

The juvenile period is marked by increasing to total independence from the nurturing caregiver of infancy—the major object of early attachment. The juvenile may continue to remain near its mother and to interact with her, but her existence is no longer pivotal to its well-being, as was the case earlier in its life. It is a time of rapid physical development, of increasing social skills and motor abilities. It is also, in general, a time when the young one acquires and tests adult patterns of behavior in order to understand the limits and tolerances imposed by its social world. The juvenile tends to enjoy a certain degree of freedom, so that it may develop social and physical skills in concert with its peers before the onset of sexual and physical maturity. Juveniles learn social responsibility and that foolish actions directed toward larger group members may bring swift and strong punishment. As at earlier ages, much is learned by observation of others in the group.

By the juvenile stage of development, males and females are doing somewhat different things. Profiles of actions and interaction reveal, on average, increasing female interest in immatures and in such activities as grooming, whereas males are more often apparently preoccupied with rough play and aggressive testing of one another and of older males. While many activities are still engaged in by both males and females, the paths of the sexes clearly diverge during this period of development.

The Subadult

The subadult period, or adolescence, is a prolonged and often stressful one for the male nonhuman primate and a brief transition for the female. A male may spend several years as a subadult, and during that time he is often behaviorally and spatially peripheral to major group activities. His increasing size makes him a less than optimal play partner for smaller, younger immatures, but his incomplete physical development prevents him from successful competition with adult males for the various items of contest in normal adult life. Some subadult males appear to be in a kind of limbo: they have to wait for full dental eruption and muscular development before they can hope to win in the daily contests of group life. Males reach sexual maturity during these years, well before dental and muscular/skeletal maturity, but social maturity must wait until all these facets of development are mature.

The female's situation is in marked contrast to that of the male. When she begins to cycle and becomes sexually receptive, she enters the adult world. When she conceives, she is firmly on the adult female path, and although she will not be physically mature (dentition, muscles, bones) for several years, she assumes the social status of an adult. Her transition from juvenile to adult may be short indeed.

The Adult

Adulthood is also a period of change. Behaviors alter with experience, and changes in group composition and structure are reflected in the life of the individual. Most, if not all, biological systems change during the mature years of life, and toward the middle years of life these changes become significant and obvious. Adulthood is characterized for both sexes by the ability to participate fully in all daily routines and reproductive events characteristic of the species. Once the female becomes an adult, she will continue to follow the cycle of motherhood until her death. Life is centered on a succession of infants, and we rarely observe a female in the wild that has lived past her reproductive years. Motherhood isn't her only preoccupation, but it is certainly a major background against which all else happens.

An adult female with one or a series of offspring is affected by them in accordance with the nature and frequency of their interactions. In some species a female's status is affected mainly by the presence of a small infant, whereas in others the effect of the status she acquires then can be long lasting. In the short run, infants may stimulate increased attention to the mother—a mixed blessing if she is very subordinate and the attentions create social tension around her. Only long-term studies such as those on chimpanzees at the Gombe Preserve in Tanzania (Goodall 1968) and on rhesus macaques on Cayo Santiago (Sade 1972) will provide us with sufficient information to evaluate the advantages and disadvantages to mothers of interactions with offspring. For many nonhuman primates there are no clear lasting bonds or interaction patterns between a mother and her mature offspring.

If a species maintains high frequency of interaction along kin lines, then the numbers of related animals and their sex, and thus their temperaments, could be very important to any individual. For example, dominant lineages among some macaques may determine reproductive success within social groups (Silk et al. 1981; Kaufman, personal communication). The nonhuman primate situation is totally different from the human condition, in which all manner of real and not real goods can be channeled through real or fictive relationships from generation to generation as well as within age grades. Adoptions, so common among humans, are rare indeed among nonhuman primates (Dolhinow and De May 1982), and no monkey or ape is able to create relationships or responsibilities by decree.

An adult male will assume various roles of power or control during his mature years. He will be far more likely to leave, or to be forced to leave, his natal group than will a female of comparable age. His foci of attention will include immatures only incidentally. Among most monkeys and apes, "fathers" exist only in the mind of the observer. Individual males may show interest in infants, but as a class adult males tend not to be significantly involved in daily infant care (Bernstein et al. 1981, Altmann 1980, Ransom and Ransom 1971, Redican 1976). Their presence in the group of course indirectly ensures a healthy rearing context. Some observers have suggested that males will attempt to destroy infants fathered by other males in an attempt to increase the subsequent likelihood of their own role as progenitor of the next set of infants in the social group (Hrdy 1974, 1977). But others have suggested that at least a significant proportion of the few well-documented infanticidal acts are more the result of abnormal or highly stressed social conditions than of species' genetically evolved reproductive strategies (Boggess 1979, Curtin and Dolhinow 1978). As a male ages, his social status changes, although the great conservatism of the primate group may slow these changes.

Boundaries of Stages of Development

Stages of development are based on both physical and social patterns, and few of either category are easily amenable to precise measurement in normal contexts. For convenience, we divide the life span into stages, but to the animal there are no sharp boundaries—not even, for example, at weaning or sexual maturity. The changes that do occur are related to only a part of the animal's social world. There are implications and changes in other parts of the animal's life, but emphasis can be placed on elements of continuity rather than on ripples of change from a few big events.

Most changes are relatively slow. Even the natal color change, signaling the end of high dependency for some primates, takes place gradually. Physical changes, as in size, coordination, dental eruption, epiphesial union, and the like, are gradual and may not be measured easily or at all by observation. Physiological markers associated with the sexual maturity of the female are perhaps the most obvious, since she will show receptivity when her hormonal development makes such behavior appropriate. Her cycles, although irregular at first, soon fall into clear patterns.

Other social behaviors that may be considered stage markers do not appear suddenly or in any convenient, easily measured surge. Because there is much learning and shaping of behavior and relationships, and because many, if not most, social events are based more on cumulative experiences than on sudden biological triggers, our definition of stages must relate to a complex mesh of both biological and social profiles. In early development social behavior relates directly to its biological substrate in that an organism reaches ability levels of performance depending on, for example, central nervous system development and related motor coordination.

It is useful to think of the life span in terms of such general divisions as early, middle, and late, or, as Sherwood Washburn (1981) suggests, periods of preparation, adaptation, and decline. The length of immaturity (early or preparation) varies among nonhuman primates. It is a period of high cost, and the longer it lasts, the greater the cost to the species. An infant requires a substantial investment of time, attention, and energy by older animals and especially by the mother. It is a period of learning and growth, and we must look into the next period of life, that of maturity, to determine whether the investment in immaturity pays off in terms of reproductive success for the species. The dependent immature must have the appropriate social context in which to grow and learn or there will be deficits in behavior that may last a lifetime. The period of immaturity has been termed the years of preparation for the tasks of adulthood.

Maturity occupies the greater part of a primate's life span. Full maturity may not begin until several years after a male reaches sexual maturity, since for him physical adulthood also includes dental, osteological, and muscular development. An individual's reproductive success is a function of that animal's adult years. For the free-ranging primate, maximal reproductive performance continues for most of the years of maturity.

When biological systems begin to decline in efficiency, a primate enters the late, aged, or decline period of life. Washburn points out that old age is best viewed as a by-product of selection for good performance at earlier ages. Since physiological systems wear at different rates, there is much individual variation in the so-called ravages of age. One fact merits emphasis: there are very few old animals alive in the field. There are far more years of decline for the human than for the nonhuman primate. The latter may have few or none at all.

Estimating Ages

It is difficult to assign accurately a number of weeks or years to specific stages of life, and it is similarly very hard to make estimates of average or maximum life-span potentials (Bourlière 1960; Bowden, ed., 1979; Bowden and Jones 1979; Caminiti 1978). A survey of the nonhuman primates indicates that the life span varies significantly among major groups. The available estimates of maximum life-span potential (Cutler 1976, 1981) are relatively meaningless because the numbers are based on animals living in captivity or they are estimates of age based on field studies of less than life-span length. In evolutionary terms and for evaluation of living species, the length of time general vigor is maintained is more important than total possible life length. It should be noted that very few, if any, animals achieve the maximum possible life span under normal conditions. In fact, few individuals even outlive their effective reproductive period (see Graham, ed., 1981). Average length of life in the wild is affected by many environmental factors that are poorly documented and are certainly not well understood. We need field studies of old animals of known age and a far more complete record of the aging processes during the years of maturity. Most estimates of age of old animals are based on physical appearance, including such features as obvious tooth wear, locomotion patterns (the so-called arthritic gait), and wrinkles—all of which may be clues to antiquity, but are not necessarily good measures.

The life spans of nonhuman primates originally estimated by Adolph Schultz in 1969 have been corrected (Washburn 1981) with data not available in 1969. The early figures uniformly underestimated the length of life of the nonhuman primates and tended to perpetuate the notion that among the living primates there was an increasing length of life expectancy comparable to an evolutionary sequence of primate evolution. We know now that, for example, gibbons do not live longer than many Old World monkeys, and that some New World monkeys live longer than any of the Old World monkeys.

Old Age

The old nonhuman primate is an anomaly, and survival time during decline from maximal performance in the wild almost assuredly is short.

Only one animal in the Gombe chimpanzee study population has been estimated to have lived more than 35 years (Teleki, Hunt, and Pfifferling 1976); clearly this female was the exception, not the rule. It is unlikely that many chimpanzees in the Gombe lived for more than 30 years. Yukimaru Sugiyama (1976) estimates that only 1 of 61 Japanese macaque females survived more than 24 years, and that approximately half of the mature animals died between 15 and 21 years of age. Similar estimates are available for some other Old World monkeys (Bramblett 1969). Skeletal remains give testimony of the rigors of life in the wild. For example, Schultz (1944) found that most, but not all, of the gibbon skeletons he described as those of fully mature animals had fractures. Washburn, who did not include younger mature individuals in his category of old, observed fractures in all old gibbon skeletons he analyzed (personal communication).

A monkey or ape's latter years are marked by decreasing strength, increased sensory deficits (such as in vision or olfaction), and the like. For a primate living where predators are a normal part of the environment (and this is true of most primates) to experience a lessening in ability to perceive and react to danger can be fatal. The old animal that finds it difficult to keep up with a moving group is not waited for. If it cannot compete for limited food resources, it will decline even faster. There do not need to be many even relatively small deficits to increase dangerously the liability to injury or fatal assault. Poor vision, even a tiny lessening of acuity, may mean a miss as the animal leaps from one branch to another, or failure to notice a nearby carnivore. In either case, the results may well be disastrous. Predators will pick off the handicapped of any age, of course, but the incidence of handicap increases with every year of advanced age.

Old age may mean different things for males than for females. The female may experience a diminution of reproductive effort as she ages, in which case she will simply not become pregnant during an increasing number of successive birth seasons. It is not necessary for her to have an infant to take an active normal part in group life. Human females experience menopause after approximately 50 years of age. Observations of some colony-living macaques show menopause to occur between 22 and 28 years of age. Primary dysfunction of the reproductive system has also been recorded among captive aged rhesus macaque males (Wolf 1981). The male that wears, breaks, or loses his large canines or whose joints and muscles prevent easy powerful action may slip to the bottom of the power structure in his group. If he is allowed to become peripheral to dominance interactions, he may remain in the group, but not in the thick of events. He may, however, be forced to a low position in conflict and sustain injury in the process. Coalitions and central hierarchies, as seen among some baboons and chimpanzees, may serve to lessen the effects of increasing age on the status of the male nonhuman primate. We need a great deal more information on the behavior of aged primates and on the sources of danger to them from both within and without the troop. Because of the similarity of many of the physiological processes of humans and the nonhuman primates, (Davis 1978, Wolf 1981), aged monkeys provide a major model for the study of many human gerontological problems.

Major Events in Human Evolution:
Changes after Our Common Ancestry with the Apes

It has been some 4 to 5 million years since we shared a common ancestor with the African apes (Landau, Pilbean, and Richard 1982, Sarich and Cronin 1976, Sarich and Wilson 1968). We have little fossil evidence to aid in our reconstruction of lifeways at that time, but we may speculate that our life spans were probably on the order of those of the living African apes (relatively long for primates unless our ancestral form was substantially smaller (Zihlman and Brunker 1979).

On the basis of probable ancestral size, an estimated length of life of from 30 to 40 years seems reasonable. Size and life span are not necessarily closely correlated, however; humans in many modern cultures, for example, may expect to live far longer than our size alone would lead us to predict. Efforts to correlate life spans with age at sexual maturity can also lead to very inaccurate conclusions. "At present the slowest-maturing apes and the fastest-maturing human beings actually may mature at the same age, yet there is no suggestion that the life spans are similar" (Washburn 1981:19).

By 3.6 million years ago our direct ancestors were walking bipedally, as evidenced by the footprints found by Mary Leakey at Laetoli (1979; Hay and Leakey 1982). Three million years ago the brains of the *Australopithecus* forms, well represented in the fossil record, were still the size of those of contemporary apes—in the range of 400 to 500 cc. On the basis of the amount and kinds of object use among living apes, it is reasonable to suggest that the appearance of tools in the early archaeological record was certainly preceded by several million years during which objects, including tools, were used. The archaeological record shows that by 2 million years ago *Australopithecus* forms were making and using stone tools (Johanson and White 1979, Isaac 1978). After that time the fossil record reveals a twofold increase in brain size, to the range of 1,000 cc. The sequence has been first bipedalism, then stone tools, and only after that increase in brain size (Washburn and Moore 1980). By 40,000 years ago anatomically modern humans had far more complex lifestyles, widening geographical distribution, and technical abilities that far outstripped those of earlier forms. Brain size, however, was the same. Our ancestors of this time span were probably not surviving more than 45 years, and a 45-year-old individual was probably very old. With the origins of agriculture some 10,000 years ago, humans increased both in numbers and in their expectation of length of life. There is no evidence to suggest that biological factors have been responsible for the changes that have taken place in human behavior during the last 10,000 to 15,000 years. Similarly, biological factors are not responsible for the differences we readily record between a living gathering/hunting society and the most technical society of our world.

Modern humans are able to live *much* longer than humans of only a few hundred years ago (Birdsell 1975, Lovejoy et al. 1977). We now regard it as normal to live past the age at which our various biological systems have decreased significantly in efficiency (March 1981). This decrease or decline begins at about age 45, but because of our technological skills, including medicine and all of the support systems of human societies, we routinely step briskly into the period of life when our ancestors were dying or dead, and our closest living relatives still are. Clearly, selection has served to maintain primates from birth to the end of what we regard as the middle years or the period of adaptation. Individuals who last well beyond those years do so only with a good deal of help from their friends.

The Nonhuman and the Human Primate

One of the most outstanding contrasts between human and nonhuman primates is the complex web of social support systems available to the human at all stages of life. These powerful and varied systems may be based on political, economic, kinship, or other elements of social life. The nonhuman primate experiences only one strong support system during its life, and that is the early tie to its mother. That one relationship is seldom supplemented or replaced, even briefly, by another major caregiver. When weaning serves to break the strong tie between the mother and her offspring, the young monkey learns to manage life on its own. It is life in a social group, to be sure, and under the aegis of adults; but no nonhuman primate has support systems in any way comparable to those of all humans as they mature and age.

If this early nonhuman primate support system changes or breaks down before the age of independence, the infant is not likely to be adopted by kin or another social subgroup. A few orphaned monkeys or apes may adopt or be adopted by substitute caregivers, but most die. The care of immature humans, in contrast, is ordinarily assumed successfully by others if one or both of the parents should die.

After monkeys and apes are weaned, they may be characterized as relatively self-sufficient. There are some coalitions among individuals for power and the attributes and perogatives of high rank, but such groups are temporary and are exceptions rather than the rule. It is possible to regard the existence of a social group as a support system for the individual monkey or ape, and in some ways it does help to ensure safety; its existence serves, for example, to space members of local populations relative to natural resources. But these species-typical patterns of interaction and grouping are not comparable to the elaborate and complex social support systems found in all human cultures.

Nonhuman primate stages of development are biologically based. Infancy is terminated by weaning and the individual's enforced need to provide its own food and to maintain social relationships. Adulthood is introduced by sexual and physical maturation. Hormones lay the bases for transitions, and no social customs herald passage from one stage to another.

The basis for differences between human and nonhuman social systems is biological. What we consider to be the uniquely human social and technological adaptations are based on cognitive abilities and the human biology that makes these abilities possible. That biology lies in the human brain. Our brain and the human language, or the ability to speak that the brain makes possible, is the basis for our human learning, and consequently of human institutions. Nonhuman primate brains differ in structure and in the functions that those structures permit. The part of the primate brain that governs monkey and ape communication is not the part that governs human language (Myers 1977).

As I said at the outset, to understand human behavior we must begin the investigation with ourselves (Washburn 1978b). Nonhuman animals have provided many necessary models for investigation of specific problems, such as biomedical ones, for which humans could not be used, and data from the studies of nonhuman primates are also of use in reconstructing our evolutionary path. Comparative studies, however, serve to delineate major biological differences between human and nonhuman primates and the social behaviors these differences underlie. Comparative studies further identify those portions of our lives that have been subject to selection during our evolutionary history.

If we seek to compare and contrast differences between human social behavior and the social behaviors of other primates, we must consider the biological differences among the various species as essential factors in those social differences. The evolutionary significance of human longevity, however, can best be appreciated by a comparison of the human condition with that of the nonhuman primate. This comparison shows clearly that the factors that have promoted the development of longevity are of recent origin and that they are social, not biological. It is the human network of social support that permits the aged to live. Old age is a very recent human phenomenon and it has come about only in some cultures, long after we developed all of the biological characteristics of modern humans.

REFERENCES

Altmann, Jeanne
   1980   Baboon Mothers and Infants. Cambridge: Harvard University Press.
Ariès, Philippe
   1965   Centuries of Childhood: A Social History of Family Life. New York: Vintage Books.
Bernstein, Leo, Peter Rodman, and David G. Smith
   1981   Social relations between fathers and offspring in a captive group of rhesus monkeys (*Macaca mulatta*). Animal Behaviour 29:1057–63.
Birdsell, Joseph B.
   1975   Human Evolution: An Introduction to the New Physical Anthropology. 2d ed. Chicago: Rand McNally.
Boggess, Jane E.
   1979   Troop male membership changes and infant killing in langurs (*Presbytis entellus*). Folia Primatalogia 32(1–2):65–107.

Bourlière, Françoise
    1960   Species differences in potential longevity of vertebrates and their physiological implications. *In* The Biology of Aging, ed. Strehler. Washington, D.C.: American Institute of Biological Science.
Bowden, Douglas M., ed.
    1979   Aging in Nonhuman Primates. Primate Behavior and Development Series. New York: Van Nostrand, Reinhold.
Bowden, Douglas M., and M. L. Jones
    1979   Aging research in nonhuman primates. *In* Aging in Nonhuman Primates, ed. D. M. Bowden, pp. 1–13. Primate Behavior and Development Series. New York: Van Nostrand, Reinhold.
Bramblett, Claude A.
    1969   Non-metric skeletal age changes in the Darajani baboon. American Journal of Physical Anthropology 30:161–72.
Caminiti, B.
    1978   The aged nonhuman primate: a bibliography. Seattle: Primate Information Center, University of Washington.
Curtin, Richard A., and Phyllis Dolhinow
    1978   Primate behavior in a changing world. American Scientist 66(4): 468–75.
Curtin, Sheila H.
    1976   Niche separation in sympatric Malaysian leaf monkeys. Yearbook of Physical Anthropology 20:421–39.
Cutler, Richard G.
    1976   Evolution of longevity in primates. Journal of Human Evolution 5:169–202.
    1981   Life-span extension. *In* Aging: Biology and Behavior, ed. James J. J. McGaugh and Sara B. Keisler, pp. 31–76. New York: Academic Press.
Davis, Roger T.
    1978   Old monkey behavior. Experimental Gerontology 113:237–50.
Dolhinow, Phyllis
    1980   An experimental study of mother loss in the Indian langur monkey. Folia Primatalogica 33:77–128.
Dolhinow, Phyllis, and Mary De May
    1982   Adoption: The importance of infant choice. Journal of Human Evolution 11:391–420.
Dolhinow, Phyllis, and Greer Murphy
    1982   Langur monkey (*Presbytis entellus*) development: The first three months of life. Folia Primatologica 39:305–31.
Fossey, Dian
    1979   Development of the mountain gorilla: The first 36 months. *In* The Great Apes, ed. David A. Hamburg and Elizabeth R. McCown, pp. 139–86. Menlo Park, Calif.: Benjamin/Cummings.

Goodall, Jane
  1967   Mother-offspring relationships in chimpanzees. *In* Primate Ethology,
         ed. D. Morris, pp. 287–346. London: Weidenfeld & Nicolson.
  1968   The behaviour of free-living chimpanzees in the Gombe Stream area.
         Animal Behaviour Monographs 1:161–311.
Graham, Charles E., ed.
  1981   Reproductive Biology of the Great Apes: Comparative and Biomedical
         Perspectives. New York: Academic Press.
Hamburg, David A., and Elizabeth R. McCown
  1979   The Great Apes: Perspectives on Human Evolution. Vol. 5. Menlo
         Park, Calif.: Benjamin/Cummings.
Hay, Richard L., and Mary D. Leakey
  1982   The fossil footprints of Laetoli. Scientific American 246(2):50–57.
Hrdy, Sara B.
  1974   Male-male competition and infanticide among the langurs (*Presbytis
         entellus*) of Abu, Rajasthan. Folia Primatologica 22:19–58.
  1977   The Langurs of Abu: Female and Male Strategies of Reproduction.
         Cambridge: Harvard University Press.
Issac, Glynn
  1978   The food-sharing behavior of protohuman hominids. Scientific Ameri-
         can 238(4):90–108.
Jay, Phyllis
  1962   Aspects of maternal behavior among langurs. Annals of the New York
         Academy of Science 102:468–78.
  1965   The common langur of north India. in Primate Behavior, ed. Irven De
         Vore, pp. 197–249. New York: Holt, Rinehart & Winston.
Johanson, Donald C., and Timothy D. White
  1979   A systematic assessment of early African hominids. Science 202:
         321–30.
Kaufman, I. Charles
  1970   Biologic considerations of parenthood. *In* Parenthood, ed. E. J. An-
         thony and T. Benedek, pp. 3–55. Boston: Little, Brown.
Kingsley, Susan
  1977   Early mother–infant behavior in two species of great ape. DODO,
         Journal of the Jersey Wildlife Preservation Trust 14:55–65.
Landau, Misia, David Pilbeam, and Alison Richard
  1982   Human origins a century after Darwin. BioScience 32(6):507–12.
Leakey, Mary D.
  1979   Footprints in the ashes of time. National Geographic Magazine
         155:446–57.
Lovejoy, C. Owen, R. S. Meindl, T. R. Pryzbeck, T. S. Barton, K. G.
Heiple, and D. Kotting
  1977   Paleodemography of the Libben site, Ottawa County, Ohio. Science
         198:291–93.

McKenna, James J.
1979a Aspects of infant socialization and maternal caregiving patterns among primates: A cross-disciplinary review. Yearbook of Physical Anthropology 22:250–86.
1979b The evolution of allmothering behavior among colobine monkeys: Function and opportunism in evolution. American Anthropology 81(4):818–40.
March, James G., ed. in chief
1981 Aging: Biology and Behavior, ed. James J. McGaugh and Sara B. Kiesler. New York: Academic Press.
Myers, Ronald E.
1977 Comparative neurology of vocalization and speech: Proof of a dichotomy. *In* Human Evolution: Biosocial Perspectives, ed. Sherwood L. Washburn and Elizabeth R. McCown, pp. 59–73. Menlo Park, Calif.: Benjamin/Cummings.
Napier, John R., and Prue H. Napier
1967 A Handbook of Living Primates. New York: Academic Press.
Ransom, Timothy, and Bonnie Ransom
1971 Adult male-infant relations among baboons (*Papio anubis*). Folia Primatologica 16:179–95.
Redican, William K.
1976 Adult male-infant interactions in nonhuman primates. *In* The Role of the Father in Child Development, ed. M. E. Lamb, pp. 345–85. New York: Wiley.
Roonwal, M. L., and S. M. Mohnot
1977 Primates of South Asia. Cambridge: Harvard University Press.
Sade, Donald S.
1972 A longitudinal study of social behavior of rhesus monkeys. *In* Functional and Evolutionary Biology of Primates, ed. R. S. Tuttle. Chicago: Aldine Atherton.
Sarich, Vincent M., and Jack E. Cronin
1976 Molecular systematics of the primate. *In* Molecular Anthropology, ed. M. Goodman and R. E. Tashian, pp. 141–70. New York: Plenum Press.
Sarich, Vincent M., and Alan C. Wilson
1968 Immunological time scale for hominoid evolution. Science 158: 1200–1202.
Schultz, Adolph H.
1944 Age changes and variability in gibbons. American Journal of Physical Anthropology 2:1–17.
1969 The Life of Primates. London: Weidenfeld & Nicolson.
Silk, Joan B., A. Samuels, and Peter S. Rodman
1981 Hierarchial organization of female *Macaca radiata* in captivity. Primate 22:84–95.

Struhsaker, Thomas T.
  1967 Behavior of Vervet Monkeys. University of California Publications in Zoology, vol. 82. Berkeley: University of California Press.
Sugiyama, Yukimaru
  1976 Life history of male Japanese monkeys. *In* Advances in the Study of Behavior, ed. J. S. Rosenblatt et al. New York: Academic Press.
Teleki, Geza, E. E. Hunt, and J. H. Pfifferling
  1976 Demographic observations (1963–1973) on the chimpanzees of Gombe National Park, Tanzania. Journal of Human Evolution 5:559–98.
Washburn, Sherwood L.
  1978a What we can't learn about people from the apes. Human Nature 1:70–75.
  1978b Human behavior and the behavior of other animals. American Psychology 33:405–18.
  1981 Longevity in primates. *In* Biology, Behavior, and Aging, ed. Sara B. Kiesler, pp. 11–29. Washington, D.C.: National Research Council.
Washburn, Sherwood L., and Phyllis Dolhinow
  1983 A comparison of human behaviors. *In* Comparing Behavior, ed. D. W. Rajecki, pp. 27–42. Hillsdale, N.J.: Lawrence Erlbaum.
Washburn, Sherwood, L., and Ruth Moore
  1980 Ape into Human. 2d ed. Boston: Little, Brown.
Wolf, John
  1981 Centers' colony of old monkeys provides research opportunities. Primate Record 9(1):3–10.
Zihlman, Adrienne, and Lynda Brunker
  1979 Hominid bipedalism: Then and now. Yearbook of Physical Anthropology 22:132–62.

2

Theoretical Dimensions of a Focus on Age in Physical Anthropology

Cynthia M. Beall

Physical anthropology sets as its task "the understanding of human evolution and of individual and population variation" (Howells 1972: 141) and uses an evolutionary theoretical model stressing the interaction of biological, environmental, and cultural factors. Perhaps more than in other subdisciplines of anthropology, age has been an important and often used variable in all subfields of physical anthropology, such as human ecology; human adaptability, growth, and development; demography; genetics; and paleoanthropology. Despite this traditional use of age as a variable, however, little thought and attention has been paid to age in a broad context. Age has been used in many compartmentalized endeavors but has rarely been used to provide a perspective or organizing principle within the life-span context.

This chapter discusses some ways in which age has been used in physical anthropology, particularly in subfields that deal with living human populations, and the consequences of this approach. It suggests that the incorporation of a life-span framework in physical anthropology could enhance the understanding of human variation, a central theoretical issue in the discipline. It particularly attends to two of the main subfields of physical anthropology that deal with living populations: human adaptability and human growth and development. The subfield of human adaptability is concerned with the ways in which human populations adapt to their environments. The subfield of growth and development is concerned with changes in size, shape, or proportion and with changes in function or complexity. These general definitions apply both before and after maturity, but they are rarely used this way in practice. Human adaptability studies generally focus on children and young adults, while studies of growth and development classically are studies of child growth and development. The major thrusts of research in these areas have been in (*a*) discovering the "normal" physiological processes, (*b*) ascertaining their range of variation, and (*c*) understanding the genetic, pathological, and environmental processes that produce the range of variation.

Central to many growth and human adaptability studies is the concept of biological age. Biological age is traditionally used by physical anthropologists to measure the extent to which an individual has proceeded along some developmental continuum from birth to maturity. Biological age may be assessed for each of several physiological systems, such as the skeletal and dental systems. These physiological systems have universal beginning and end points (i.e., birth or conception and mature status) and measurable, irreversible sequential stages. This concept of biological age assumes that the same amount of development occurs in each individual no matter how long it takes. Skeletal age is the classic example of a biological age measure. A series of changes in shape occurs in a relatively fixed sequence in certain bones, such as those in the hand and wrist, until adult shape and function are attained. An X ray of the bones of the hand and wrist may be read and a "skeletal age year" or maturity score assigned on the sole basis of the individual's level of development (Roche 1978). This score or skeletal age year is the biological age. It is assessable for all people in all populations before skeletal maturity, and all children with the same degree of skeletal development are considered to have the same skeletal (biological) age regardless of their chronological ages.

Since all populations undergo the same developmental processes culminating in the same mature state, biological age alone cannot be used in comparative studies. In order to evaluate and compare individuals and populations, it is necessary to refer these biological developmental sequences to a nonbiological ordinal scale or index that is also universally applicable. Chronological age has provided that measure.

"Chronological age" refers to the time elapsed since birth. When it is possible to ascertain the date of an individual's birth, chronological age is calculable according to a standard calendrical system selected by the investigator, in practice the Western calendrical system. The result is an independent variable that provides an essential element of standardization for the collection, reporting, and comparison of data. Chronological age increases progressively at a regular pace, is irreversible, and is not influenced by environmental or genetic variation. For these reasons, population comparisons routinely use chronological age as an independent variable even when elapsed chronological time is not the subject of interest. (Chronological age is sometimes even used as a surrogate for biological age.)

Analysis of the correspondence between biological and chronological age has been fundamental to the study of human adaptability, growth, and development. Such analysis is typically accomplished by means of a reference population in which the chronological age equivalents of biological ages are established. In such a population, children are grouped by chronological age, and the central tendency of development for a system such as the skeleton is established for each chronological age. For example, the representative level of development among children of 9 chronological age years is assigned the skeletal age year of 9. In other situations, anyone with that level of skeletal development is assigned a skeletal age year of 9. If he were chronologically 7 or 11 he would be considered advanced or delayed in his skeletal development relative to the reference population. This somewhat narrow technical use of chronological and biological age before maturity has provided a basic research tool for the study of human variation. It has demonstrated that individuals and populations pass through the same physiological developmental stages at widely varying rates and that at a given biological age there is tremendous variation in chronological age (and vice versa). Once such human variation is documented, the aim of the physical anthropologist is to explain this variation within an evolutionary and adaptive framework.

Age at menarche is a classic illustration of the manner in which variation in chronological age exists for a given biological age (here a single event). Information on age at menarche is available from hundreds of populations, and the median age at which populations of young women arrive at this biological developmental stage ranges from a low of 12.3 chronological years to a high of 18.4 (Eveleth and Tanner 1976). Because of the abundance of information on this phenomenon, a number of underlying patterns have been discerned (Johnston 1974; Eveleth 1979). For example, Asians generally reach menarche earlier than Northern and Central Europeans, and within a single society women from higher socioeconomic backgrounds have a younger median age at menarche regardless of the population median (Eveleth 1979). Both genetic and environmental factors influence the timing of this biological event. Among the various environmental factors, the influence of variation in nutritional status has been the subject of many studies. Undernutrition during childhood delays age at menarche, while overnutrition accelerates it. These findings may help to explain other observations, such as late age at menarche in girls of low socioeconomic status or in those with many siblings, by suggesting that these factors may exert their influence via nutritional status. Thus an appreciation of variation in sociocultural as well as nutritional environmental factors enhances the understanding of variation in the chronological age at menarche. Interest in explaining the mechanism underlying this variability has in turn led to the development of a controversial explanatory hypothesis concerning the overall control of age at menarche (Frisch and McArthur 1974, Frisch 1980, Malina 1980).

This use of an age dimension has been widely applied for many years. It has provided an understanding and an appreciation of the variety of patterns and paces of growth and development during the stages of the life cycle before maturity. Maturity, however, occurs relatively early in the life cycle. One of the latest maturing of the frequently used biological age systems, the hand-wrist area of the skeleton, attains mature status near the end of the second decade in Western populations, that is, early in the context of a total life span of seven or eight decades. Mature stature is also attained around that time in Western populations. Thus the traditional focus on growth and development up to young adulthood excludes the largest portion of the life span. There are important theoretical and scientific as well as practical medical reasons for the interest in the early portion of the life span when events take place at a rapid pace and environmental factors may exert lasting effects. These are the processes that produce adult variation, and they are thus integral to an understanding of processes during adulthood. At the same time this rather exclusive focus on events up through young adulthood essentially relegates the older adult and aged stages of the life span to a residual category of marginal or no theoretical interest. It assumes tacitly that all adaptation, growth, and development have occurred before young adulthood or that the adaptations of young adults represent those of all adults. Furthermore, it conceptualizes young adulthood as an end product rather than a stage in an ongoing process. The traditional theoretical perspectives of physical anthropology have, in effect, been age parochial. There is a relative dearth of comparative data on the later stages of the life cycle, although there is growing evidence of continued growth, development, and adaptation throughout the life span, of population differences in these processes, and of important relationships among various contiguous and noncontiguous stages in the life span. Adoption of a life-span orientation explicitly acknowledges the importance of these processes that occur beyond the arbitrary end point of mature status, that is, of the process of aging.

The Western biomedical literature contains ample evidence of morphological and anatomical change throughout adulthood (see, for example, Finch and Hayflick 1977). Virtually all physiological systems manifest an age-related decline or involution in size, function, or integration throughout adulthood. In many populations a common pattern of continued change in some organ systems, such as the skeleton, is found throughout the life span (Garn 1970). In many other organ systems, such as the cardiovascular, there is clearly wide individual and population variation in the pace at which these processes occur, a phenomenon termed "differential aging" (Bourlière 1970). Currently, however, there is no available overall measure of this process that is analagous to the biological age measures used before maturity. That is, there is apparently no constant, measurable amount of adult development that everyone experiences before death. Therefore the approach to the measurement of biological age during adulthood has focused on descriptions of changes or differences in morphology and function associated with chronological age as reflections of biological age (see discussion in Costa and McCrae 1980). The available data derive principally from samples of Western industrial populations. These data, plus the few available for nonwestern populations, indicate that the absolute levels of the changes and differences in these variables which reflect biological age (such as blood pressure, grip strength, weight, visual acuity) as well as those related to chronological age differ markedly among populations (e.g., Bourlière 1970). These data strongly suggest that similar variation in additional traits will be found once systematic comparisons are undertaken.

The importance of understanding the full range of possible manifestations of age-related changes in adult functional capacity is illustrated by adult blood pressure. Extensive work, in particular among nonwestern populations, demonstrates the inaccuracy of the once widely held view that an increase in adult blood pressure is a universal phenomenon of

aging. Among horticulturalists of Amazonia and New Guinea, for example, adult blood pressures do not rise (Sinnett and White 1973; Oliver,
Cohen, and Neel 1975). Specific factors underlying this variation are not
yet clear, although dietary and lifestyle variables are implicated. It is
clear, however, that a rise in adult blood pressure is not an inevitable
concomitant of the passage of time. The same may be true of other
supposedly inevitable declines in function that are accepted as normal in
the West. Studies of the biological experience after maturity of populations in varying environments analagous to those undertaken by students
of child growth and development are essential further steps toward a full
characterization of the biological aging process. Currently it is often
unclear whether certain phenomena related to chronological age are universal or normal or pathological or specific to certain environmental or
other factors. Theories of human growth, development, and adaptability
and of the evolution of the life span itself must explain as many of the
manifestations of normal biological aging as possible—yet until we are
aware of the possible range of normal and abnormal variation, we do not
know what we are trying to explain.

Another aspect of age changes in adult morphological and functional
capacity is the way they impinge on individuals' participation in their
culture. Theoretically, functional capacity of one or more physiological
systems may decline so far that performance of certain activities in standard fashion is no longer feasible. The possible cultural responses are
myriad, and include chronological-age-related norms for economic tasks
(e.g., retirement age), formal assessment of individual capacities (e.g.,
tests of visual acuity for retention of a driver's license), and informal
assessment of ability to perform certain subsistence tasks and the like.
The transitions between culturally defined age categories may thus be
viewed in the context of underlying biological changes. Such so-
ciodemographic characteristics as household composition may also be
viewed this way. For example, it might be hypothesized that the elderly
who live alone have higher levels of function in some physiological
systems than those who live with adult children. Culture does not merely
respond to these biological changes, however; it may also influence the
rate at which they occur. Smoking, for example, may adversely affect
pulmonary function as well as alter chest morphology (Borkan et al.
1981). The traditional Eskimo hunting way of life required high levels of
physical activity and physical fitness; yet once a man's son became a
skilled hunter, so that he could select items from his son's catch and

reduce his own hunting activity, a rapid deterioration of physical condition ensued (Shephard 1978). This example further illustrates the necessity of analyzing biological changes throughout the life span with reference to the appropriate cultural context.

The life-span perspective also directs attention toward another group of potentially important sources of variation within populations: events in previous stages of the life span. To a certain extent, a particular phenomenon of adult growth, development, or adaptation may represent a continuation of an earlier pattern or an outcome of an earlier adaptation. Indeed, attempts to explain and understand variation in adult form and function may be misleading or inaccurate when they are undertaken without reference to possible influences that originated earlier in the life span and whose biological outcomes are expressed during adulthood. The importance of understanding the relationships among stages can be seen from a number of studies. Although none covers the entire life span, they demonstrate the utility of explicitly considering the succession of life-span stages as interrelated rather than as discrete entities. For example, the phenomenon of catch-up growth, a period of rapid growth following the end of a period of restriction (Tanner 1978), is illustrative of the connections between stages. It has been argued that there is an association between early growth patterns and the biological aging process, with accelerating growth before maturity associated with a shortening of life expectancy. Studies of fatness and obesity demonstrate a continuity in size not only between life-cycle stages but also between generations (Garn 1980; Garn, Bailey, and Cole 1980). Maternal prepregnancy fat levels, for example, influence offspring size at birth, which in turn is claimed to be "the most important single determinant of individual growth during the first seven years of life" among normal U.S. term infants (Garn, Shaw, and McCabe 1977:1049). Birth weight is also associated with variation in the chance of surviving infancy (e.g., Van Valen and Mellin 1967). Studies of fatness and obesity in particular have been concerned with describing and understanding fatness at various stages of the life cycle and its relationship to fatness during previous or subsequent stages. These studies have been guided in great part by the concept of a critical period of special vulnerability, and argue that the age of onset of obesity is an important variable that influences the nature and degree of obesity. Information on the later stages of life contains other suggestive examples of continuity between life-cycle stages, such as the influence of adolescent diet on young adult blood pressure (Valadian, Berkey, and

Reed 1981). Additionally, there is evidence that a child's blood pressure relative to that of chronological age peers remains stable throughout childhood and adolescence and into adulthood (Blumenthal 1978). This continuity is referred to as tracking or canalization, a phenomenon that is mentioned most often in the literature on physical growth of children but that is also applicable to other systems and life-cycle stages.

Findings such as these not only illustrate continuity between life-cycle stages, they also direct attention toward the need to identify the underlying mechanisms that produce biological variation. A. Roberto Frisancho, Stanley Garn, and Werner Ascoli (1970) have shown that chronic malnutrition slows growth and skeletal and pubertal development among Central American children. During adolescence, however, in response to stimulation by the hormones of puberty, there is an improvement in skeletal age (but not in height), with the result that the individual quickly reaches skeletal maturity (and thus has limited potential for further height increase) but does so at a height below the norm for populations that do not experience chronic malnutrition. This integration of data from several life stages illustrates the mechanism for the widely observed phenomenon of short adult height in undernourished populations by noting continuity of one feature (rate of height growth) in juxtaposition with change in another (rate of skeletal development).

Another variation in an adult characteristic which may be better understood with reference to earlier stages of the life cycle is that in age at death and its relation to exposure to childhood diseases. Survivors of periods of high childhood mortality during the late 1700s and early 1800s in the Connecticut River Valley enjoyed greater life expectancy than their unstressed counterparts, apparently as a result of a developmental strengthening process (Meindl and Swedlund 1977). Further examples include variation in the reproductive success of women who live at high altitudes in North America and in pulmonary capacity of men at high altitudes in South America, both dependent on the developmental age at exposure to high altitudes (Frisancho et al. 1973, Weinstein and Haas 1977). Among girls born in Boston during the 1930s, those with relatively high concentrations of animal protein in their diet during adolescence tend to have a more successful reproductive experience (Valadian, Berkey, and Reed 1981). Thus adaptation to a stress such as chronic malnutrition, disease, high altitude, or low levels of dietary animal protein at one stage of the life span may influence biological characteristics in subsequent stages of the life span.

While such analyses are somewhat infrequent, they demonstrate the powerful theoretical potential of a broad life-span perspective and suggest that the origins of some adaptations and variations that occur after maturity may lie in earlier experiences (see also Falkner 1980, Garn 1980, Plato and Norris 1980). By restricting its focus to the period before maturity and young adulthood and then by underemphasising the possible relationships among stages, physical anthropology traditionally has artificially constricted its scope and may have elaborated a distorted understanding of human growth, development, and adaptability.

Aging has been defined as a loss of adaptive capacity (Shock 1977, Cowdry 1952). Physical anthropologists interested in human adaptability possess a sophisticated set of models and techniques to analyze adaptive capacity (see, for example, Baker, ed., 1977; Damon, ed., 1975) yet have so far largely overlooked the opportunity to bring them to bear on the later stages of the life span. A model consisting of several components, including (a) age-related biological changes after maturity, (b) influences before maturity, (c) influences after maturity, (d) the interactions of a, b, and c, (e) age-related changes in adaptive capacity, and (f) the environment, yields a complex, new, and fascinating perspective on the time period of the life span after maturity. It might be argued, for example, that populations that inhabit—that is, are chronically exposed to—extreme environments enjoy a slower rate of loss of adaptive capacity than populations that are not so exposed, since it would be more immediately dysfunctional to lose adaptive capacity in a chronic stress situation. Alternatively, it might be argued that such systems are subject to more wear and tear and thus may suffer a faster rate of loss of adaptive capacity. It might be hypothesized, for example, that factors that delay or accelerate growth and development before maturity delay or accelerate the loss of adaptive capacity. The concept of the universality of the loss of adaptive capacity could itself be addressed. The relationships between changes in adaptive capacity and the cultural notions of social age categories, age-normative behaviors, the division of labor, dependency, status, and so on are important biocultural questions that could be addressed by means of this model. These ideas are based on our current understanding of human population–environment interactions, which, as indicated earlier, may or may not be somewhat skewed. Further research into these interactions throughout the life span may result in honing or qualifying or elaborating the currently used models.

There are numerous techniques to measure adaptation to a wide range of stresses, such as heat, cold, and altitude, which have generally been applied to young adults and occasionally to adolescents and children (see, for example, Little and Hochner 1973, Frisancho 1980). Application of these techniques to a broader age range would not be difficult and the rewards great in terms of our enhanced understanding of the relationship between human populations and their environments.

Studies of the whole life span, however, do pose some problems not encountered in studies of child and young adult growth, development, and adaptation. One of these problems is the need to consider historical context. Cohort differences in exposure to varying environmental influences produce secular trends (and occasional reversals thereof) which complicate the study of continuities among life-cycle stages by exaggerating or obscuring age differences and age changes. For example, 30-year-olds may be taller than 70-year-olds because the former were taller at maturity, the latter have lost stature, or both. New analytical techniques for partitioning aging and secular trend phenomena in cross-sectional samples must be added to those now available (e.g., Hertzog, Garn, and Hempy 1969; Himes and Mueller 1977). Semilongitudinal and longitudinal samples (measured more than once so that individual rates of change may be ascertained) are likely to receive greater emphasis (e.g., Garn 1980, Friedlaender and Rhoads 1982).

Another problem is to select or devise measures that are feasible and meaningful throughout the lifespan. The rates of change with age and the ranges of variation at any age differ for many variables at different life-cycle stages, and these differences complicate the analysis and interpretation of data. Another complicating factor is the partitioning of illness and aging phenomena. These and other conceptual and methodological challenges will require innovative research designs and hypotheses.

The life-span approach emphasizes description and analysis of the patterns of change and continuity in age-related biological phenomena from conception to death. It puts these phenomena in a broader context and suggests new research methodologies and designs. It points out areas where knowledge is woefully lacking and where the approach and interests of the physical anthropologist could make a substantial contribution to general knowledge about biological phenomena and the interrelationship between human populations and cultures and their environments and human biological variation.

The two subfields of physical anthropology emphasized here are not unique in the use of the age variable, either chronological or biological.

Indeed, it is pervasive. Studies of archeological and fossil human populations, for example, routinely explore the biological characteristics of the remains and, by analogy with some contemporary reference population, estimate the individuals' chronological age at death. In this case biological age is used as an index of chronological age, and accuracy depends on the validity of the assumption of a similar pattern and rate of biological change during elapsed chronological time in the two populations. Secular trends in certain features of the contemporary population may alter the interpretation of age in the archaeological population (Trotter and Peterson 1967). In addition, studies of demography and genetics also routinely use chronological age as an index variable to study fertility and mortality patterns, population structure, and the actions of natural selection on human populations. Age-specific mortality patterns have an obvious influence on life expectancy and are modified by biological, environmental, and cultural factors. Indeed, a great deal of our understanding of the phenomenon of aging derives from age-specific mortality patterns and their changes through time.

The evolution of the human life span, with its characteristic stages and maximum life-span potential, is a major theoretical and research question, requiring input from each subfield. Whether aging is a programmed process resulting from natural selection for such a stage in the human life span or whether it is a by-product of natural selection for other essentially human characteristics is an issue of great import for our study of the whole subject of the life span and aging (Weiss 1981). Knowledge about the essential biological characteristics of our species' life span and about the environmental and cultural factors that may modify these characteristics is essential for this endeavor. (See also Dolhinow, chap. 1 of this volume.) The contributions of each subfield of physical anthropology will be essential in order to develop a comprehensive theory of the characteristic human life span, that is, one that addresses both the ultimate causes of the evolution of the life span and the proximate causes of the manifested biological processes.

REFERENCES

Baker, Paul T., ed.
   1977   Human Population Problems in the Biosphere: Some Research Strategies and Designs. MAB Technical Notes no. 3. Paris: UNESCO.
Blumenthal, S.
   1978   Precursors in childhood of primary hypertension in the adult. Annals of the New York Academy of Science 304:28–32.

Borkan, G. A., R. J. Glynn, S. S. Bachman, R. Bosse, and S. T. Weiss
  1981   Relationship between cigarette smoking, chest size, and body size in health-screened adult males. Annals of Human Biology 8:153–60.

Bourlière, Françoise
  1970   The Assessment of Biological Age in Man. Public Health Papers no. 37. Geneva: WHO.

Costa, Paul T., and Robert R. McCrae
  1980   Functional age: A conceptual and empirical critique. *In* Second Conference on the Epidemiology of Aging, ed. Suzanne G. Haynes and Manning Feinleib. Bethesda, Md.: U.S. Department of Health and Human Services.

Cowdry, E. V.
  1952   What is aging? Panel discussion. Journal of Gerontology 7:452–63.

Damon, A., ed.
  1975   Physical Anthropology. New York: Oxford University Press.

Demirjian, A.
  1978   Dentition. *In* Human Growth, ed. Frank T. Falkner and J. M. Tanner, vol. 2. New York: Plenum Press.

Eveleth, Phyllis B.
  1979   Population differences in growth: Environmental and genetic factors. *In* Human Growth, ed. Frank T. Falkner and J. M. Tanner, vol. 3. New York: Plenum Press.

Eveleth, Phyllis B., and J. M. Tanner
  1976   Worldwide Variation in Human Growth. Cambridge: Cambridge University Press.

Falkner, Frank T., ed.
  1980   Prevention in Childhood of Health Problems in Adult Life. Geneva: WHO.

Finch, Caleb E., and Leonard Hayflick, eds.
  1977   Handbook of the Biology of Aging. New York: Van Nostrand Reinhold.

Friedlaender, J. S., and J. G. Rhoads
  1982   Patterns of adult weight and fat change in six Solomon Islands societies: A semi-longitudinal study. Social Science and Medicine 16:205–16.

Frisancho, A. Roberto
  1980   Human Adaptation: A Functional Approach. St. Louis: Mosby.

Frisancho, A. Roberto, Stanley M. Garn, and Werner Ascoli
  1970   Unequal influence of low dietary intakes on skeletal maturation during childhood and adolescence. American Journal of Clinical Nutrition 23:1220–27.

Frisancho, A. R., C. Martinez, T. Velasquez, J. Sanchez, and H. Montoya
  1973   Influence of developmental adaptation on lung function at high altitude. Human Biology 45:583–94.

Frisch, R. E.
1980 Letter to the editor. Annals of Human Biology 7(4):387.
Frisch, R. E., and McArthur, J. W.
1974 Menstrual cycles: Fatness as a determinant of minimum weight for height necessary for their maintenance or onset. Science 185:949–51.
Garn, Stanley M.
1970 The Earlier Gain and Later Loss of Cortical Bone. Springfield, Ill.: Charles C. Thomas.
1980 Continuities and change in maturational timing. *In* Constancy and Change in Human Development, ed. Orville G. Brim and Jerome Kagan. Cambridge: Harvard University Press.
Garn, Stanley, M., S. M. Bailey, and P. E. Cole
1980 Continuities and changes in fatness and obesity. *In* Nutrition, Physiology, and Obesity, ed. R. Schemmel. Palm Beach: CRC Press.
Garn, Stanley M., Helen A. Shaw, and K. D. McCabe
1977 Birth size and growth appraisal. Journal of Pediatrics 90(6):1049–51.
Hertzog, K. P., Stanley M. Garn, and H. O. Hempy
1969 Partitioning the effects of secular trending and aging in adult stature. American Journal of Physical Anthropology 31:111–15.
Himes, J. H., and W. H. Mueller
1977 Aging and secular change in adult stature in rural Colombia. American Journal of Physical Anthropology 46:275–80.
Howells, W. W.
1972 Physical anthropology. Yearbook of Physical Anthropology 16:141.
Johnston, F. E.
1974 Control of age at menarche. Human Biology 46(1):159–71.
Little, M. A., and D. H. Hochner
1973 Human Thermoregulation, Growth, and Mortality. Addison-Wesley Module in Anthropology no. 36. Reading, Mass.: Addison-Wesley.
Malina, R. M.
1980 Letter to the editor. Annals of Human Biology 7(4):387.
Meindl, R. S., and A. C. Swedlund
1977 Secular trends in mortality in the Connecticut Valley, 1700–1850. Human Biology 49(3):389–414.
Oliver, W. J., E. L. Cohen, and J. V. Neel
1975 Blood pressures, sodium intake, and sodium-related hormones in the Yanomamo Indians, a "no-salt" culture. Circulation 52:146–51.
Plato, C. C., and A. H. Norris
1980 Bone measurement of the second metacarpal and grip strength. Human Biology 52(1):131–49.
Roche, A. F.
1978 Bone growth and maturation. *In* Human Growth, ed. F. Falkner and J. M. Tanner, vol. 2. New York: Plenum Press.
Shephard, R.
1978 Physical Activity and Aging. Chicago: Yearbook Medical Publishers.

Shock, Nathan W.
1977 System integration. *In* Handbook of the Biology of Aging, ed. Caleb E. Finch and Leonard Hayflick. New York: Van Nostrand Reinhold.

Sinnett, P. F., and H. M. White
1973 Epidemiological studies in a total highland population, Tukisenta, New Guinea. Journal of Chronic Diseases 26:265–90.

Tanner, J. M.
1978 Fetus into Man: Physical Growth from Conception to Maturity. Cambridge: Harvard University Press.

Trotter, M., and R. R. Peterson
1967 Relation of diameter of adult femur to age in American whites and Negroes. American Journal of Physical Anthropology 27:246.

Valadian, Isabelle, Catherine Berkey, and Robert B. Reed
1981 Adolescent nutrition as it relates to cardiovascular disease and reproductive capacity later in life. Nutrition Reviews 39(2):107–11.

Van Valen, Leigh, and Gilbert W. Mellin
1967 Selection in natural populations 7: New York babies (fetal life study). Annals of Human Genetics (London) 31:109–26.

Weinstein, R. S., and J. D. Haas
1977 Early stress and later reproductive performance under conditions of malnutrition and high altitude hypoxia. Medical Anthropology 1:25–54.

Weiss, Kenneth M.
1981 Evolutionary perspectives on human aging. *In* Other Ways of Growing Old, ed. Pamela Amoss and Stevan Harrell, pp. 25–68. Palo Alto: Stanford University Press.

Part Two / Age and Society

3

Age, Generation, and Social Structure

Meyer Fortes

When we speak of age or aging in the context of personal or social life in a modern Western society, what we have in mind is chronological age calculated by reference to a dating system. This approach is well documented in Binstock and Shanas' *Handbook of Aging and the Social Sciences* (1976). In the nonwestern, preliterate, preindustrial societies on which anthropologists have in the past mainly concentrated, the case is different. As is apparent from such reviews of the anthropological data as Gulliver's (1968), Goody's (1976), Kertzer's (1982), and Foner and Kertzer's (1978), chronological age is seldom formally recognized in societies of this type. The idea that status (e.g., legal majority), occupational roles (such as those discussed in Riley 1976), claims on society (e.g., retirement benefits), and many other incidents of normal personal and social life should be regulated by a calculus corresponding to our schemes of chronological-age-linked rules is totally lacking in preliterate tribal culture. But age and aging as observable and experienced natural processes are universal; and the way they are incorporated into tribal forms of social structure or invested with cultural value and significance is a topic of central relevance for anthropological theory. It is interesting to look back over the past quarter century—one natural generation, according to a widely accepted convention, but at least three academic

99

generations ago—to S. N. Eisenstadt's seminal comparative study
(1956). Though much has been added to the ethnographic record since
then, Eisenstadt's cross-cultural comparison yielded fundamental theoretical insights. His hypothesis that the way in which the variable of age
is incorporated into social structure is directed by the way in which what
he aptly describes as "citizenship"—that is, broadly speaking, the status
in society at large that confers politicojural rights and duties as opposed to
familial rights and duties—is achieved and maintained is a key to some of
the most confusing problems in this field.

Cross-culturally viewed, the first question is how the universal biological substructure of aging is dealt with. Anthropologists see aging as
incorporated into social structure by way of the individual life cycle.
Perceived by both observers and actors as beginning with conception and
ending only with death, it is invested with customary values and meanings and subject to social control throughout its course. Theories about
sex and procreation that reflect norms of parenthood in its jural and moral
no less than in its physiological aspects, and that imply doctrines of a
religious character about the soul and personality, are found in all human
societies. But what is here relevant is that the life cycle is made up of
stages of *maturation* or growth along the gradient of biological age, as
Cynthia Beall terms it (in Chapter 2 of this volume). The cross-cultural
evidence is that stages of maturation are identified, named, culturally
defined, and built into the social structure in all societies. The number of
stages that are so recognized—Shakespeare's well-known seven are an
instance—varies from society to society; but as such dramatic manifestations of this universal practice as initiation and nubility ceremonies remind us, the cultural recognition of any stage of maturation takes note not
only of biological signs (such as first menstruation) but of achieved and
expected capacities, skills, and potentialities, as well as of such imputed
conditions as ritual purity and impurity. "He is ready for a following
sibling" is a remark often made by Tallensi about a newly weaned toddler
who is toilet trained and is happy to play by himself or run around with
other children. Another infant of apparently the same chronological age
but retarded in maturation would not be so described. As our own laws
governing the registration of births, deaths, and marriages and our religious customs of baptism, circumcision, and confirmation emphasize
and cross-cultural evidence amply supports, what the social incorporation
and cultural validation of maturational stages signifies is not only recog-

nition but *authorization*—to join the cattle herds, to marry, to sit with the elders, and so on.

What must be emphasized is that stages of maturation over the individual life cycle are not determined by or coterminous with chronological age. Age in the latter sense is established by a cultural apparatus, a dating system that is independent of and neutral in regard to both the biological substructure and the social incorporation of maturational stages. Criteria and norms of chronological age imposed on these stages in Western societies occur not mainly because the apparatus is available and dominates our thinking about maturation but because the laws that define and determine the rights and duties of citizenship demand it. Young children worked in British coal mines 150 years ago because the law, or more exactly the state, allowed them to be so employed, and they stopped doing so when the state prohibited such labor by individuals under a certain age, regardless of their stature, strength, state of health, or intelligence. Today parents are in breach of the law if they do not ensure that their children, again regardless of physical or mental capacity, attend school until the age of 16.

Western-trained anthropologists often project interpretations of chronological age on maturational field data, partly out of habit but mainly to relate their observations to the models of the life cycle that guide members of Western societies in the conduct of their lives. Writing about the socialization of Tallensi children, I felt obliged to establish age-related maturational norms, arrived at by roundabout inquiries or sheer guesswork, in order to fit my observations to the accepted models of social and psychological development in our society (see Fortes 1938; and see also Rabain 1979, passim). And this practice is typical. Yet the terminology of chronological age is likely to be indirectly if not directly misleading, as in the studies of so-called age-grade and age-set organization in tribal societies, to which I shall return presently.

A no less ambiguous conflation of actors' concepts and observers' constructs appears in the ways generation differences are interpreted in terms of age. Kertzer (1982) discusses this difficulty in the context of elucidating the proper genealogical connotation of the generation concept, as in anthropological usage in family and kinship studies. He makes his point by contrasting this formally correct usage with the metaphorical extension of the generational model to depict successive phases of historical change in social, political, and cultural movements in the manner popularized by Karl Mannheim (1952) between the wars. I have reservations about his criticisms, as I shall presently explain. But the issue to which they lead him is of cardinal significance in the anthropological study of age and generation. There are many situations in which relationships by generation conflict with relationships by birth order, which we gloss as age, and institutionalized measures for resolving the contradictions that ensue are found in most societies.

Fieldwork constantly brings up instances, as I found among the Tallensi. I recollect one morning meeting a youth whom I guessed to be about 20 scolding a small boy, who might have been about 6 or 7, for letting the goat he was herding stray. When I asked the young man why he did not wallop the boy, he answered, looking quite shocked, that he couldn't do that. "Don't you know he is my father?" he said. It transpired that the child was the son of his grandfather's youngest wife, therefore his classificatory father. Similar contradictions due to polygynous marriage over a long stretch of years, Kertzer observes, are common, and are often protracted to later generations by the lineage principle.

The Tallensi resolve the problem by ranking individuals by generation in the context of family and lineage relations, by order of birth in interlineage or political relations (see Kertzer 1982, Fortes 1945:225). My friends Teezeen (aged about 70) and his classificatory father Nyaangzum (about 50) neatly exemplified this system. A Tallensi man is allowed to marry a widow of his patrilineal grandfather provided she is not his own grandmother, and that was how Teezeen inherited Nyaangzum's mother before Nyaangzum was weaned. Thus it came about that Teezeen brought up his classificatory father, who in due course assumed his jurally proper role as head of their branch of the lineage. Then Teezeen, as the oldest man by birth order in the clan, was elected to the office of head of the local clan assembly. Thus in all internal affairs of the lineage, such as marriage and sacrifices to the lineage ancestors, Nyaangzum was supreme by virtue of genealogical reckoning, whereas in the affairs of the clan, such as the management of the Boghar cult (see Fortes 1945:110–15), Teezeen was the leader by virtue of his "age" superiority. Both insisted that this division of authority raised no problems as the internal and external affairs of the lineage were necessarily distinct. The pattern is common and widespread, and not only among the Tallensi. Contradictions between generation order and birth order are cited as leading to the bending of rules of age-set allocation in East African age-set systems (see Baxter and Almagor, eds., 1978:26) in order to place individuals in appropriate slots in the system.

The Tallensi exemplify this apparent contradiction in other ways, too, notably in the fundamental jural rule that no man can achieve jural autonomy—become *sui iuris*—until his father dies. I happened to call on the chief of Tongo (aged about 55) when a delegation from a neighboring chief was with him. The visitors had come to solicit the hand of one of his daughters in marriage. The chief thanked them and explained that he did not "own himself," as his father was still alive. Marriage is an internal affair of the lineage, not a clan concern, he reminded them, and therefore was subject to his father's jurisdiction, not his own. Would they kindly go to put their plea to his father? The old man was in fact nearly senile, so the decision would certainly de facto be made by the chief, but it would have no jural validity unless it was formally approved by his father. I have records of adolescent boys who had to adopt roles for which they were totally unprepared by knowledge or experience, because the deaths of their fathers had left them the jurally autonomous, formal heads of their natal families.

Such contradictions between age and generation in family relationships are of course not uncommon in Western societies. In second or third marriages, after the divorce or death of a spouse, the birth of children may come many years after the birth of children of a first marriage. Thus a man's youngest offspring may be born about the same time as his first or even second grandchild by an earlier son or daughter. I know of several such cases, in one of which son and grandson went to the same school and grew up together as close friends and companions. We do not nowadays expect such situations to produce problems of personal or social adjustment. We have no classificatory kinship institutions and, in particular, no rules that prescribe respectful, let alone avoidance, behavior in relation to parents or classificatory parents. Moreover, neolocal residential arrangements enable individual offspring to move out to their own dwellings at marriage. Of course if hereditary property or rank were at stake, the situation might be different. A man's oldest son might resent the birth of a half brother twenty-five years younger if it meant that the estate or title he expected to inherit and pass on to his son might be bequeathed to the half brother.

The case of Teezeen and Nyaangzum is not unique among the Tallensi. And there was one important and characteristic division of loyalties between them. They had grown up with different "mates" (*taab*), their contemporaries of other families and lineages. Lifelong friendships are thus created which are independent of kinship ties or genealogical generation.

What are the theoretical implications of these observations? They are already adumbrated in Eisenstadt's study and are more explicitly drawn out in the review articles by Riley, Kertzer, Foner, Keith, and others alluded to earlier. The first and most essential point is that genealogical generations are uniquely created in the family nucleus of parents and children. The succession of the generations thus brought about is the essence, the sine qua non of the reproductive process, first for the physical replacement of each generation but second and more fundamentally for its social and cultural replacement by the next generation. But behind the continuity of society and culture thus ensured lies a split. It is now accepted that the relations between parents and their children of the same sex are fraught with deep ambivalence. Parents must cherish their children to ensure their own replacement, but they see them—and are seen by their children—as threatening rivals, their oedipal enemies. Open or covert and varying greatly in expression in different cultural environments, this seems to be a universal law of human social life (see Fortes 1974). And where there is a classificatory kinship system, this pattern of intergenerational relations is likely to be extended outside the nuclear family to collateral kin.

Equally widely accepted is the corollary that beneath the solidarity and amity that mark the relationships of siblings, especially those of the same sex, when they confront their parental generation or the outside world we always find the deep divisions of sibling rivalry, which mirrors the rivalry between successive generations. The universality of these intrafamilial cleavages is attested in myths, religious doctrines and prohibitions, and such more down-to-earth ways as the residential separation of successive generations and of successive siblings (as among the Nyakyusa; see Wilson 1951, Fortes 1969:243–44). We ourselves are constantly reminded of them in the works of our poets, novelists, and dramatists, not to speak of our Bible. Nor need we go back to the *Oedipus* trilogy of Sophocles. Shakespeare's *King Lear* makes use of a variant of the same theme. It is poignantly and profoundly examined in Dostoevski's *Brothers Karamazov;* and it appears almost undisguised in Trollope's best-known novels and in those of other Victorian novelists. And a lesson that all these literary portrayals, as well as the ritual and other relevant customs of such peoples as the Tallensi and Nyakyusa convey, is this: these propensities are intrinsic to the human family structure and thus pose for every society problems of how they can be disciplined and mobilized for constructive social purposes.

It should be noted that *age,* whether chronologically reckoned or reducible to relative order of birth, is an adventitious factor in family structure and indeed in the relations of generations in the domestic domain (see Fortes 1969:95–100). A parent is a parent, a sibling is a sibling regardless of age; nor are stages of maturation significant except insofar as procreative sexual relations are possible only between individuals who have reached puberty and insofar as a woman's fecundity ceases with the menopause. In short, my father is my father whether he was 20 when I was born or 60, and my sibling of three months is no less a sibling than is a married brother or sister.

Generations are brought into being by the combination of conjugal and reproductive relations that is the core of every kinship system, be it that of Bushmen and other hunters and collectors at one end of the scale of social organization or of our Western society at the other. The concept of a generation and of a sequence of generations is a function of kinship relations and is therefore specifiable by reference to genealogical connections. These considerations emphasize that the process of ranking, reckoning, and grouping individuals by generations is wholly distinct from that of ranking, reckoning, and grouping people by either stages of maturation or the equivalents of age. In classificatory systems, as I have suggested, the principles of the unity of the lineage and the equivalence of siblings (see Fortes 1969:76–80) enable the generation model to be extended so widely as to provide the basis for regulating social relationships in an entire tribal community, as for instance among Australian aborigines. The domestic domain is thus stretched to serve as the basis of the politicojural domain, so that inter- and intragenerational relations, as opposed to maturation or age, are effective in political and jural affairs as well as within the family. The East African age-grading or age-set institutions, to which I shall return presently, fall into place in a wider comparative perspective if they are dealt with on the lines of this model.

I mentioned earlier the tendency among anthropologists to translate what are from the actor's point of view generational categories into observers' age categories (see, e.g., Goody 1976). This tacit tribute to our habituation to thinking in terms of chronological age, and indeed to seek to chronologize all manner of events and occurrences, suggests to me that the metaphorical use of a generational model in historical and sociological studies of cultural and social change is not unreasonable. It strikes me as an apt imagery by means of which to depict continuities and discontinuities in a community's social and cultural life over a stretch of time. It seems to come intuitively to hand, as it is within the framework of the succession of generations that all humans acquire their cultural heritage and learn to perceive their society. Mediated from earliest infancy by the natal family, the society readily takes on a generational form to the individual, and it is commonly accepted that attitudes deployed in social relations outside the family—such as with peers or authority figures—and toward norms and values of societal origin are laid down in the intra-familial socialization process. To describe the interplay of continuity and discontinuity in, say, a political ideology or an intellectual movement or an aesthetic tradition in generational terms reflects the universal human experience of filial familial generations replacing and so continuing the parental generation, but being also likely to turn against it in rivalry and even hostility.

In any case, it is by their fruits that historical and other applications of the generational model should be judged. And an excellent example is at hand in the Fall 1978 issue of the journal *Daedalus*. The generational model is applied with impressive skill, scholarship, and insight in all the contributions. Those of Laura Nash (1978), Matilda White Riley (1978), and Noel Annan (1978) deserve special mention as having a direct and illuminating bearing on my argument. Annan's demonstration of the power of the generational concept in effectively shaping studies of social and cultural movements over a stretch of time is masterly.

As these articles indicate, old age does not deprive individuals of their generational status and may even enhance it. In preindustrial societies the decline in economic and reproductive capacity that comes with advancing years does not deprive the old of their kinship status. For, like orphaned young, they are not segregated, but remain members of their families, lineages, and associations. This does not mean that they are invariably treated with what we should regard as benevolence or deference (see Keith 1980). Whether or not it is a response to economic or demographic necessity, Eskimo senilicide (like infanticide in precolonial Tikopia and premodern Japan) is not felt by the people themselves to be shameful or heartless. It is the same with such "retirement" practices as the withdrawal of the Fulani family head from the family camp after finally distributing his herd among his sons and handing over the camp to his

oldest son. Living uncomfortably outside the camp is not felt as degradation—though it is understood as the culmination of intergenerational rivalry—but rather as a kind of reinfantilization, a return to the jural and
economic dependence of childhood. Relinquishing to his inheriting son
the two critical indices of paternal authority, the control of the herd and
the right to father children, does not make him a pariah (see comments in
Goody 1976). These ostensibly victimized old people are so treated in
virtue of the rights and responsibilities their kinship status allocates to
them. Among many peoples, in Africa, Asia, and Oceania, old age, even
senility, does not deprive a person of either jural or, what is likely to be
more important, ritual authority and responsibility, though such responsibilities are likely to become nominal and symbolic, with the effective
roles being delegated to brothers, sons, or nephews (see Mendonsa
1982:chap. 6).

What must be stressed is that concepts of chronological age do not
come into these customs and practices. Old age is perceived as a stage in
the maturational life cycle marked by declining physical and mental
powers but very often counterbalanced by high generational status. The
Tallensi are not unique in regarding grandparenthood as the finest
achievement possible in any lifetime and more than compensating for the
inevitable infirmities of old age (see in this connection Nash's [1978]
remarks about the same attitudes in classical Greece).

Contrast these attitudes and values with what happens in societies in
which the life cycle is defined in chronological rather than maturational or
generational terms. I take an example from a somewhat unexpected quarter. The Skolt Lapps of Finland, though still retaining their cultural identity and territorial autonomy, now form part of a modern industrial and
commercial nation-state. Alcohol, tobacco, gambling, and above all
snowmobiles and motorcycles have become the primary interests of the
younger men (younger women emigrate). But financing these interests
and addictions is not possible by local wage labor. The main source is the
pension income of the older members of a household, which is awarded
by the state to military veterans and to men and women who have reached
retirement age. Three out of four households have such income. So old
parents are valued especially for the pension income from which alloca-
tions are made for the purchase of snowmobiles for their sons. The sons
generally use the vehicles recklessly, without regard to the heavy costs of
upkeep, which are met by their pensioner parents. The parents refrain
from exercising control for fear of alienating their sons (Ingold 1976).

What is at issue is clear. Pensions are awarded by the state not on the basis of kinship, family, or generational status but on the basis of the rights and duties of citizenship, that is, of membership in the political community. The criteria are objective and independent of maturational or generational conditions: chronological age and completion of service to the state. And the case of the Skolt Lapps—which is far from unique (see Keith 1980)—reminds us of the degree to which the rule of the state impinges on the life of the individual and of the family. This, of course, is something we are so inured to that we take it for granted. The politico-jural regulation of our lives in terms of chronological age constrains us from birth to death and in all our activities—personal (e.g., age of consent), economic (age of entry into and retirement from the productive system), civic (age of majority), moral (age of criminal liability), and educational (obligatory age for school entry and minimal age for school leaving). The details have been spelled out in many publications, as in the papers by Riley (1976) and her colleagues (Riley, Johnson, and Foner 1972).

None of these activities has anything to do with ability, capacity, state of maturation, or genealogical generation. This fact is brought home to us by the frequent evidence of discrepancies between actual performance and age-linked expectations of achievement created by the numerous norm-fixing institutions that politicojural demands impose on our social system. The IQ symbolizes this phenomenon most graphically. It emphasizes not only how central age-linked norms are to our political life (as in controversies about racial levels of intelligence) but also how they intrude into individual and family situations. In England the name of a burglar or murderer who is under 16 may not be divulged when he is on trial, and the agonies of parents who learn that their child is subnormal intellectually (by IQ or educational measurement) are familiar to teachers and doctors. Age-linked norms of career attainments and of physical and mental health, even of intimate personal relationships, as in the spheres of marriage and sex, are constantly invoked.

Clearly these age-linked institutions and practices depend in Western countries on literacy, numeracy, and the techniques of science. But these are only the necessary cultural instruments for implementing what is a fundamental requirement of our political and legal order. To be sure, chronological norms, thought, and judgment permeate every aspect of our culture and social life. A birth certificate is an indispensable credential for establishing a person's basis of citizenship and consequently for identifying his or her age-linked rights and duties and claims on society. And at the other end of the life cycle, a death certificate recording age at death and testifying to its cause is mandatory for the complete termination of the person's life. Marriage certificates, records of criminality, of disease, of achievements, all significant events in a life cycle are age-specified. And so it is with everything that makes up our material environment and with the facts of history.

I am aware, of course, that what I have been describing is not confined to Western societies. Dating systems and age-linked stipulations for status attainment have been and are found in Muslim and other nonwestern societies and were known in antiquity; I shall return to this topic later. What I am stressing here is the contrast between generation and chronological age as elements of social organization and of cultural values. Whereas a generation and a sequence of generations are family-generated (the terminological overlap is illuminating), age specification is politico-jurally institutionalized. Generational organization subsumes the ostensible discontinuities between successive generations in a framework of overall continuity. Age selection, by contrast, operates atomistically, with the formally isolated individual as the unit of reference, and leaves the matter of structural continuity or discontinuity in society to the nonfamilial institutional order. This contrast reflects the opposition between the family as the core of the domestic domain and the politicojural framework of the total society, which in its most differentiated and developed form is the state. Family and polity, or in more general terms kinship and the state or its equivalent, are at the opposite ends, so to speak, of the axis of social structure, tending sometimes to pull against rather than complement each other. Though the state has, in our type of society, absorbed many of the traditional nurturing and socializing functions of the family, it has not taken over the primary familial function of physically producing each generation and beginning the socialization process.

It is instructive to compare what happens in some Israeli kibbutzim, where the kibbutz, as a local political community, endeavors to take over the child-rearing and socialization tasks shortly after a child's birth, leaving to the parents only the maintenance of affective relations with offspring. There is much recent evidence, however, that the parental family is reasserting its right to autonomous existence and some responsibility for rearing its children (see Spiro 1980). Needless to say, kibbutz child rearing is distinctly age-oriented.

At the other end of the scale are such simple hunting and gathering societies as the Kalahari Bushmen and the Australian aborigines. Among these peoples kinship and polity are fused and kinship institutions, norms, and values are paramount. Significantly, these people do not recognize chronological age. But the claims of the politicojural order are asserted, often in ritual terms, in such institutions as initiation ceremonies, which remove boys from the family and transform them into actual or potential adults and authorize girls to be married and exercise their reproductive sexuality (see Richards 1956, Tuzin 1980). Initiation ceremonies resolve the rivalrous tensions that underlie the relations of successive generations in the family by incorporating the filial generation into the polity as cocitizens of their parents. Such ceremonies, often in association with circumcision and other mutilating rituals, are common also in more complex pastoral and agricultural societies, where these rivalries are acute (see, for instance, La Fontaine 1967, on the Gisu).

There is an interesting Ashanti sidelight on this subject. Traditionally the Ashanti held a public nubility ceremony for a girl, celebrating her attainment of menarche and often associated with her betrothal (see Rattray 1927:69–87). Thereafter she was held to have reached sexual maturity and to be entitled to marry and have children. Had she become pregnant before the ceremony, she and her lover would have been deemed to have committed a crime against the political community and would have been banished or even put to death.

It was well known that girls were not all equally developed at the time of their first menstruation, some being buxom and well grown while others still looked like young children. Chronological age being still unrecognized among the majority of Ashanti, they of course did not connect menarche with age. By 1945, however, the significance of chronological age as a marker of status had become known through the practice of registering pupils in schools and as a result of some colonial administrative regulations. Literate and semiliterate men began to keep notebooks in which, among other entries, ages of children and dates of family events were entered. On being permitted to see typical notebooks, I found references to nubility ceremonies of daughters and nieces recorded as being at the age of 16. I learned then that it had become customary in some quarters for newly nubile girls to be recorded as being 16 years of age though their dates of birth were unknown. One explanation given to me was that women aged 16 and over were classed as adults liable to the equivalent of a head tax by colonial law. The association of chronological age with requirements of external institutions based on the colonial political system was thus becoming customary.

The concept of a date by numbering a year by reference to a historical year of origin, corresponding to our usage of B.C. and A.D. or to the Muslim A.H. or classical Rome's A.U.C (*ab urbe condita*), is not found in the traditional cultures of Africa or other continents. This was brought home to me when I revisited the Tallensi in 1963. A number of young clerks and others in literate occupations asked me for the dates of my earlier visits. They explained that they had been told they were born in the dry or wet season or just after the Golib or the Da'a festival or whatever of the year of my first or second residence at Tongo, but, of course, had no birth certificates or other evidence of exact dates. They could now, they said, be able to tell exactly how old they were.

A dating system, as this example shows, must have a point of anchorage outside a society's ongoing structure and routines of social life. It relates a society to an externally validated frame of time. That is why our Western dating system can be adopted by peoples of the most diverse origins and ways of life. From within a society a dating system becomes relevant only if it becomes instrumental to the political and legal order or to cultural pursuits of a scientific nature. Where dating systems are lacking, lapses of time that we reckon cumulatively in years or decades or centuries are reckoned in terms of a span of generations, as in the book of Genesis. But it is important to realize that lack of a dating system does not mean lack of a calendar. The concept of a year, based on recognition of the recurring cycle of the seasons and sometimes associated with observed movements of conspicuous stars and planets (e.g., the Pleiades), is probably universal among humankind. Universal cultural markers are seasonal religious festivals, at harvest or sowing time for agriculturalists or at times of ecologically determined transhumance among pastoralists. Significantly, these are normally tribal or national festivals, not family or kin-group celebrations. A famous African one is the Ashanti Odwira, described and discussed by Rattray (1927:chap. 12). The Tallensi perceive the year as made up of one rainy season and the following dry season, each year being inaugurated by the Golib sewing festival, at the beginning of the wet season, and divided in two by the dry-season harvest festivals (Fortes 1970). Fundamentally the same pattern is familiar enough to us from studies of ancient Greek and Roman and Hebrew and Muslim calendars (see *Encyclopaedia Britannica* 1965, vol. 4, s.v.

"Calendar"). And, of course, our own calendar conforms in essentials to the same pattern.

Furthermore, all such calendars recognize and identify divisions of time spans within the year—lunar months and often other periods. The Ashanti, for example, divide the year by months and weeks. The seven-day weeks are overlaid with a six-day cycle of auspicious and inauspicious taboo days that together produce a twenty-one-day half cycle and a forty-two-day full cycle (see Rattray 1923:115), the first day of both units being a taboo day. These are the occasions for the solemn Wednesday and Sunday *adae* ceremonies, in which the ancestors and the divinities of every politically discrete community are commemorated or worshiped with sacrifice and libation (see Rattray 1923:86–120). *Adae* ceremonies continue to be strictly observed even by Christian and highly educated chiefs (Fortes 1969:152), and the forty-two-day cycle remains important for fixing times for many rites of passage.

These calendars, however, like those of the Greeks, the Romans, and the Hebrews, do not serve the purpose of dating events and so being of use for fixing chronological age. They have a purely internal structural relevance. Tallensi often told me about the punitive expedition of 1911 which finally subdued the Hill Talis. Many of them who had lived through it could describe the state of the crops at that time, but none of my informants could do better than guess, and that pretty wildly, at how many years ago it had happened. The usual answer to an inquiry on this point was to cite a stage of maturation: a woman would say, "Well, that was before I had sprouted breasts"; a man would say, "That was when I had just reached puberty" or "just got married" or "started to hoe regularly." Typically, my friend Kurug of Pusega, in response to a question, declared casually that old Deemzeet, whom I guessed to be in his sixties, was "over a hundred." Similarly, in Ashanti individual ages were unknown among nonliterates. Hence in the demographic study my colleagues and I carried out in 1945 (Fortes et al. 1954) we had to set up a grid of well-known events and occurrences for which dates could be ascertained from official and published sources, so that dates of birth could be approximately fixed by reference to it.

Let me repeat: dating systems and the recognition of chronological age which depends on them are irrelevant if they are not critical for political or legal rights and duties, that is, for citizenship status. Among the Ashanti and the Tallensi citizenship was traditionally derived solely from authentic lineage membership; it was even denied to individuals of slave descent (see Fortes 1969:263). In Ashanti, high political office could be held by able men and women of any age provided they were of the right descent. Among the Tallensi, men of mature years were preferred, provided they were of the right descent (see Fortes 1945:82). It is worth noting that hereditary succession in European royal families is also tied to descent and generation without regard to age, whereas strict rules of citizenship and of minimal age govern eligibility for the presidency of the United States.

The evidence of Mediterranean antiquity is of particular interest for my argument. The Judeo-Christian Bible is full of lengthy genealogies and numerous references to the succession of generations but contains no exact chronological age references. Indeed, the notions of age we meet with in Genesis remind me of experiences among the Tallensi in the 1930s. It was often said of old men and women that they had probably lived 100 years since their birth, as in the example I have previously given. To emphasize the miracle of Isaac's birth, his parents are said to have been 90 or more years of age—in obviously poetical round numbers. Nowhere in the Bible are we told the exact age of David or of Jesus at crucial times in their careers, though their genealogies and hence generational rank are meticulously recorded. And it is the same with other biblical personalities.

In Homeric and fifth-century Greece, Laura Nash's previously mentioned paper (1978) tells us, "numerical age is meaningless, except in the designation of life expectancy." In contrast, she observes, "genealogical identity (stage of life) [i.e., generational rank] is easily recognizable." Men born at the same time, she notes, are identified with one another in a peer group. And the greatest happiness to be hoped for is to live long enough to have grandchildren—a sentiment that would be applauded by Tallensi and Ashanti. Thus a generation is defined as the time between the birth of a son and that of a grandson. It is a picture fully reminiscent of what we find in contemporary preindustrial societies.

In Rome, by contrast, a calculus of chronological age seems to have played a part in social life from early times. This form of reckoning was obviously connected with the special prominence of legal and political institutions in Roman society. The status of citizen (*civis*) was, from early times, defined not by criteria of kinship and descent (as in the Athens of the fifth century B.C.) but by legal and political enactments. As early as the third century B.C. civic obligations and eligibility for many offices of state were linked to chronological age. Thus men became liable for military service at age 17 but could not hold the office of *quaestor* before the age of 28 or the consulship until the age of 37 (see Heitland 1909, 3:193). Chronological age also figures prominently in the law of persons. Thus a male *sui iuris* who had not reached puberty had to have a legal guardian (*tutor*). As to the determination of puberty, W. W. Buckland comments (1947:90): "In the time of Gaius it was disputed whether this was to be taken at a fixed age or determined by the actual physical development of the person concerned." In later law the accepted rule was that the *tutela* should end at 14 for boys and 12 for girls. And many other features of Roman private law link status, rights, and duties to chronological age.

Comparing these Roman data with Nash's account of early Greek ideas, we are led again to the conclusion that chronological age becomes significant when the political and legal framework takes precedence over familial and kinship relations for determining citizenship. Further evidence is found in the development of the English law of civic status. As Alan Macfarlane has shown (1978:chap. 4), the concept of the individual as an autonomous legal personality deriving citizenship not through family or kinship ties but in his own right goes back to the thirteenth century. One indication of the force of this concept is the significance found attached to chronological age in the fixing of legal rights and duties. Thus Sir Frederick Pollock and F. W. Maitland (1905, 1:40), writing of the "legally constituted classes" of the thirteenth century, comment that "the lay Englishman, free but not noble, who is of *full age* . . . is the law's . . . typical person" (my emphasis), full age being 21. And again, "Whether the wardship of a woman was to endure until she attained the age of twenty one or was to cease when she attained the age of fourteen [the legally marriageable age] seems to have been a moot point" (p. 320).

There is no need to add further examples to establish my main point. Aging is a natural process of individual maturation that runs its course in society between two poles of social structure. At one pole is the domain of social reproduction, normally centered in some form of family organization. Every family system fulfills its end through the succession of the generations of parents and children, be it narrow, like ours, or ramified lineally and collaterally, as in many nonwestern societies. Thus arises the generational calculus that is the basis of social and personal relations primarily in the domestic domain but capable of being extended to wider ranges of social life. In this context maturational stage is significant but chronological age is neither culturally encoded nor relevant to social life.

But the family, however constituted, and its ramifications in the diverse kinship systems of humankind are embedded in society, may indeed be thought of as existing for the sake of society. For it is the family's reproductive performance that maintains a society in existence over time.

And this is where the second pole of social structure comes to the fore. Every individual is not only a member of a family and a generation but also a citizen, subject to rules and constraints and bearer of rights and duties that represent the force of society as a whole, as against family and kinship; that are, in other words, of political and legal origin and work with sanctions different from the affective and moral norms that operate in the familial domain. Societies vary from our own system, in which the spheres of the politicojural domain and the domestic or familial domain are structurally quite distinct, to those of the many nonwestern peoples in which these spheres overlap to a greater or lesser degree. For us there is no necessary connection between being a kinsman and being a citizen, whereas in many traditional African and other nonwestern societies one can be a citizen only by virtue of kinship or descent credentials.

What I am suggesting is that recognition and consideration of chronological age as opposed to maturation and generation depend on the differentiation between the politicojural and the domestic domains of social life. Strip the individual of kinship status—that is, let the identity of the person's parent or child or spouse or sibling be irrelevant to the granting of citizenship, with all its economic and other concomitants—and what remains to serve as a criterion for social classification other than sex, local association, and chronological age?

Since no society can reproduce itself except through the agency of some form of family, a key issue is the acquisition of the right to exercise reproductive sexuality. This is a conspicuous issue in systems of generation and age-set organization, as the recent discussions of East African and other systems makes clear (see Foner and Kertzer 1978; Baxter and Almagor, eds., 1978:Introduction).

The peoples among whom these systems of social stratification are found had neither the institutions nor the cultural apparatus to date events or reckon chronological age before colonial administration and modern schooling reached them (see Abrahams 1978:41). Hence, as I remarked earlier, the terminology of "age grades" and "age sets" is likely to be misleading. Chronological age is in fact an ethnocentric observer's construct that does not correspond to the way the actors see the system. The basic framework of all "age-set" systems is, as we would logically expect, the generation sequence, the crucial rule being that successive genealogical generations of fathers and sons must be separated. But a generational division may be subdivided into more closely contemporary age sets (I shall follow the current convention to save circumlocution) often (though not invariably) with the proviso that brothers must belong to separate divisions. Yet the jural, moral, and economic rules and norms that prevail in the internal affairs of a generation grade or set are clearly modeled on the ideals of siblingship. Agemates are defined as equals, entitled as of right to share food and drink and possessions in the same way that they share the privations of work, war, or their group life. There are systems in which this rule of equality is carried to the extreme of obliging married men in junior sets to share the sexual services of their wives with their agemates—a custom reminiscent of the adelphic polyandry that prevails in some parts of Tibet.

Since generation and age sets are extradomestic organizations of boys, youths, and men, the ideals of fraternal equivalence and amity, which in the reality of family life are subject to the strains of intersibling rivalry, are dramatized and enforced at the level of society at large, as moral values that are vital for the existence of society, not merely for the family or kin group. Thus age sets in this respect represent a means of drawing intersibling rivalry away from the family, where it is potentially destructive of both the productive and the reproductive tasks required of it by society, by subjecting the individual as individual, not as kinsman, to the objective discipline of the political and jural order. Age-set organization can be seen as a way of asserting that a person's obligations to society, as citizens in the politicojural domain, are distinct from and opposed to those he has as a kinsman, and superior to them. He is, in other words, defined as subject to legal and political regulation of society, be it, as often happens, couched in terms of religious rules rather than economic requirements or military defense; and this definition is seen as opposed to the morally binding sentiments of mutual trust and interdependence that mark family and kinship relations. At the same time, as I have earlier implied, fraternal solidarity is emphasized by age-set organization as a social value that transcends the family. Society, it might be said, insists that fraternal siblings are all equal to one another and must love one another willy-nilly, and shows them how this rule can be implemented, while at the same time making room for the fact of sibling rivalry. And this organization is especially important where, as in most African societies, there is so much overlap between the familial and the politicojural domains that family loyalty and citizenship duty are often in danger of clashing. The absence or rarity of age-set organization in societies with a highly developed descent-group structure, first noticed by Eisenstadt (1956) and frequently confirmed by later investigators (see Baxter and Almagor, eds., 1978:Introduction), is understandable. Where membership in a descent group determines citizenship at birth, siblingship is subordinated to and mobilized in the service of the descent principle, for it is both the source and the model of the internal segmentation on which the stability of the descent group and its solidarity vis-à-vis the outside world rests. Not age or its parallels but generation is the basis of its internal stratification. In external relations, the descent group is a corporate jural and political unit in a statelike system (see Fortes 1969:chap. 14).

What we are here concerned with is alternative forms of politicojural institutions. Both age-set and generation-set organizations, on the one side, and the combination of corporate descent groups and statelike social structure on the other serve to establish for the individual the status of what Eisenstadt called citizenship, in contradistinction to kinship and family status. But in these societies the politicojural domain and familial domain are not wholly differentiated. Citizen status and kinship status are interconnected in ways that have long been obsolete in Western societies, where the domains are wholly separate. There is no room, or perhaps it might be more correct to say no need, in such preliterate, preindustrial societies for a calculus of chronological age to establish and regulate citizenship. Generation and age-set organizations can be seen as a sort of halfway house.

As Eisenstadt perceived and the recent reviews I have quoted confirm, however, what is most important is that age-set organization resolves and mobilizes for the services of society the tensions and potentials for conflict intrinsic to the relations of successive generations of fathers and sons. As I have already noted, if there is one rule that is apparently universally followed in systems of age-set stratification, it is the rule that fathers and sons must never belong to the same set. There are systems in which they are assigned to successive sets, as in the familial generation sequence, thus placing this family structure under political and jural regulation in a framework of extrafamilial social order. But there are other systems in which father and son must be separated by two or more generations, as among the Guji, one of the Oromo-speaking Ethiopian groups (see Hinnant 1978), who separate father and son sets by five generations. Parental authority and filial subordination, which tend almost invariably to clash within the tight limits of family and kin group, are, under the aegis of citizenship, placed in a legitimate and accepted hierarchy. What is often described as the gerontocracy, entrenched in the governmental or religious supremacy of senior age sets, is better understood as the transposition to the societal level of the generational authority of fathers, and a key factor is the control vested in the senior age sets of the right to marry, that is, to exercise legitimate procreative sexuality.

It is this right that is primarily at stake in the rivalry of successive generations in the family. Transposed to the politicojural domain in the age-set hierarchy, it is toned down to orderly aspirations that will be satisfied at the appropriate time. What happens then is that the age set that has earned this right tends to disperse as each member marries and assumes the productive and reproductive responsibilities of family life. This step marks the end of the crucial transition from adolescence to adulthood. The withholding of the rights of marriage and of procreative sexuality are easily understood as the obverse of the incest taboo, the core of which is to prohibit the mixture of generations, not the mixture of stages of maturation (that is, ages), since old men often marry women young enough to be their daughters or even granddaughters. But son may not marry mother or daughter father—these relationships being understood in the classificatory sense. It is absolute compliance with this rule that marks the attainment of adulthood. Thus is the circle completed. The age-set organization removes the individual from the family at an early prepubertal stage of his maturation (ideally) and the family claims him back again at a stage when he is required to play his part in the productive and reproductive processes and is physically and socially mature enough to do so. At that stage his membership in his age set may well become largely of ritual and symbolic significance. Generation and age sets as such seem rarely, if ever, to have corporate legal, political, administrative, or economic roles and capacities, as Evans-Pritchard long ago pointed out. But this does not make generations and age-set systems less political in significance, simply because by incorporating the individual into the order of society as a citizen, the age-set system creates a status that remains with him throughout his life. It is in fact more usual for a boy's father or substitute father to take the initiative and certainly the responsibility of having him initiated into his first age set than for this task to be undertaken by a superior age set collectively—as if, one might say, it is the father's duty to hand him over to society as citizen. He is thus bound to serve the purposes of maintaining and perpetuating the society even at the cost of personal fulfillment within his natal family.

Age-set institutions are regularly portrayed as being concerned directly only with the life cycle of males, and in fact females are not often correspondingly organized. As Paul Baxter and Uri Almagor point out (1978), this fact reflects the rule that women are rarely politically and jurally autonomous in tribal societies. Before marriage they are generally in the jural power of fathers or uncles. After marriage they become jural dependants of husbands or fathers-in-law, and even when they attain the comparative freedom of the menopause they are likely to remain to some extent jurally dependent on male heads of families or lineage elders. This situation confirms the conclusion that generations and age sets are concerned with the political and jural status of males, not with their family status.

There is one aspect of the age and generation structure of society that deserves at least a passing comment. How do individuals perceive and interpret their own progress through the life cycle in relation to this dimension of the social structure? It would be rash to generalize on this subject. All the stages of maturation from birth to old age, and the attributes of role and status associated with them, coexist in every society at any given time and are therefore perceivable and knowable by all members of the society. What seems to happen in nonwestern societies is that individuals at all stages look forward, in childhood and youth eagerly, at later stages with equanimity or even pride, to what we would describe as step-by-step aging. The emphasis is not on the physical changes of aging but on their social and cultural accompaniments. It is about the time when he will be initiated or join the cattle herders or start proper farming that the small boy daydreams; it is the nubility ceremony that will lead to her marriage that his sister anticipates eagerly; it is parenthood and economic independence that the young men of what are in some tribes designated as warrior age sets hope to achieve; and it is to eldership and grandparenthood, with their political and ritual responsibilities and privileges, that men in the middle stages of the life cycle aspire, even if their progress lands them in the apparent ignominy of the forcible retirement exemplified by the Fulani. It is, in other words, the major transitional stages that mark critical maturational attainments or shifts in role or status or social personality (as indicated by Foner and Kertzer 1978) that are aspired and looked forward to. The idea that one might fear or resent growing up or growing old does not evidently occur in traditional preliterate, preindustrial societies.

REFERENCES

Abrahams, R. G.
  1978 Aspects of labor, age and generation grouping, and related systems. In Age, Generation, and Time, ed. Paul T. W. Baxter and Uri Almagor, pp. 37–68. New York: St. Martin's Press.
Annan, Noel
  1978 "Our age": Reflections on three generations in England. Daedalus 107(4):81–110.
Baxter, Paul T. W., and Uri Almagor, eds.
  1978 Age, Generation, and Time: Some Features of East African Age Organizations. New York: St. Martin's Press.
Binstock, Robert H., and Ethel Shanas, eds.
  1976 Handbook of Aging and the Social Sciences. New York: Van Nostrand.
Buckland, W. W.
  1947 A Manual of Roman Private Law. Cambridge: Cambridge University Press.
Eisenstadt, S. N.
  1956 From Generation to Generation: Age Groups and Social Structure. Glencoe, Ill.: Free Press.
Foner, Anne, and David Kertzer
  1978 Transitions over the life course: Lessons from age-set societies. American Journal of Sociology 83(5):1081–1104.
Fortes, Meyer
  1936 Ritual festivals and social cohesion in the hinterland of the Gold Coast. In Fortes, Time and Social Structure and Other Essays. London: Athlone Press, 1970.
  1938 Social and psychological aspects of education on Taleland. In Fortes, Time and Social Structure and Other Essays, pp. 201–59. London: Athlone Press, 1970.
  1945 The Dynamics of Clanship among the Tallensi. London: Oxford University Press.
  1969 Kinship and the Social Order. Chicago: Aldine Press.
  1970 Time and Social Structure and Other Essays. London: Athlone Press.
  1974 The first born. Journal of Child Psychology and Psychiatry 15:81–104.
Fortes, Meyer, et al.
  1954 A demographic field study in Ashanti. In Culture and Human Fertility, ed. Frank Lorimer. Paris: UNESCO.

Goody, Jack
1976   Aging in nonindustrial societies. *In* Handbook of Aging and the Social
        Sciences, ed. Robert H. Binstock and Ethel Shanas. New York: Van
        Nostrand.
Gulliver, Philip H.
1968   Age differentiation. International Encyclopedia of the Social Sciences,
        vol. 1. New York: Collier-Macmillan.
Heitland, William E.
1909   The Roman Republic. 3 vols. London: Cambridge University Press.
Hinnant, John
1978   The Gudji: *Gada* as a ritual system. *In* Age, Generation, and Time, ed.
        Paul T. W. Baxter and Uri Almagor, pp. 207–44. New York: St.
        Martin's Press.
Ingold, Tim
1976   The Skolt Lapps Today. Cambridge: Cambridge University Press.
Keith, Jennie
1980   "The best is yet to be": Toward an anthropology of age. *In* Annual
        Review of Anthropology 9:339–64.
Kertzer, David
1978   Theoretical developments in the study of age-group systems. American
        Ethnologist 5(2):368–74.
1982   Generation and age in cross-cultural perspective. *In* Aging from Birth
        to Death: Sociotemporal Perspectives, ed. Matilda White Riley,
        Ronald Abeles, and Michael Teitelbaum. Boulder: Westview Press.
La Fontaine, J. S.
1967   Parricide in Bugisu: A study in intergenerational conflict. Man n.s.
        2:249–59.
Macfarlane, Alan
1978   The Origins of English Individualism. Oxford: Basil Blackwell.
Mannheim, Karl
1952   The problem of generations. *In* Essays on the Sociology of Knowl-
        edge. London: Oxford University Press.
Mendonsa, Eugene L.
1982   The Politics of Divination: A Processual View of Reactions to Illness
        and Deviance among the Sissala of Northern Ghana. Berkeley: Univer-
        sity of California Press.
Nash, Laura L.
1978   Concepts of existence: Greek origins of generational thought. Daedalus
        107(4):1–22.
Pollock, Sir Frederick, and F. W. Maitland
1905   The History of English Law before the Time of Edward I. 2 vols. 2d
        ed. Cambridge: Cambridge University Press.
Rabain, Jacqueline
1979   L'Enfant du lignage: Du Sevrage à la class d'âge. Paris: Payot.

Rattray, Robert S.
1923 Ashanti. Oxford: Clarendon Press.
1927 Religion and Art in Ashanti. Oxford: Clarendon Press.
Richards, Audrey I.
1956 Chisungu: A Girl's Initiation Ceremony among the Bemba of Northern Rhodesia. London: Faber & Faber.
Riley, Matilda White
1976 Age strata in social systems. *In* Handbook of Aging and the Social Sciences, ed. Robert H. Binstock and Ethel Shanas, pp. 189–217. New York: Van Nostrand.
1978 Aging, social change, and the power of ideas. Daedalus 107(4):39–52.
Riley, Matilda White, Marilyn Johnson, and Anne Foner
1972 Aging and Society. Vol. 3: A Sociology of Age Stratification. New York: Russell Sage Foundation.
Spiro, Melford J.
1980 Gender and Culture: Kibbutz Women Revisited. New York: Schocken.
Tuzin, Donald F.
1980 The Voice of the Tamberan: Truth and Illusion in Ilahita Arapesh Religion. Berkeley: University of California Press.
Wilson, Monica
1951 Good Company: A Study of Nyakyusa Age Villages. London: Oxford University Press.

4

Age and Kinship: A Structural View

David Maybury-Lewis

Anyone who has taken an interest in kinship theory is bound to have a feeling of *déjà vu* when the subject of age arises. Aging, like copulation and procreation, is physiologically given. It is indeed one of the "facts of life," though not normally one that we feel an obligation to explain to our children, perhaps because it takes place so publicly. Yet it is treated in a wide variety of ways by different societies. This variability poses a problem familiar to students of kinship: if a biological given that is universal among humankind receives cultural treatment that varies from place to place, how are those cultural variations determined? The biological constants are insufficient to account for the variations in their cultural use, which must therefore be explained in some other way.

General theories of kinship, and therefore explanations of specific kinship systems, have been hampered by two sorts of problems. The first is disagreement over the nature of kinship systems themselves. Debate still rages over the extent to which kinship systems stay, or are intended to stay, close to the biological facts of life. Are they systems of terms intended to express genetic relationships (which may on occasion be extended beyond the strict genetic limits) or are they taxonomies modeled on genetic grids? If one subscribes to the first view, then it follows that whatever affects the biological relations between individuals in a society is going to be reflected in their kinship system. A biological or even a sociobiological theory of kinship is therefore a possibility. If one subscribes to the second view, as I do, such theorizing is less relevant. If, as I believe, kinship in the general sense has to be thought of as a system of communication, rooted in a genealogical metaphor, then we are faced with a different and even more difficult task. This is the second kind of problem in kinship theory to which I alluded above—the difficulty of determining why societies have one type of metaphorical kinship system rather than another. The study of age and age sets confronts a similar problem and should seek similar solutions.

It has been pointed out again and again that age is a basic principle of social categorization, like kinship or sex (most recently by La Fontaine, ed., 1978; Baxter and Almagor, eds., 1978; and Keith 1979). Some of the differences between these principles, however, are worth noting. First, they differ in their systemic aspect. Since Lewis Henry Morgan's work in the nineteenth century, anthropologists have been properly impressed by and preoccupied with the systematics of kinship, governed by terminologies that were identifiably kinship terminologies. It is true that the modern tendency is to argue that we have overdone it; that kinship systems are not necessarily all that systematic and that in any case all of them are fuzzy at the edges. Nevertheless, if we compare what has been done on kinship with what is being done on age and sex, the contrast is striking. I argue that societies certainly do treat age and sex systematically, if occasionally with ambivalence amounting to schizophrenia, but we do not yet speak of sexual systems or age systems (except when we refer to age-set systems, a point to which I shall return). The difference seems to be that all societies institutionalize some sort of kinship system, but not all societies explicitly institutionalize a sexual or an age system. This may prove to be a blessing for those who are interested in the comparative study of sex or age, for they are less likely to treat sexual or age systems as things apart from the rest of society, a tendency that has bedeviled kinship studies.

Another difference between sex, kinship, and age lies in the relative stability of these principles as conceptual and social markers. Sex is the most stable. Individuals are normally and automatically ascribed to their sex by virtue of their physical characteristics. Most societies recognize the possibility of some indeterminacy or even change in an individual's sex, but this is usually minimal. The flexibility and variation occur in the area of sex roles rather than in their ascription to one sex or the other. The kinship status of an individual is not so immediately given by his or her genealogical ties. Most societies recognize a great deal of flexibility and change in this area. Age is the least stable. The age of an individual is constantly changing, so that the use of age as a marker is fraught with special problems.

Age-set systems are one solution to this problem, for they arbitrarily and conventionally fix people's ages and thus facilitate the use of the age marker to set up social groups. Africa, particularly East Africa, has been the classic area of reference for students of such systems, because of the incidence and significance of age-set systems there and also because of the good descriptions of them available in the literature (see Stewart 1977:15–24). But the peoples of Central Brazil studied by my students and me also have elaborate age-grade and age-set systems, and a comparison of these systems with the East African ones is instructive. I am sadly aware, however, that my readers are likely to know something about the East African systems and equally unlikely to know anything about the Central Brazilian ones, so I shall start by describing the latter.

The systems I am referring to are, or were, found among the Gê-speaking peoples who live on the high plateau of Central Brazil. The Northern Gê peoples can be easily distinguished from the Central Gê on linguistic grounds. They consist of a number of tribes ranging from the Kayapó (see Bamberger 1979, Turner 1979, and Vidal 1977), who total nearly 3,000 people divided into eight or more independent communities, to the Suyá on the Upper Xingú River, who have been reduced to a single community of about 150 inhabitants (Seeger 1981). The eastern peoples among the Northern Gê, such as the Ramkokamekra (Nimuendaju 1946) and the Krĩkatí (Lave 1979), live in small villages about 100 strong set in dry savannah country. The western peoples, such as the Kayapó, live in communities that are on the average twice as large and are located in the jungles of southern Pará and northern Mato Grosso.

The Central Gê are now comprised of the Sherente (Maybury-Lewis 1979a), numbering some 800 people divided among four or five communities, and the Shavante (Maybury-Lewis 1967, 1979a), who total approximately 3,000 in communities of about 200. They live in savannah country with some access to forests along the rivers.

Traditionally all of these tribes lived by hunting and gathering, supplemented by agriculture, which varied from being a minor activity, as it was among the Shavante when I studied them in 1959, to a major source of subsistence, as it is for all of them now and has been for some of them for perhaps a century.

All of them are reported to have or to have had age-grade or age-set systems. For the moment I shall refer only to two Northern Gê systems. One of these systems was found among the more easterly of these tribes. The Ramkokamekra had it, though it has now vanished, and so did the Krĩkatí, who have replaced it by a naming system. But the details of the system are well described by Curt Nimuendajú (1946:91–95) and we can therefore use it as one of the instances in our comparison. The other Northern Gê system to which I shall refer is found farther west, among the Kayapó. I shall also refer to a third system, found among the Central Gê. It has almost vanished among the Sherente but is still functioning among the Shavante.

Peoples such as the Ramkokamekra and the Krĩkatí initiated all the eligible boys in the community at ten-year intervals. The newly constituted age set (which I shall call A) would thus consist of boys whose ages roughly covered a ten-year span—for example, from 8 to 18. It would have its own meeting place at one of the four "corners" of the circular forum in the center of the village. This place would be vacated by a senior age set, which moved to a new location, displacing another age set, whose surviving members would move into the center and join the age grade of "elders" (see Figure 1). Ten years later the next age set (B) would be initiated, but it would enter the forum on the *opposite side,* leaving the members of age set A (in their twenties) still at their original corner. Ten years later another new age-set (C) would displace A, who would move down to the southern corner of their side of the forum. The members of A would be in their forties when D was initiated, but they would remain in their southeastern meeting place. Finally, the survivors of A, now in their fifties, would move into the center to join the elders when E was initiated.

Age sets sometimes sponsored their own ceremonials and were often ranged against each other as eastern and western age-based moieties, with age sets A and C opposing age sets B and D. Nimuendaju thought that the age sets had originally constituted the groups that went on war parties or on communal hunting expeditions. During the 1930s there were no more war parties and communal hunting had become a rare and insignificant activity, so that the age sets when he was there were largely engaged in ceremonial activities. Such activities, particularly log racing, are still

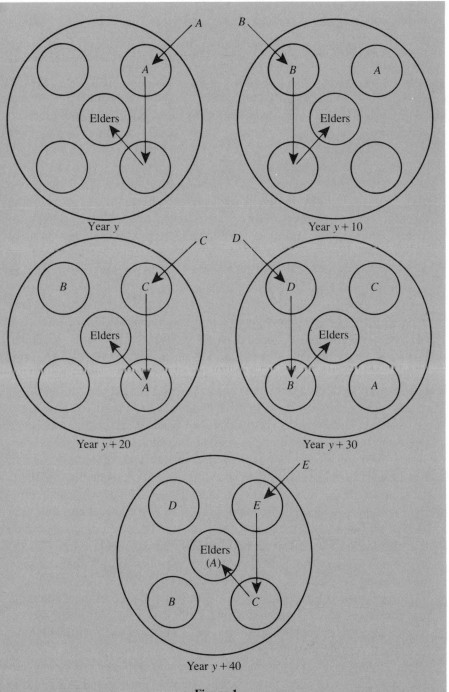

Figure 1

carried out by these peoples today, but their age-set systems have disappeared. Jean Lave (1979) has shown that, among the Krīkatí at least, the progressive individualization that accompanied their change to an economy based on small farming coincided with the disappearance of the age sets and their replacement by a naming system. The Krīkatí now refer to name-based categories of people where previously they would have turned to agemates.

The Kayapó have a system of age grades rather than age sets (Bamberger 1979:134–38; Turner 1979:205–6). Both males and females are classified from birth to death in a series of categories, progression through which depends on events in the individual's life, such as onset of menstruation, male initiation, birth of first child, becoming parent of more than one child, and so on. This system of age grades and the relationships established through it is specifically seen by the Indians as the antithesis of kinship. Men were expected to join their age mates in the center of the village, where, according to Kayapó tradition, eastern and western men's houses, analogous to the eastern and western age moieties of the other Northern Gê, faced each other. But internal politics exploded this symmetry even before acculturation set in. Factions tended to form, pitting one society of agemates against another and leading to such frequent splitting of villages that today no Kayapó community still has both men's houses. Instead Kayapó villages appear to formalize a dichotomy between two opposing sets of agemates or between the mature men's age grade and the younger men's age grade as replacements for the moiety system of opposing men's houses which used to operate in the forum. In fact Lux Vidal suggests (1977:195–98) that a branch of the Kayapó have reorganized the opposition between mature men and younger men, forming them into two moieties composed of men of various age grades who are led by two complementary village chiefs. This system is very much like the traditional one described for the Ramkokamekra and Krīkatí, where two age-based moieties, containing members of different age sets, were led by age-set officials (Nimuendajú 1946:93).

An age-set system was also a vital feature of the life of the Central Gê and continues to be so among the Shavante. The principles of the system differ, however, from those of the two Northern Gê systems I have described. Among the Shavante (Maybury-Lewis 1967:105–37, 338–39) all the eligible boys in a community are initiated at five-year intervals into named age sets that cycle through the system in a prescribed order. Table 1 shows the system at the moment when the boys of age set G are initiated

Table 1. Age-set system of the Shavante

Age grade	Age set	Approximate age of assumption of position
Mature men	A	
		42–47
	B	
		37–42
	C	
		32–37
	D	
		27–32
	E	
		22–27
	F	
		17–22
Young men	G	
		12–17
Boys in bach- elors' hut	H	
		7–12

and become "young men." At the same moment the young men of age set *F* move up and join age sets *A–E* in the mature men's age grade. Meanwhile a new age set, *H*, enters the bachelors' hut, where its members will live, slightly set apart from the village, for the next five years. The boys are normally 7 to 12 years old when they enter the bachelors' hut and 12 to 17 years old when they are initiated and become young men. Five years later, when they are 17 to 22 years old, their age set will move up to join the mature men. Five initiations later, age set *H* (whose members will now be between 42 and 47 years old) will become the senior age set in the system, *F* will be the young men, and *G* will be in the bachelors' hut. Five years after that the system will return to the position diagrammed in Table 1. The boys entering the bachelors' hut will be members of age set *H* and so on. At this moment the survivors of the *H* group we have been following are from 47 to 52 years old. These few elders will help their "agemates" (the boys in *H*) to construct their new bachelors' hut and generally associate themselves with their own reincarnation. By this time, of course, the old members of *H* have long ceased to come together *as an age set* for any purpose, so that the induction of a group of boys into their age set really does breathe new life into it.

The principles of alternation and complementarity which we have noted among the Northern Gê are also evident in the Shavante system. The bachelors' hut is built at the extremity of one of the arms of the village semicircle. At each initiation the new bachelors' hut is constructed at the extremity opposite that of the previous one. There are two meeting places in the middle of the village, one for the mature men and one for the young men. The relative positions of these meeting places are also reversed at each initiation. Meanwhile many ceremonies require log races to be run in connection with them, and these races normally take place between age moieties; that is (refer again to Table 1), they pit men from age sets A, C, E, and G against men from age sets B, D, F, and H.

The Shavante spoke of their age sets as warmaking groups, as hunting groups, even as groups that worked together in the gardens. Yet I noticed that hunting and gardening were hardly ever explicitly undertaken by agemates, and the rare war parties were not constituted by age set either. The point about age sets was that they stressed togetherness, and Shavante attached this general value to any specific activity that they were talking about. This sense of solidarity could be clearly observed in ceremonial activities; one could see age sets and age moieties performing one ritual or another every day. Shavante were quite explicit about this solidarity to be found in age sets, inculcated by the age-set system and expressed in ritual. They contrasted it with the divisive tendencies of descent groups and tried to counterbalance a moiety system based on one with a moiety system based on the other.

The Sherente once had an age-set system that was probably very similar to that of the Shavante. When Nimuendajú visited them in the 1930s he reported that their culture was in a state of collapse because their system of age sets had become a system of men's associations which was in turn obsolescent. I was happy to be able to show that Sherente culture was still very much alive thirty years later (Maybury-Lewis 1979a:219–21). Their age-sets, however, had indeed become men's associations, and these groups functioned only to bestow names on females. The vital core of Sherente culture when I visited them was a factional system based on patrilineal descent groups and expressed through the kinship terminology in a binary matrix, as if the kinship-based moieties were still functioning.

We cannot properly understand these age systems unless we can see them as part of their total social context. I therefore need to say something about Central Brazilian social and cultural organization. These peoples first attracted attention because of their dual organization, as discovered

and reported by Nimuendajú (1939, 1942, 1946). The nature and significance of what he discovered have been much debated, and this is not the
place to go into those arguments. It is enough to say that the dual organization found among the Central Brazilian peoples is not a matter of
exogamous moieties, for they are not found among the Northern Gê and
are not everywhere present among the Central Gê. Recent work done in
central Brazil indicates a different view of this striking and characteristic
feature of their social organization (see Maybury-Lewis 1971, 1979b).

All of these peoples make a sharp division between the sexes. The
symbolic and social functions of men are clearly distinguished as being
antithetical to those of women. These distinctions are reflected on the
ground in the fact that the center of the village is thought of as a male
sphere opposed to the periphery of the village, which is a female sphere.
In the center there are men's houses or men's meeting places. These
places are contrasted with the huts at the periphery, which, although they
are the dwellings of men and women alike, are thought of as preeminently
a female sphere. Females grow from childhood to maturity at the periphery and stay there, often in the same household throughout their lives.
Men, on the other hand, start off at the periphery in childhood and are
then separated from it during the period of initiation in order to be
reintegrated into the society at the center. All political and public matters
are brought up, discussed, and (formally at least) decided at the center by
the men. In fact, as I argued in regard to the Shavante (Maybury-Lewis
1967:179), no matter can become a public issue unless and until it is
taken up in the men's forum, and this is generally true for all of the
Central Brazilian societies. The central male world is therefore also the
place where all the public affairs of the community are conducted. What
happens in the peripheral, female world is of only domestic concern.

The public affairs of the community include a great deal of ceremonial
activity, which is carried out largely by men at the center. Such male
groups may occasionally be accompanied by female associates, but the
participation of women does not alter the fact that it is the male groups
that are seen to perform the ceremonies. The exclusion of women from
the center, however, is not absolute. They are not categorically prohibited
from approaching the men when they are attending a meeting in the center
of the village or from entering the men's house (in those societies that
have men's houses), though they rarely do so. Even when the men are
performing esoteric ceremonies or using instruments that women are
theoretically prohibited from seeing, there is not the same categorical

prohibition on female approach as there is in some other parts of the world.

The most important Shavante ceremony, for example, is the *wai'a,* during which initiated men have sexual intercourse with selected women and then go on to seek contact with the spirits. During the *wai'a* performed at initiation, it is the newly initiated men that have intercourse with the women. Afterward the men dance round the village, while the women are obliged to stay inside the huts. Women may not in theory see the dance or the ceremonial items that men brandish while they dance, and men speak luridly of the gang rape that would be the punishment for women who flouted this prohibition. Yet most women have seen part or all of the ceremony, and the women who have just had intercourse with the men are actually painted in the male paint styles and accompany the men who dance around the village. The point is that women are not *supposed* to see this ceremony. Men establish this rule unequivocally but do not seem to mind much whether the women actually observe it or not.

This situation demonstrates a fundamental principle of central Brazilian culture. The male world is the social world and the focus of the symbolic life of the community. It is this world that is at center stage. Men are considered to be the only fully social beings. They enter this social world by means of initiation and through the names that are bestowed on them.

Names distinguish humans from animals, giving each human a social persona and linking him or her to other people. Central Brazilians consider that there are two separate aspects to each individual personality. There is the social self, inculcated through names, and the physical self, which is acquired biologically. The distinction is more important for men than for women, because the social aspect of a man will eventually be perfected through initiation and will enable him to take part in the public and ceremonial life of the community. He will eventually achieve a bifurcation between his social persona, with its corresponding roles at the center of the community, and his physical person, which functions at the periphery. No such sharp separation will ever be achieved by women, whose social potentialities will remain undeveloped at the periphery.

Among the Northern Gê the central forum is not only a political place where the public affairs of the community are decided, but also a ceremonial place where the social dramas of the community are played out. In many of these societies men belong to different groupings and moiety systems by virtue of their names and their age sets or age grades, and it is through this name- or age-based dual organization that community rituals are performed to emphasize complementarity, balance, and harmony. Conflict and disharmony, meanwhile, are associated with kin groups and kinship ties. All the Northern Gê are cognatic and uxorilocal, so that males at the periphery come together in informal domestic clusters. A man is said to belong to such groups through his physical self. That whole aspect of his persona and of society which is built out of such relationships is relegated to the periphery, where, according to the prevailing ideology, it is secondary and trivial. The energy and attention of the society is focused on harmony at the center, while an attempt is made to control disharmony by banishing it to the periphery, where it is ideologically unimportant.

The Central Gê take a different approach. They do not have name-based or age-based ceremonial moieties at center stage. Instead they have patrilineal descent groups, though they still maintain uxorilocality. Their dual organization therefore operates, sometimes with moieties, sometimes without, at both the center and the periphery. Descent groups and moiety systems do not have separate and contrasting functions. Instead they reinforce each other in the same general domain. Similarly names are associated with, instead of contrasted with, descent groups, which operate at all levels of the system.

The Central Gê seek the balance and harmony that we have come to expect in the dual organization of this part of the world not by contrasting name- or age-based ceremonial moieties with kin-based political groups, but by seeking to establish an equilibrium between different sorts of binary institutions. On the one hand they have moieties or two-section systems constructed out of lineage-based factions, and on the other hand they have sporting moieties and particularly age moieties. Names are associated with the first dichotomy, which is, in the minds of the Indians, a model of conflict. That conflict model, however, is counterbalanced by institutions that are, in the minds of the Indians, models of complementarity. These are the moieties based on age sets. The Indians are both eloquent and explicit about this contrast, which they see as permeating their society because it is immanent in the universe.

Central Brazilian dual organization can thus be seen as an ideology of equilibrium derived from a theory of cosmic harmony, in which human societies of necessity participate since they too are part of the scheme of things. Of course the Central Brazilians are not alone in believing (or insisting) that there is harmony in the universe and that this harmony stems from the interaction of opposing principles that dialectically establish the balance of things. The idea is so firmly rooted in the great philosophical schemes of the East and also in much of Western philosophizing that it may even be for this reason that the Central Brazilians were once considered so anomalous. For if this is also a central tenet of central Brazilian philosophy, then we must admit that such ideas can be independently developed by societies much less technically sophisticated than our own. Yet the remarkable thing about Central Brazilian societies is less that they have developed these philosophies than the extent to which they have succeeded in living out their beliefs. Their dual organization is not a smoke screen, as Claude Lévi-Strauss once suggesed (1952), but rather an ideology. Like the "cold" societies that Lévi-Strauss brilliantly discussed in *La Pensée sauvage* (1962), the Central Brazilians see themselves, their past, and their future contained in categories that are immutable and impervious to change. The paradox they face is that they insist on the timeless nature of their systems while at the same time struggling hard to protect them from erosion.

If we consider Central Brazilian age systems in the light of their social theory and social action, then the comparison with the East African systems offers some instructive similarities and contrasts. In both areas the military role of the systems has been stressed, and in both areas this emphasis is now being questioned. I have already mentioned that Shavante war parties were not recruited by age set, and Baxter and Almagor have pointed out a similar exaggeration of the military functions of age sets in East Africa (1978:2–3, 17–20). The belief that Central Brazilian age sets were "originally" or "mainly" military organizations stems from a misunderstanding of the way the Indians themselves talk about them. They stress that initiation, the men's house(s), and the age-set or age-grade systems train men to be men. These institutions define what it means to be a man in those societies. Warfare is also seen as an expression of manliness, but by no means the only one. Shavante men gave constant displays of their manliness by running with racing logs (Maybury-Lewis 1967:245–47), singing around the village, and above all singing by night to show that they were alert and could do with little sleep—and these activities (unlike military expeditions) were carried out by age sets. It is this training for and definition of manhood that the Central Brazilian age systems have in common with the East African ones. It could hardly be otherwise in societies that have age systems, yet it would be absurd to claim that age systems are essential for such preparation.

The Central Brazilian and East African systems differ sharply, however, in the effect of age systems on property rights. The East African literature stresses that the system helps older men to control cattle and women for as long as possible, denying them (and thus fully responsible manhood) to their juniors, who are kept waiting for long periods of time. This aspect of the system is insignificant in Central Brazil. The Indians do not compete for individual control of critically important resources such as cattle. There is some tension between the older men, who take a disproportionate share of the women in polygynous marriages, and the younger men, who may be left without eligible spouses; but this tension is mitigated by the fact that women marry earlier than men do. Young men thus normally start cohabiting in their late teens with girls who are little more than child brides. Moreover, the promotion to the formal status of mature men comes relatively quickly in Central Brazil without the formal retirement of the elders or their social relegation in any way. Thus, while there is some tension between senior and junior age sets, it cannot be said that the age system as a whole is an important instrument of gerontocracy.

It is not surprising, then, that the Central Brazilian age systems appear to have fewer overt political and legal functions than the East African ones. Yet this contrast may be more apparent than real. As Baxter and Almagor point out (1978:15–16), there is a tendency for serious disputes in East Africa to be moved out of the age-set sphere and into the courts or into the patrilineal area, where descent groups compete with each other. When disputes are adjudicated there, the elders who must resolve them never appeal to the ideals of age-set solidarity as they sit in judgment. This situation exactly parallels that of the Central Gê: the Shavante ruefully admit that the competitive kin-based moieties usually triumph over the harmonious age-based ones. Meanwhile the recent history of the Sherente shows that their factional moieties have survived a century of acculturation, whereas their age-set system has virtually collapsed. In Central Brazil, as in East Africa, men tend to fade out of age-set activities and devote themselves to kin-based politics. Among the Kayapó, who made a tremendous effort to prevent the formation of kin-based factions, the result seems to have been that factionalism has taken over the age-grade systems. It seems therefore that in East Africa, where the political and legal functions of the age-set system are explicitly recognized, they nevertheless give way eventually and invariably to the real politics of descent groups. Similarly in Central Brazil the age systems were supposed to be apolitical, indeed the very antithesis of politics. The whole emphasis on moieties, particularly age moieties, was an attempt to counter and to neutralize political factionalism. Yet in the end the politics of descent groups triumphs or, as in the Kayapó case, the antipolitics of the age system is undermined.

Both the Central Brazilians and the East Africans are preoccupied with the divisive effects of kin-based politics. In Central Brazil, however, age systems are seen as devices to counteract the solidarity of kin groups. Men are inducted into them by surrogate fathers in demonstration of the fact that age systems are the antithesis of kinship systems and that surrogate fathers are an alternative to the divisive solidarity of the tie between fathers and sons. This distinction between real fathers and surrogate fathers parallels the distinctions between fathers and patrons of firestick sponsors discussed by Paul Spencer (1976) for the Masai-speaking peoples, but in East Africa the preoccupation is with the maintenance of senior (paternal) authority and the control of the tensions this emphasis creates between fathers and sons.

This difference between the Central Brazilian and the East African systems is connected with another important contrast. In East Africa age systems are often conceived on a generational model that seeks to institutionalize specific relationships between paternal and filial age sets. In Central Brazil there is no such preoccupation. There is no specific relationship between the age set of a father and that of his son, and a father may have sons scattered through several age sets. There is thus an explicit coordination of the age-set system with the kinship system in East Africa, whereas in Central Brazil the two systems are seen as distinct and antithetical.

The Central Brazilian systems therefore cast doubt on Eisenstadt's general thesis, set forth in *From Generation to Generation* (1956), that age systems serve as a mechanism to link the family with society and are therefore found in societies where the family is neither a functional isolate nor integrated into the society by other means. The thesis is in any case imprecise, for it is not clear what the criteria are for establishing the isolation or integration of the family. Central Brazilian societies, however, have developed numerous ways of linking individuals and families to the society at large, through kinship, through kinship-based moieties, through moieties whose recruitment does not depend on kinship, and through naming and name-based groups and moieties, and they have also developed quite elaborate age systems.

While questioning Eisenstadt's thesis, I nevertheless endorse his approach, which is to try to consider age systems in their total social context. It is clearly futile to try to account for them by their specific functions. It is not essential that they be military societies or property-holding corporations. They cannot be satisfactorily explained by the tasks they perform, such as hunting or gardening or ceremonial activities. It is even difficult to argue that they are political or economic necessities where they are found, though they usually have political and economic functions.

Certainly one must start the elucidation of age systems by a careful analysis of the properties of the systems themselves, but this is only a first step. To leave the analysis there, as Kertzer (1978) suggested, would be unsatisfactorily formal and "intellectualist." The second step is to examine age systems in the context of wider systems of ideas, institutions, and actions. When we take this step in regard to Central Brazil, we can see that the age systems there are poorly understood if they are analyzed in terms of their systematic properties or of their functions—even of their functions taken in the broadest social context.

Instead I have argued that a proper understanding of the age system of Central Brazil must include the ideology behind them. It must take account of the fact that the Central Brazilians use age as a principle to fashion an elaborate social theory and also as a principle of organization to set up institutions derived from that theory. Once we understand how age enters into the world view of the Central Brazilians, how it informs their ideas about time and space as well as people, how it is used in combination with other principles, such as kinship and naming, to create institutional arrangements, then we are in a position to complete the program that Evans-Pritchard adumbrated in *The Nuer* (1940). After his pioneering analysis of the Nuer lineage system and its relationship both to the local ecology and to Nuer ideas about time and space, he admitted that he had been "unable to show a similar interdependence between the age-set system and the political system" (1940:264). Yet it is only when the relations between these systems are understood, and the interrelationship between age and other principles of thought and action as well, that we can hope to make a satisfactory comparative analysis of age systems.

This demonstration has focused, for the sake of simplicity and clarity of exposition, on age *systems*. An investigation of age systems has the additional advantage that it is carried out in societies that have given explicit attention to the matter of age. Their ideas about age are therefore more clearly expressed. But what is true for age systems also holds, a fortiori, for the study of age and aging in general. This observation brings me back to my opening remarks about the parallel between the study of kinship and the study of age. The data from central Brazil show very clearly how age and kinship are combined with other principles to generate social action. The contrast with East Africa is instructive because it demonstrates that quite different results are obtained when similar principles are combined in different ways and for different purposes. The comparison highlights the way in which age and kinship are combined with other principles to generate both social theory and social action. I suspect that this is a universal phenomenon that deserves more intensive study in areas whose social theory and social institutions may seem less exotic than those of central Brazil, or even those of East Africa. It follows that there cannot, in any useful sense, be a general theory of age, any more than there can be a general theory of kinship. Such theories could only be general theories of society—which is why they are so elusive. But, in the meantime, a better knowledge of such interconnections within well-studied societies will certainly tell us a great deal more about the universally experienced and poorly understood phenomenon of age.

REFERENCES

Bamberger, Joan
    1979   Exit and voice in central Brazil: The politics of flight in Kayapó soci-
            ety. *In* Dialectical Societies: The Gê and Bororo of Central Brazil, ed.
            David Maybury-Lewis. Harvard Studies in Cultural Antropology, vol.
            1. Cambridge: Harvard University Press.
Baxter, Paul T. W., and Uri Almagor, eds.
    1978   Age, Generation, and Time: Some Features of East African Age Orga-
            nizations. New York: St. Martin's Press.
Eisenstadt, S. N.
    1956   From Generation to Generation: Age Groups and Social Structure.
            Glencoe, Ill.: Free Press.
Evans-Pritchard, Sir E. E.
    1940   The Nuer. Oxford: Clarendon Press.
Keith, Jennie
    1979   The ethnography of old age: An introduction. Anthropological Quar-
            terly 52(1):1–6.

Kertzer, David I.
1978   Theoretical developments in the study of age-group systems. American Ethnologist 5(2):368–74.

La Fontaine, J. S., ed.
1978   Sex and Age as Principles of Social Differentiation. New York: Academic Press.

Lave, Jean
1979   Cycles and trends in Krĩkatí naming practices. In Dialectical Societies: The Gê and Bororo of Central Brazil, ed. David Maybury-Lewis. Harvard Studies in Cultural Anthropology, vol. 1. Cambridge: Harvard University Press.

Lévi-Strauss, Claude
1952   Les structures sociales dans le Brésil central et oriental. In Indian Tribes of Aboriginal America, ed. Sol Tax. Selected Papers of the XXIXth International Congress of Americanists. Chicago: University of Chicago Press.
1962   La pensée sauvage. Paris: Plon.

Maybury-Lewis, David
1967   Akwẽ-Shavante Society. Oxford: Clarendon Press.
1979a   Cultural categories of the Central Gê. In Dialectical Societies: The Gê and Bororo of Central Brazil, ed. Maybury-Lewis. Harvard Studies in Cultural Anthropology, vol. 1. Cambridge: Harvard University Press.
1979b   Kinship, ideology, and culture. In Dialectical Societies: The Gê and Bororo of Central Brazil, ed. Maybury-Lewis. Harvard Studies in Cultural Anthropology, vol. 1. Cambridge: Harvard University Press.

Maybury-Lewis, David, organizer
1971   Symposium: Recent research in Central Brazil. In Verhandlungen des XXXVIII Internationalen Amerikanistenkongress (1968), 3:333–91. Munich: Klaus Renner.

Nimuendajú, Curt
1939   The Apinayé. Washington: Catholic University of America Press.
1942   The Šerente. Los Angeles: Southwest Museum.
1946   The Eastern Timbira. Berkeley: University of California Press.

Seeger, Anthony
1981   Nature and Society in Central Brazil. Harvard Studies in Cultural Anthropology, vol. 4. Cambridge: Harvard University Press.

Spencer, Paul
1976   Opposing streams and the gerontocratic ladder: Two models of age organization in East Africa. Man 11(2):153–75.

Stewart, F. H.
1977   Fundamentals of Age-Group Systems. New York: Academic Press.

Turner, Terence
1979   Kinship, household, and community structure among the Kayapó. In Dialectical Societies: The Gê and Bororo of Central Brazil, ed. David

Maybury-Lewis. Harvard Series in Cultural Anthropology, vol. 1. Cambridge: Harvard University Press.

Vidal, Lux
1977 Morte e vida de uma sociedade indígena brasileira. São Paulo: HUCITEC, University of São Paulo.

5

Age in the Fortesian Coordinates

Eugene Hammel

Age is a measure of elapsed time. It is most often considered as an attribute that explains the condition of persons, collectivities, or other entities in a developmental process. Individuals, objects, social organizations from the family to total societies—all can have ages. The concept of age can be applied also to things that are thought not to change, as in the phrase "a concept of justice of great antiquity." It is important to distinguish the lapse of time from the attributes that may accompany that lapse. Age is also an attribute of social relationships: a contract can have an age, as can a marriage. Some aging processes go from a start to a finish, like individual lives. Others may never end, or may never have begun, as various notions of the history of the universe would have us believe. Still others may be cyclical, as yet other notions of the universe claim. Age, then, *is* time. As time, it has manifold implications for the study of social structure and human behavior. The implications are usefully manifold because time, although superficially a simple variable, is capable of combinatorial elaboration and expression on various scales.

In the anthropological context, age has long been used to speak of individual persons and of whole societies, or even of humankind entire in the secular (i.e., noncyclical) processes of life and of evolution. In its application to persons, age must be a concept as old as humankind. In its

141

application to humankind age is at least as old as Thucydides. In more recent applications to humankind, at the hands of Darwin and his successors, age begins even earlier. (One can ponder the richness of "age" in these last three sentences.) It was Meyer Fortes that pointed out (1949) that some social units run on a cyclical clock, and that the secular ages of persons in such units give to the unit of their membership itself an age, a position in its cycle of development. Like most very fundamental ideas, this one was not foreign to experience, but its meaning for social structure had not been articulated. Indeed, it even enjoyed independent reinvention (Hammel 1961). In its most general sense, the concept is simply that the age of some social units is a function of the ages of their members. Age, then, is a variable associated with entities of varying position in taxonomies of objects—for us, persons, social relationships, social groups, social categories (whether of native or of analytical identification).

Measurement

The primary thrust of this paper is to urge attention to two aspects of the ages of pairs of persons involved in social relations: their actual ages in the sense of elapsed time since birth and their relative ages, that is, their ages relative to each other. Before proceeding, however, I set forth some general principles.

Age can be measured in numerous ways, not all of which need be numerical in the strict sense, and it can be measured in more than one way at the same time for the same object of interest. The first distinction in this regard has already been mentioned—whether aging is a cyclical or a secular process. If aging is cyclical, as in the repetitive renewal of households, the time scale on which the age of households is measured is modular, going from zero to some point in time, then reverting immediately to zero for the next cycle. If aging is secular, as in the lives of individuals, the time scale on which age is measured goes from zero to some maximum but does not repeat again from zero for the same unit. When there are many units in a secular aging process, following one another in time, one may of course speak metaphorically of cyclical aging in the sense that the course of development is repeated again and again, but by different units. Indeed, in the ordinary cycle of household development, it is more the repeatedly occupied dwelling place or the "house" in a genealogical sense that shows a cyclical pattern, while successive families constituting the line of inheriting households show repetitions of closely similar secular aging patterns. The easy metaphorical transition from observed secular courses of development to an idealized cycle is analytically productive but can be misleading, as we shall see.

The second distinction to be observed is that age can be measured both on ordinal and on interval scales, and on each with varying degrees of refinement. Let us first take ordinal measurement of age, since it is common in all societies in discussing individuals, and since it is the only measure of individual age in some societies.

The commonest ordinal measure of age for individuals is birth order. Within a sibling set, this is a relative measure. If A is born first, B second, C third, then A is older than B, who is older than C. This measure has transitivity, since if $A > B$ and $B > C$, then $A > C$. Across sibling sets birth order is an absolute measure. If A is firstborn in the sibling set $[A,B]$ and C is firstborn in the set $[C,D]$, then A and C are "the same age" in this sense, as are B and D, and A is "older than" C. Obviously, some care must be taken in the interpretation of these relative age statements across sibling sets. A can be older than C in this sense (being a firstborn son while C is a second-born son) even if A was born a century later than C. The absolute ordinal measurement of age has meaning only against an analytical grid on which particular ages established by a relation within some set (here siblings) are felt to have important associated characteristics across sets, that is, no matter which sibling set they occur in. Thus, for example, we might expect firstborn children to have particular personality characteristics, regardless of the sibling set into which they are born.

Ordinality of age can be cruder in measurement than birth order (in the sense that it distinguishes larger blocks of time as measured on an interval scale of years). An important measure of age in all societies, for example, is generation, arising from the parent-child link. This measure, too, is transitive within a descent line. If A is the parent of B and B the parent of C, then A is older than B and B older than C, and thus A is older than C. But this measure can be used absolutely, too. If D is also the parent of E, then A and D are both parents, and B and E are both children; but some care must be taken in thinking of A as parent and E as child, since it makes no difference to their comparison in some senses if E was born before A. Similarly we should observe that in this use of absolute projection onto an analytical grid, B is both a parent and a child, an occurrence that should surprise no ethnographer familiar with the confusions of the life course.

Much the same problems can arise if age is measured in other common, ordinal ways—infant, child, adolescent, adult, or primary school pupil, high school pupil, college student, and so on. The two major issues that have arisen in discussion are whether societies that do not have calendars can reckon age, and whether the absolute projection of relative age within sets of linked persons is legitimate. On the first, of course such innumerate societies can reckon age—in birth order, in generation, in age grades variously defined, in descriptive maturational stages, and so on. On the second, it should be clear that extension of within-set concepts across sets is analytically useful and thus legitimate, but that some care must be exercised to avoid losing control of the metaphor. David Kertzer (1982) has criticized and discussed at length the metaphorical usage of "generation" by Karl Mannheim and his followers. "Generation" is variously used. It can mean an ordinal age relationship in filial steps between persons actually linked by consanguinity, lineal or collateral. This is its central meaning and etymologically its root, derived from the Indo-European word having to do with giving birth. It can be used in absolute extension, to mean relative age groups, whether directly linked by kinship or not, as in the phrase "the generation gap." Further, it can be used with the relativity of intergenerational differences scarcely noted, as in the phrase "the Beat Generation," denoting persons presumably sharing certain life experiences by virtue of contemporaneity and cultural exposure. Kertzer properly details the logical inconsistencies of such metaphorical usages. Nevertheless, they are all measures of some kind of age; the differences reside in whether the scale of age is individual, societal, or historical.

Ordinal measures are applied to units larger than individuals, as well. Households in our own culture can be "new," "established," or "empty nests," and any native speaker of English would recognize these designations as placing households in an order, according to their developmental state. A household is older in its empty-nest stage than it was when it was new, and in the absolute extension of these terms, any empty nest is older than any new household, even though the new household may be in this century and the empty nest in the last, and even though of two households that were new in 1956, one may have emptied later while the other was still new.

Measurement of age on interval scales is so familiar as to require little methodological discussion. Doris Mayer pointed out at the conference, however, that the existence of an absolute calendrical age scale can provide a firm base for anxiety about the development of individuals (and, I might add, of other units). A mother whose concept of her child's age is only that he is beginning to walk is not worried that he is two years old at that point. Conference discussion also noted that calculation of ages on calendrical scales is fundamentally a device of governments in establishing universalistic criteria for status—for example, in implementing conscription.

Problems of understanding the implications of age differences between persons or units in particular relationships and of those between persons only conceptually in the positions of such relationships—the problems introduced by generalizing absolutely from relative links—do not disappear when age is measured more finely, as a calendrical variable. Demographers, for example, may compare the fertility of married women ages 20–24 to the fertility of those same women (or at least their survivors) when they are aged 25–29. They will no doubt discover that fertility declined. On the other hand, they can compare the fertility of two sets of women, aged 20–24 and aged 25–29 contemporaneously, and here they might easily discover that the older women have higher fertility within the respective five-year spans. Or they could compare the fertility of women ages 20–24 in 1930 and in 1950, and there they would surely find (in the United States) that fertility had increased. Demographers are much occupied with teasing out the differences among these different kinds of age—the ages of individuals measured on the scale of their own life clock, yielding age effects; the ages of sets of individuals measured on the clock of a succession of such sets, yielding cohort effects; and the ages of sets of individuals measured on a historical clock of their society, yielding period effects. These kinds of age are not always distinguishable, even in principle. Failure to admit the possibility of their effects, however, can give rise to serious errors of misinterpretation.[1]

Suppose one examines the patterns of professional activity among scientists alive in some year, according to their ages. One may well discover that the very youngest scientists are moderately productive, the middle-aged ones very productive, and the old ones only moderately or even less productive. One could easily ascribe these differences to the personal aging process. On the other hand, one might examine just the older scientists and discover that although they had begun their own lives

---

1. The literature on this topic is vast, and is to be found in demography, history, economics, anthropology, and psychology. Some suggested starting points are Riley 1976, Baltes 1968, Cohn 1972, Mason et al. 1973, Pressat 1972, Ryder 1965.

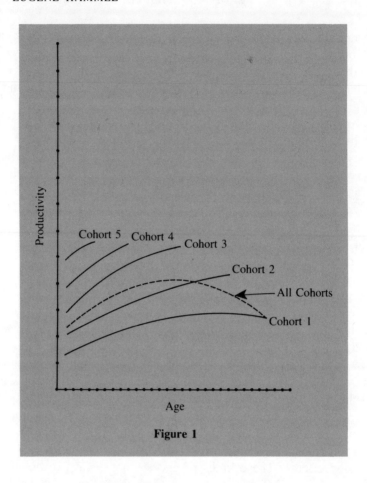

Figure 1

with relatively low productivity, they had increased it steadily through-out, never actually showing a decline. The differences first isolated in examination of the totality of the data could be the result only of a steady improvement in the productivity of successive groups of scientists begin-ning their professional lives, each such group increasing from its own unique starting point. Since information on the older scientists is avail-able only for people who were born a long time ago, their lower produc-tivity is a function of their date of birth, not of their age (see Figure 1). Indeed, a recent study of the productivity of academic chemists shows a pattern very much like this one; cohort effects can be mistaken for age effects (Hammel 1983).

A Bivariate View of Age

My intention here is not to chronicle examples of the naming and use of individual and social age, or to show their workings in a particular society, or to explore further the potential confusions of age, cohort, and period effects, as important as these matters may be. Rather, I wish to expand and refine two ways we look at age as a variable, expressing some things that all of us know but have often ignored in our analyses. I introduce two clumsy acronyms for two important concepts distinguishing absolute age (ABSAGE) from relative age (RELAGE). ABSAGE is the age of an individual or social unit on some scale of months, years, named age grades, or any such scale. RELAGE is the difference between the ABSAGE of two persons or units in some social relationship, on such a scale. ABSAGE and RELAGE are the Fortesian coordinates of my title. Both have consequences for individuals and groups, and for each other; that is, technically, the axes of age need not be orthogonal.

ABSAGE is the simpler of the two. A familiar effect of ABSAGE is the relationship between the age of a conjugal union (often itself a function of the ABSAGE of one or both of its members) and the developmental position of the household founded on it. Similarly, the ABSAGE of all members establish the productive and consumptive patterns of households, their dependency ratios, and in some societies their political influence. Generally, social position, alignment in networks, and other important behavioral attributes of households are determined or constrained by their age structure in the ABSAGE sense.

A less familiar example has to do with the ABSAGE of entry into particular relationships, for example, of individuals into marriage. Families with wives who married young are likely to have more children than otherwise comparable ones in which the wives married later. The child-bearing and child-caring periods in such families will be longer. The duration of the family-building period and the number of children have consequences for the behavior and self-conception of parents and for the position of the household in the larger society. If early marriage is the rule, concepts of sex-role behavior may be expected to be concordant, either as cause or as effect. In times of rapid social change, severe role conflicts may emerge, for early marriage commits many individuals to long married lives, and they cannot always easily alter their behavior. Such problems are now important to many Americans who were born in the 1930s and married in the 1950s. Families based on early marriage will also ramify more rapidly (at any given level of age-specific fertility rates) than will those based on later marriage, since they will produce, on the average, more children. Such relationships between age at marriage and the ramification of lineage structures are important in some societies, particularly if there is much intrasocietal variation in age at marriage. Early age at marriage is more likely to ensure the presence of heirs, a matter important in some societies, but it may also produce too many for some purposes, with consequences for the division of resources and even the creation of social classes or occupational groups formed by the disenfranchised. The implications of differential fertility and thus, in this instance, of the effects of age-related phenomena for local political structures are also important.

Long childbearing spans mean wide temporal spans in sibling sets. The RELAGE patterns between siblings in a set of wide span are quite different from those in a sibling set of narrow span. Socialization patterns can vary accordingly, sometimes with some children in quasi-adult roles vis-à-vis much younger siblings. Wide spans of this kind also have implications for the kinship system and its terminological consistency. Where siblings can differ markedly in age, it is easy for kin of very different personal ages to be members of the same formal genealogical generation, and for members of different formal genealogical generations to be of the same personal ages (see also Kertzer 1982). Such inconsistencies would be small but common between persons who were collaterally close, but might be extreme (although less common, because of random variation along chains of kin) between persons who were collaterally distant. Terminological systems in which explicit elder/younger distinctions were obligatory would be particularly affected, because of differences between generational and age criteria for naming.

RELAGE has more complex consequences and is less straightforward. Consider first the Fortesian coordinates laid out in the ordinary Cartesian way (Figure 2). The bivariate point to be plotted in this graph is a dyad of entities engaged in some social relation, usually role incumbents, although supraindividual units could be treated similarly. In the examples to follow, the points of the plot are considered to be cross-sectional data, those dyads observed at an instant in time; they are not (unless so indicated) successive observations of the same dyad.[2]

2. I am indebted to Kenneth Wachter for pointing out the potential ambiguity attendant on not making this specification explicit.

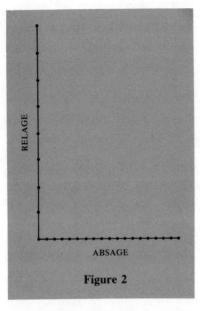

Figure 2

To plot such points we must define the axes first. In a marriage, for example, RELAGE can be the difference between the ages of the spouses (or their ratio), while ABSAGE can be the age of one of them, or the average of both ages, or the age (duration) of the marriage. There must be a convention about how to compute RELAGE, which is here taken as a difference between two ABSAGES, and a convention about which ABSAGE (of the dyad or of one of its members) is selected. In regard to marriages, we might always take RELAGE as ABSAGE(husband) minus ABSAGE(wife) and ABSAGE as ABSAGE(husband); these definitions are entirely arbitrary, although particular choices might be motivated by theory or by convenience in further manipulation, as in making most differences come out positive rather than negative. Suppose we adopt the definitions just given and plot some number of contemporary marriage dyads in a hypothetical society in which quite young women have their first marriages with much older men and then successively marry younger men as they become widowed; quite young men begin their married lives as the husbands of old widows and then marry successively younger women. We can call this the Tiwi model, if we like (Hart and Pilling 1960). At any one time the marriage dyads may be plotted as in Figure 3. Notice that the sloping line describes an ideal linear relationship between the two kinds of age. Obviously, in any empirical situation there would be scatter about this

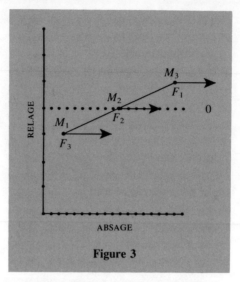

Figure 3

line. Notice also that although any set of contemporary marriage dyads might fall on the line, any marriage dyad observed over time moves horizontally to the right, the age difference between spouses remaining constant as the husband's age increases. The horizontal arrows indicate such time-series movement. Notice also that successive marriages of individuals move along the sloping line in different ways. The points F_1, F_2, and F_3 describe the successive marriage dyads for a woman, beginning in her tender youth, married to a much older and absolutely old man, then a second marriage to a man her own age, then a third marriage in her old age to a younger and absolutely young man. Conversely, the points M_1, M_2, and M_3 show the successive marriages for a man.

In modern Europe the relationship is more like Figure 4. The points F_1, F_2 and M_1, M_2 can be interpreted as first and second marriages of a man and of a woman. In earlier centuries the relationship was probably more like Figure 5, since widows had lower remarriage rates than widowers, and since widowers usually married women younger than themselves. These graphs just say that the age relationship between bride and groom can be expressed as a straight line in terms of intercept and slope. Of course, the relationship between RELAGE and ABSAGE need not be linear; these are just a hypothetical examples.

For some dyads and the interpretation of behavior, the relationships between RELAGE and ABSAGE are certainly not so simple. The importance of RELAGE may vary with the value of ABSAGE, and presentation of the

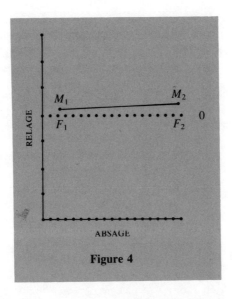

Figure 4

data should reflect this fact. I attempt to show it graphically here, but it should be understood that my aim is to exposit the idea of this dependence between RELAGE and ABSAGE, not to develop a notational system. To keep matters simple, discussion is restricted to positive values of RE-LAGE, that is, in the marriage example, where husband is older than wife.

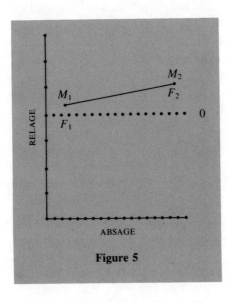

Figure 5

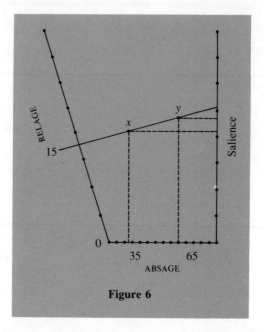

Figure 6

In Figures 6 and 7 the axes of RELAGE and ABSAGE are not at right angles, and there is a third axis of implied interactional salience onto which the [RELAGE,ABSAGE] bivariate point is projected. Values of RE-LAGE and ABSAGE are plotted at right angles to their respective axes, and implied interactional salience is read at right angles to that axis. Suppose a set of marriages in which the husband is 15 years older than the wife (Figure 6). When the wife was 20 and the husband 35, the physiological differences between them by virtue of age would be relatively small, but when the wife was 50 and the husband 65 they would be much greater. The salience of those differences for sexual relations or caretaking would be greater at higher ABSAGES. In Figure 6, both point *x* and point *y* lie on the line for RELAGE values of 15, but *x* is for ABSAGE 35 and *y* is for ABSAGE 65. The projected point on the salience scale for *y* is higher than the point for *x*. On the other hand, the power differential between the spouses might diminish or reverse as they aged; Figure 7 expresses this relationship. Here the power of the husband consequent on his seniority decreases as the age of both spouses increases. Points *x* and *y* again lie on the line for RELAGE value 15, *x* for ABSAGE 35 and *y* for ABSAGE 65; the projected point on the salience scale declines. The same kind of graph would express the importance of age differences between siblings in most societies.

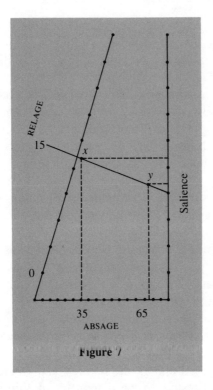

Figure 1

Both of these examples rest on the rate of biologically and socially relevant change at different points in the individual life span. These kinds of change affect different kinds of social dyads differently. Spouses may grow apart, siblings may grow together as they age (or the reverse); the aging of individuals can have important effects on the networks of interpersonal relationships in which they participate. There is, of course, nothing new about that as an observation. My point is only that such shifts can be described in a reasonably abstract way, permitting us to make more general, cross-cultural statements about the importance of age.

Some Real and Imagined Examples

By now it is well known that the disparity in spouses' ages has implications for the consanguineal structure of affinal relations, where endogamy is not totally proscribed (see Hammel 1976 for a review, formalization, and microsimulation results). To summarize briefly, consistent differences in spouses' ages at marriage, so that on average the husband is older than the wife, or the reverse, increase the probability that a man will marry a matrilateral and a woman a patrilateral cross-cousin. The demography of marriage creates a genealogical network of a particular kind, and this genealogical network forms a latent social one that could be called into play in the manipulation of social ties and the elaboration of symbolic forms. Whether such latent networks emerge as real social and cultural phenomena, and under what conditions, deserves serious analytical attention.

Edmund Leach's work on the structural implications of unilateral relationships (1951) suggests that we may expect countervailing obligations to accompany the movement of spouses along a continuum of social groups. These obligations can easily be social as well as material (see also Salisbury 1956). In particular, we might imagine that relations of clientage might accompany those of affinity; certainly such a coupling would not be foreign to our own Western exerience.

Consider, for the sake of this argument, the possible role that the demography of marriage might have played in the development of European mercantilism. In the Middle Ages and Renaissance, marriages were rather strictly controlled among the nobility and emerging bourgeoisie. Much of the control rested on the demonstrated ability of the intended groom to secure a living, through either access to usufruct or the exercise of a trade. Marriage of males was thus delayed to some degree beyond their physical maturity. The marriage of females may have been delayed to some extent by the need to accumulate dowry, but the evidence suggests that there was a fairly consistent disparity in age at marriage—not large, but consistent, with husbands older than wives by at least five years. Some unilateral alliances of families or lineages or septs or other groupings must have resulted from this circumstance. Marriages were often broken by the death of one spouse, more frequently the husband, since he was the older, but sometimes the wife. Broken marriages must have been even more frequent in the early stages of the Renaissance, when Europe was devastated by periodic plagues. When marriages were broken, more surviving widowers remarried than surviving widows. Widowers seeking a second mate in the population would be more likely to find one younger than themselves than older, simply because of the shape of the age pyramid; there were always more younger women than older women. The more severe the mortality crisis, the farther below themselves in the age pyramid they would have to go to find a spouse, and the average disparity in age between spouses would be exacerbated by this additional competition for wives. The probability of occurrence of unilateral chains of kin, linked by consanguinity as well as affinity, would be enhanced. Trust based on kinship is a fertile ground for the development of mercantile relations, as Burton Benedict (1968) has shown from modern ethnographic data. These (admittedly speculative) demographically induced patterns of social relations can only have assisted the growth of the modern world economic system.

The implications of age as a variable for politics are not exhausted by this flight of sociological fancy. Age, as we know, is a correlate of and often a prerequisite to the acquisition of important social goods in all societies. Access to strong drink in this country is limited by law to those of a specified age. Its importance has been diminished by the advent of other sources of pharmaceutical satisfaction, but these things cost money, and access to money is still regulated by age, even if only by the age necessary to attain the strength to rob. Genital sex involving more than the self, long a socially controlled source of personal satisfaction, is difficult of acquisition before puberty. There are of course many other limits on access to satisfaction. Kinship, class, caste, a myriad of ascribed characteristics keep the many from enjoying the perquisites of the few. Acquired characteristics—education, the proper use of language codes for particular purposes, and many others—are not easy to master; they take time, thus age. The perpetual revolt of the young and aspiring against the mature and established is a revolt of the have-nots against the haves. But of all the prerequisites to status in any society, age is the most generous. It is of course itself constrained in its effects by the magnitude and distribution of existing resources, and by the ratios of magnitude of adjacent age groups in the population structure. But against this ground of expected benefit, constrained by the parameters of resource supply and demographic demand, time is the most egalitarian of barriers. They also receive who only stand and age. Nothing is denied the aspirant simply by virtue of current age, not even death. The gradual accomplishments achieved by virtue of aging are a different form of the "trickle effect" (Fallers 1954), giving each person an illusion of mobility.

These democratic benefits of the aging process are subject, however, to serious demographic perturbations that can pit one age class against another in ways that deny the inherent equalizing effects of the process. Fluctuations in fertility and mortality play havoc with the ratios of generations and cruel tricks with the life chances of those who precede or follow on. Too many babies at one point means wholesale adaptation of social institutions in succession—first nursery schools, then primary schools, then high schools, then colleges, and ultimately nursing homes. Too few babies, by comparison, mean that the young must ultimately produce much wealth to support the old. The sins of one generation are thus visited on the next. In our own recent history the carelessly restrained reproductive behavior of the marriage cohorts around 1950 created just such an age bulge in the population, and it has been moving through the age structure quite like a pig in a python's peristalsis, all but wrecking every institution it touched.[3] The unwitting reaction of these babies is now to deny the originally sinful their golden years, as the social security system totters into bankruptcy.

Conclusion

That age is an important attribute of individuals in social organizations and that their lives are much conditioned by it has long been recognized. Our use of age as an analytical variable has been limited by the crudity with which we have measured, manipulated, and compared it, and by our failure to give sufficient attention to second-order effects of age. This paper is but a simple excursion that clarifies and presents a few points:

1. Ages are ages, whether measured on ordinal or other scales.
2. In a taxonomy of inclusions, of individuals in social units and of social units in higher-level units, age at any level has implications for the age of the including unit.
3. Some ages are absolute, others relative, comparing two persons or units in social relationship.
4. Relative and absolute ages of persons in some dyad are *both* important, and they interact in their effects on social relations.
5. Relative ages can be abstracted metaphorically, idealized from their direct intradyadic context to more general form, but with inherent difficulty.
6. The *age structures* of populations and of sets of persons engaged in dyadic relationships have systemic consequences for social action.

3. I am obliged to Harold Wilensky for the original of this pungent observation, made between whiffs of tear gas at Berkeley in the 1960s.

They may create latent social structures capable of symbolic elaboration, and they may affect the nature of accession to social benefits.

Most of the interesting systemic or structural effects of age-related phenomena will be stronger and more frequent in the kinds of societies anthropologists usually study than in modern nation-states. The sharpness of age effects arises from the small size of such "anthropological" societies, in two ways. First, in small societies kinship is more often a central organizing principle, kinship networks are more dense, and thus age-dependent effects on kinship have greater salience. Second, the smaller a society, the more subject it is to random fluctuations in the demographic rates that create the biological links on which kinship systems are most often based. The effects of these inevitable perturbations through the age structure on kinship and thus on social relations can be quite extreme. Indeed, small societies must be anything but stable in their kinship structures over time. We may profitably regard the systems of symbols and mutual expectations that are the culture of kinship as adaptive mechanisms to cope with the vagaries of demographic structures. Recognizing the effect that demographic rates, through the age structure, can have on social relations, and the ways in which these relations are handled symbolically, will enhance our understanding of the role of culture as an interpretive and adaptive schema.

REFERENCES

Baltes, Paul B.
  1968 Longitudinal and cross-sectional sequences in the study of age and generation effects. Human Development 11:145–71.
Benedict, Burton
  1968 Family firms and economic development. Southwestern Journal of Anthropology 24:1–19.
Cohn, Richard
  1972 On interpretation of cohort and period analyses: A mathematical note. *In* Aging and Society, vol. 3: A Sociology of Age Stratification, ed. Matilda White Riley, Marilyn Johnson, and Anne Foner, New York: Russell Sage Foundation.
Fallers, Lloyd A.
  1954 A note on the "trickle effect." Public Opinion Quarterly 18:314–21.

Fortes, Meyer
  1949   Time and social structure: An Ashanti case study. *In* Social Structure, ed. Fortes. Oxford: Oxford University Press.
Hammel, Eugene A.
  1961   The family cycle in a coastal Peruvian slum and village. American Anthropologist 63:989–1005.
  1976   The matrilateral implications of structural cross-cousin marriage. *In* Demographic Anthropology, ed. Ezra Zubrow. Albuquerque: University of New Mexico Press.
  1983   The productivity of chemists and mathematicians at the University of California. Program in Population Research Working Paper no. 11. Berkeley: University of California, Program in Population Research.
Hart, C. W. M., and Arnold Pilling
  1960   The Tiwi of North Australia. New York: Holt, Rinehart & Winston.
Kertzer, David
  1982   Generation and age in cross-cultural perspective. *In* Aging from Birth to Death, ed. Matilda White Riley, Ronald Abeles, and Michael Teitelbaum, vol. 2. Boulder: Westview Press.
Leach, Edmund R.
  1951   The structural implications of matrilateral cross-cousin marriage. Journal of the Royal Anthropological Institute 81:23–55.
Mason, Karen Oppenheim, William M. Mason, H. H. Winsborough, and W. Kenneth Poole
  1973   Some methodological issues in cohort analysis of archival data. American Sociological Review 38:242–58.
Pressat, Roland
  1972   Demographic Analysis. Chicago: Aldine.
Riley, Matilda White
  1976   Age strata in social systems. *In* Handbook of Aging and the Social Sciences, ed. Robert H. Binstock and Ethel Shanas. New York: Van Nostrand.
Ryder, Norman B.
  1965   The cohort as a concept in the study of social change. American Sociological Review 30:843–61.
Salisbury, Richard
  1956   Asymmetrical marriage systems. American Anthropologist 58:639–55.

6

Age in Cultural Economics:
An Evolutionary Approach

Rhoda Halperin

This chapter considers age as a variable in the cross-cultural analysis of economic processes in history and anthropology. It is an exploratory theoretical piece, designed primarily to use age as a stimulus for revealing questions about the analysis of economic processes in different types of societies and to tie these questions to some of the larger theoretical issues in cultural economics. By "cultural economics" I mean a cross-cultural comparative science of the economy, the major aim of which is to understand how economic processes function and change over evolutionary and historical time. Cultural economics deals with livelihood processes in cultural systems—all systems, small and large, preindustrial and industrial.

Age is a critical variable for our understanding of economic processes in any culture. Individuals in all cultures grow old, change their productive tasks, and later change their involvement in economic processes. The social units within which individuals produce, distribute, and consume their livelihood change, and thus age with time. The fact that age has been treated only serendipitously in anthropological studies of economic

I thank Ken Kensinger, David Kertzer, Jennie Keith, and Christine Fry for their comments and suggestions. For research assistance and great patience with typing I thank my graduate assistant, Richard Kurz, and our department secretary, Kay Klein.

processes is both a testimony to the relatively primitive state of the art and a reflection of our own culture's denial of inevitable aging processes (Myerhoff 1978). Aging processes are as much a part of culture as production or distribution processes, and they are linked in variable and intricate ways in different cultures.

Traditionally, what I designate as "cultural economics" has been called "economic anthropology," the study of small-scale, preindustrial, precapitalist, kin-based economies, their systems of exotic trade and exchange, their ways of organizing land and labor, their marketplaces and forms of money. Traditionally, too, economic anthropology has always been part of the larger scientific study of anthropology, particularly cultural anthropology. Because the distinctive feature of economic anthropology has been its emphasis on economic processes in cultural systems, the name "cultural economics" seems more appropriate for the field (Halperin 1982). The term "economic anthropology" is unsatisfactory because it suggests a rather unhappy marriage between economics and anthropology and not a comparative scientific enterprise. By contrast, the term "cultural economics" reflects the range of economic processes and cultural contexts anthropologists commonly study in the 1980s. Anthropologists join economists, development sociologists, and historians in studying economic processes of all sorts—not only small-scale primitive economies, so important for establishing baseline data, but also developing village economies in the Third World and segments of industrial-world economies, among them modern health-care systems and multinational corporations (Wolfe 1977). Given the wide-ranging concerns of cultural economics, the anthropological investigation of the relationship between age and economic processes is by no means confined to preindustrial societies, but includes modern industrial and postindustrial economic formations as well.

The analysis of age as a variable in economic processes depends greatly on the type of society under consideration. Before meaningful comparisons can be drawn, either for processes of aging and life course or for processes of livelihood, a framework within which comparisons can be carried out must be established. The perspective I will take is an evolutionary one. Generally, as cultures evolve from preindustrial egalitarian societies to highly stratified capitalistic systems, age becomes less an independent variable that shapes such economic processes as the division of labor for production than a dependent variable that is controlled by economic processes, and to some extent by technological processes as well.

I use "age" in several ways in this chapter. In some instances the term refers to demographic age distribution, in others to individual chronological age, in still others to life-cycle stage as culturally defined, or level of physical functionality. This last is particularly important in determining contributions to subsistence in societies that rely solely or primarily on human muscular energy. I would have liked to be consistent and use the word "age" with a single meaning, but the data and the nature of our language do not allow me to do so. Nevertheless, I think the general argument that age shifts from an independent to a dependent variable in the organization of production and distribution still holds, regardless of the specific meaning or meanings of age employed. Within evolutionary types it is possible to find patterns that delineate the relationships between age and fundamental processes of production, distribution, and consumption. To propose an evolutionary framework is not to exhaust the range of evolutionary types. It is to attempt to organize some questions that may lead to the addition of more detailed qualitative and especially quantitative data to an otherwise primarily descriptive and anecdotal ethnographic record concerning age and the economy in human societies (Nag 1973:10).

If we assume that the quality as well as the quantity of an individual's contribution to the livelihood of a household, a village, or a nation varies over time, then the task becomes one of explaining the variation. Who works, for how long, at what sorts of tasks in different societies? What does an understanding of the variation tell us about production processes? If we know the answers to these questions, our understanding of economic processes in different cultures is greatly enhanced, and we can begin to ask some further questions. Why, for example, are the elderly marginal in our own economy and key resources in others? What kinds of institutions and ecological settings in different cultures create economic importance for certain categories of individuals at particular points during the life course? Given the increased and increasing longevity of populations in industrial societies (Fries 1980), what are the economic implications, theoretical as well as practical, of long-term dependency of the old on the young?

Conceptualizing time is critical for understanding age and economic processes. As individuals age, their economic relationships in such social units as households, villages, and cities change. The social units themselves exist in historical time and therefore change ecologically, demographically, and technologically. In a sense, then, to pose the question of age as a variable in any cultural process is to inquire about time and social structure. Recognizing that the cross-cultural examination of age and economic processes presents many of the same problems as the study of any process in cross-cultural perspective, I will examine the theoretical possibilities for a more precise understanding of processes of production, distribution, and consumption which derive from dealing with issues concerning age and the life course in an evolutionary framework.

An Evolutionary Framework

If aging processes are universal in human societies, so are processes of gaining a livelihood. The intersection of these two basic processes demands attention not only because individual producers and consumers must go through their life courses, grow old, and change the nature of their productive efforts, but also because production units themselves change with time and thus mature in some societies within an individual's lifetime, in others over many generations. Households age, and so do villages, cities, and nation-states.

Age touches every facet of economic life, but the way it does so varies from culture to culture. The way in which production units and laboring individuals change with age depends on the political, technological, and ecological contexts within which the units operate. In cultures that are demographically small, technologically simple, and politically egalitarian, age functions with sex as one of the two determinants of the division of labor in society. In most preindustrial cultures, age statuses function alongside those of kinship; often the two overlap to set patterns of labor division. In more complex and politically stratified social systems, age is only one of many principles that divide labor and it is subordinate to social class.

In part, the failure of ethnographers to deal with age as a variable in economic processes is a theoretical issue and relates to some of the ongoing debates in economic anthropology. Problematic conceptualizations of the nature of production processes have made it as difficult to deal with age as with sex. I have argued elsewhere, for example, that to confine production to hunting and gathering activities alone in band-level societies results in a totally inadequate understanding of the division of labor by sex (Halperin 1980). I suspect that the same could be said of age.

Farming is not the only productive task connected with the maintenance of livelihood in agricultural societies, yet discussions of the division of labor in such societies often remain confined to activities surrounding cultivation (see Nag 1976). In the long run, a focus on age as a variable will provide some of the longitudinal data we need in order to understand the changing relationships between processes of production, distribution, and consumption, and will bring some of the diachronic considerations that have always been part of the craft of archaeology and ethnohistory into the mainstream of cultural anthropology.

I begin with egalitarian societies with hunter-gatherer and horticultural technologies and ask the general questions: How do people at different ages participate in the subsistence effort? What kinds of contributions do people make? I then deal with ranked and stratified societies, first chiefdoms and then state-level societies with increasingly larger and more complex political units. By organizing the ethnographic material in this way, we can ask a series of questions: Once human societies become sedentary, how does age affect economic organization in general and the division of labor in particular? What is the relationship of population size, the age pyramid, and the function of age in the overall economic organization of preindustrial societies? How does the development of the state and class stratification affect the economic roles of people of different ages?

It should be noted that technology alone does not suffice to classify cultures as similar or different. Societies with horticultural technologies, for example, differ enormously along a range of variables, among them population size, resource base, and degree of political centralization and ranking. At one end of the continuum, egalitarian horticultural societies, such as those in the Amazon basin, exhibit economic processes that in many respects are similar to those of hunter-gatherers. At the other end of the prestate continuum are such horticultural societies as the Trobrianders, with much larger populations and an economic organization closer to that of preindustrial states. Most peasant producers in nation-state systems practice some form of horticulture. In some cases, peasant horticultural production units are small households, more simply organized than horticultural production and distribution units at the chiefdom level. The latter may comprise a clan, a group of clans, or a whole village population. The implications of the size of the production unit for the allocation of tasks among people of different ages need further analysis, with controls for technology.

In all horticultural societies, the use of root crops or grains results in closer birth spacing (Draper 1975, Kolata 1974). With sedentarization and increased population size, certain infectious diseases, such as measles, mumps, rubella, and small pox, begin to become significant. In the long run, nutritional well-being tends to go down, fertility rates go up, life spans shorten, and infant mortality rates increase (Cockburn 1971). In the short run, however, there is some evidence that children and old people fare better in a sedentary context than they do as members of a nomadic foraging culture. Nancy Howell reports, for example, that !Kung families that in the 1960s were burdened by the sick or handicapped or by many children or elderly had a tendency to congregate at Bantu cattle posts. Healthy !Kung tended to gain weight on the high-calorie diet provided there (1979:50). It should be noted, though, that the !Kung contact with the Bantu pastoral agriculturalists involves the !Kung in relations with a culture that is several steps up the evolutionary ladder. How do these patterns affect age as a principle of economic organization? More precisely, how do these factors affect the proportions of young and old in the population and in turn the allocation of people among economic activities? We know that prolonged survival of incapacitated individuals, young or old, is less likely in nomadic than in sedentary populations (Dunn 1968:224).

Egalitarian Societies

Egalitarian societies are the oldest, smallest, and technologically most simple societies in the human cultural experience. Subsistence in egalitarian societies commonly consists of hunting and foraging in demographically small nomadic bands of extended families that cluster together or split apart according to the seasonal availability of resources. For most of our existence on earth as *Homo sapiens,* we lived as hunter-gatherers. Contemporary examples include the Eskimo, the Kalahari !Kung, and the Tiwi of Australia. Some societies that practice rudimentary extensive horticulture (sometimes referred to as slash-and-burn or shifting agriculture) also manifest egalitarian social structures. Small semisedentary villages relocate approximately every five years to replenish the soil and take advantage of new sources of meat and vegetables. Examples include some tropical horticultural groups in the Amazon basin which combine hunting, fishing, and gathering with horticulture. Demographically, these small-scale horticultural societies are comparable

in many ways to foraging bands. Politically, semisedentary horticulturalists are egalitarian. Consensus arrived at without specialized political
roles is the hallmark of egalitarian societies (Leacock 1978:249).
Egalitarianism means that no individual or group has differential access to
resources—that is, no ranking or class stratification, and thus no potential
for control or monopolization of scarce resources. In these societies, the
egalitarian social structure ensures itself by rules of reciprocity and redistribution manifested by food sharing and resource management so that
all members of the group have equal access to available food. In times of
scarcity everyone goes without. To understand the role of age in the
economies of egalitarian societies, we must take these important definitional features into account.

I realize that to classify hunter-gatherers and horticulturalists together
in this way is somewhat unusual in anthropology. Suffice it to say that in
order to understand economic processes in different types of societies it is
necessary sometimes to group societies and cultures by some criteria
other than economic ones. Political organization (if defined independently of subsistence strategy) tends to reflect the allocation of resources and
overall demographic adjustment much better than does a categorization
according to technology. The use of political criteria to group cultures
also allows for the analysis of differences in economic processes in societies that are technologically alike but ecologically, and often demographically and politically, different. The Indians of the Northwest Coast
of North America are an example. The Kwakiutl are technologically
hunter-gatherers, but demographically they are large because of their
extremely abundant maritime environment. Politically they are by no
means egalitarian and are therefore not comparable to most small-scale
egalitarian hunter-gatherers. They look much more like ranked horticulturalists such as the Trobrianders, and therefore, for evolutionary
purposes, must be treated as such (Fried 1967).

An evolutionary framework requires a whole complex of interacting
elements that result in a cultural unit. Most anthropologists have treated
the Northwest Coast Indians either as unusual hunter-gatherers (Netting
1977) or as an aberrant exception, and have not attempted to deal with the
institutional, ecological, and technological variables that make them understandable in a comparative evolutionary framework. Because cultural
ecology has not coordinated technology with social and political structure, the Northwest Coast has remained an anomaly. Marcel Mauss
(1966) and later Abraham Rosman and Paula Rubel (1970, 1978), al-

though not focusing on ecological variables or on an evolutionary framework, noticed the similarities between Northwest Coast and Melanesian exchange systems. Rosman and Rubel have called these "potlatch" societies. An evolutionary framework can explain the similarities between Kwakiutl and Trobriand chiefs, including, perhaps, their age requirements. Because population size and its resource base figure so importantly in shaping the relationships between age and economic organization, a clear and precise evolutionary framework is particularly essential for our purposes.

Hunter-Gatherers

We find some contradictory or at least highly variable data on the life span of hunter-gatherers. Frederick Dunn tells us, for example, that by modern European or American standards, the life expectancies of hunter-gatherers are low, but they compare favorably with those of displaced hunter-gatherers, many subsistence agriculturalists, and poor urban peoples in the tropics (1968:224). Richard Lee reports that of 466 !Kung Bushmen in the Dobe area, no fewer than 46 (17 men and 29 women) were over 60 years old, a ratio that compares favorably with the percentage of elderly in industrialized populations (1968:37). Howell (1979:35) describes an 82-year-old man whose hunting days were long since over, but who still had the ability to walk long distances when the group moved and who could still collect much of his own food. This is an interesting statement for several reasons. It indicates the viability of an elderly man, and exemplifies the flexibility of the sexual division of labor. Older males take on the female task of food collecting. Lee further says that adolescents assume adult responsibility late in life; the young are not expected to provide food regularly for the group until they are married (between the ages of 15 and 20 for girls, five years later for boys); approximately 40 percent of the population in camps contribute little to the food supply.

Biesele and Howell (1981) present a somewhat different view of the contributions of the elderly in !Kung economy. They say that older men and women make up the core of a !Kung camp. Because of their long-term association with a particular waterhole, the old maintain steward-like control over water and food resources in a region. They are resource managers who control rights to *the* critical resource: water. The aged also are repositories of essential technical knowledge concerning seasonal fluctuations in local resources, animal behavior, and the like. The elderly pass on their accumulated knowledge as part of their stewardship of gathering areas and hunting grounds. Thus their status can be seen as directly related to their economic contribution. In order to exploit the Kalahari environment effectively with the technology at their disposal, the San need the elderly's detailed knowledge of plant and animal life (Biesele and Howell 1981:84).

Elderly !Kung engage in decision making, and senilicide is rare. Lee says: "Long after their productive years have passed, the old people are fed and cared for by their children and grandchildren. The blind, the senile, and the crippled are respected for the special ritual and technical skills they possess" (1968:36). Lee describes four elders at one waterhole who were totally or partially blind. Apparently this handicap did not prevent their active participation in decision making and ritual curing. The !Kung allocate work to young and middle-aged adults; children, adolescents, and the elderly lead a life of leisure (Lee 1968:36). Patricia Draper (1976:216) says that for both ecological and technological reasons, !Kung food-getters must be grown adults. They must be old enough to be sufficiently knowledgeable about the locations of the various plants and animals, but not too young or old to walk 16 kilometers or more a day, often while carrying at least one child in addition to the harvest.

In a later volume Lee (1979:263) presents some interesting and problematic patterns of age and productive effort. He arranges 28 Dobe adults into three age categories, old (60+), middle-aged (40–59), and young (20–39), and says that work effort declines with age, from 38 percent workdays for the young to 29 percent for the old. Lee also says that overall the men work harder than the women in all age groups. The middle-aged men work the hardest, with young and old men contributing equally. The hardest workers among the women are the young, and the work effort declines much more dramatically with age. The problems, I think, derive from several points. First, Lee's definition of workday is confined to "a day in which one person collected food for the camp or a day in which one man went hunting." By restricting production to hunting and gathering, Lee excludes the tasks of getting water and preparing food, both time-consuming activities performed almost exclusively by women. Water procurement becomes more difficult as the dry season progresses, and groups must travel greater distances from the waterholes to gather food (Draper 1975). Lee's data on age also reveal a key point about the division of labor by sex. As the area around the permanent waterholes becomes hunted out, in order for men to be working so consistently they must be engaging in women's work (Halperin 1980)—that is, in gathering, an activity much easier to perform when a man is either a young and inexperienced hunter or too old and debilitated to hunt (see also Biesele and Howell 1981).

The subject of food taboos in relation to age is extremely interesting, for age significantly affects consumption patterns. For the !Kung, food taboos apply to younger people in the various stages of reproductive life. These taboos are often relaxed at the cessation of childbearing. The prohibition on the consumption of ostrich eggs is a case in point. The eggs are reserved for the very young and the very old, and are prohibited to people of both sexes who are actively engaged in reproduction. The belief system says that ostrich eggs make reproductively active people crazy if they eat them; older people are said to be past the danger of having their minds affected by the rich food (Biesele and Howell 1981:90). An alternative explanation may be that since eggs are soft food, they may be reserved for people who have difficulty chewing hard food, especially when grinding monongo nuts with mortar and pestle may be inconvenient—in short, the very young and the elderly.

The abundant environment of the Australian Tiwi hunter-gatherers is another case in which viable producers are relieved from active production roles. All males between the ages of 14 and 25 absent themselves from food-production units for long periods of the year. After the age of 20 the young men do contribute to household food production, but C. W. M. Hart and Arnold Pilling point out that "only a very well-off tribe could afford to allow so much time off from food production to all its young hunters" (1960:95). Since Tiwi women contribute substantially to subsistence from a very young age, doing the great bulk of the food-getting (Goodale 1971:38–39, 169), the division of labor by sex, created in large part by matrilineal kinship, early bethrothal, and polygyny, combined with the abundant maritime environment, permits the leisure not only of male youths, but of males in general. Were the Tiwi living in the Arctic, the leisure of young male producers would be out of the question, at least for most periods of the year.

Complementing the Tiwi data is a study by F. G. G. Rose (1960) of the Groote Eylandt aborigines of northern Australia, a maritime food-collecting group that "almost always [had] meat (protein) of sea origin" (1960:82). Here the distribution of the food was carried out primarily by older men. Arguing that polygyny is an economic necessity, Rose shows (1960:87) that the incidence of polygyny among women varies considerably with age. He has suggested that rates of polygyny are high for women in their childbearing years because the demands on women are greatest at this point in the life course. Rose also argues that monogamously married women tend to die out sooner because women have difficulty supporting themselves without the help of cowives. While his data are extremely limited, his ideas merit testing with the use of diachronic and cross-cultural data.

The Eskimo represent a famous situation opposite that of the !Kung and the Tiwi. E. Adamson Hoebel has argued that senilicide was general among the Eskimos because they were unable to sustain the old in times of stress (1954:76–79). Citing numerous anecdotes illustrating requests for death from old people, Hoebel states that senilicide, invalidicide, and suicide are manifestations of the same postulate that underlies infanticide: a harsh life with a small margin of safety. People who cannot contribute their full share to productive activities forfeit the right to live (1954:76).

The Eskimo and the !Kung Bushmen undoubtedly represent two extremes of scarcity and abundance among hunter-gatherers. In abundant environments the data describing the relatively small contributions of the very young and very old may be more of a testimony to the bountifulness of the habitat than a statement about age as a variable in the subsistence strategies of hunting and gathering societies. Such extreme differences do raise questions about the relationships among seasonal resource fluctuations, overall adaptive strategies, and the variability of roles for young and old in egalitarian societies. If we combine these data with our knowledge that, in general, malnutrition (patent and perhaps even borderline) is rare in well-adapted hunter-gatherer populations because of diverse dietary resources, the Eskimo are indeed atypical.

In sum, the role of age in egalitarian hunting and gathering societies is more a function of resources available than of any other variable. Whereas ecology does not seem to affect the overall egalitarian division of labor by sex among hunter-gatherers, environmental scarcity or abundance does limit the number of nonproducing consumers, young and old, a society can afford, in both the long and the short run.

Egalitarian Horticulturalists

Egalitarian horticultural societies consist of small village populations. Many, such as those in the Amazon basin, are semisedentary populations living in villages that relocate every five or six years. The Cashinahua of lowland South America are one example (Kensinger 1975). Young or newly settled villages may coexist in a single culture with older, more mature ones with full-blown gardens near the end of their productive cycle. New villages require a great deal of energy to clear and plant the new gardens as well as to maintain a viable level of subsistence in the village by hunting and gathering until the gardens have begun to produce. Once the gardens have come into production, gathering subsides. The longer a group stays in an area, the more uncertain hunting becomes. At the other end of the village life cycle, resources may be hunted and gathered out and the soil less productive. Thus just before the village moves the population may be so nutritionally stressed that mortality rates rise. As different subsistence activities become more or less prominent, the division of labor will change.

The division of labor by sex changes as males and females age. For both males and females, age may reverse traditional economic roles as they are defined by sex. For example, the Mundurucú of the Brazilian Amazon basin have different expectations of women at different points in the life course. During childbearing years, women are supposed to be basically passive in almost all domains. Retiring and demure behavior is the norm; male company is not sought, and men and women occupy separate physical and social domains. By contrast, postmenopausal women can sit anywhere, with men or with women, and men will defer to an older woman by making room for her. Older women may also speak freely and with credence and authority that may influence people's behavior (Murphy and Murphy 1974:105–6).

A comparable case is that of the Machiguenga, a horticultural group in southeastern Peru. Orna and Allen Johnson's (1975) analysis of male–female relations and the organization of work among the Machiguenga is interesting not because they pay any explicit attention to age as a variable in the division of labor, but rather for the questions about age and economic organization which can be derived from their careful and detailed analysis of the division of labor by sex. Like the Mundurucú and many other lowland South American groups, the Machiguenga derive their subsistence from slash-and-burn agriculture combined with hunting and collecting.

Among the Machiguenga, men's work is far more physically demanding than women's work. Men work long, strenuous hours in gardens and at other tasks, with few interruptions. Men expend an average of 3.3 calories per minute in manufacturing activity and 4.5 calories per minute in garden labor; women expend an average of 1.6 calories per minute (Johnson and Johnson 1975:643). One obvious question, of course, is how many hours, on the average, do men and women work?

If these data are indeed accurate (and I suggest that the energy requirements of gathering have perhaps been underestimated), then the question is: What is the relationship between age and an individual's productive life in this society? When can a man no longer hunt? Do men work fewer years than women? Do men die younger? Do men at some point take on women's tasks? Do they switch from producers to distributors and finally exclusively to consumers? To what degree does the physical nature of the work task impose limitations on people in different stages of their life courses? These questions have been asked most often in regard to women of childbearing age. We know, for example, that cultures deal very differently with the same biological processes when it comes to allocating work tasks around reproduction. How flexible can cultures be when it comes to the division of labor by age? Does the biology of aging impose some of the same kinds of limitations on work in all cultures or do cultures vary just as much in their ways of allocating work to the elderly, for example, as they do in allocating work to childbearers?

Dorothy Hammond and Alta Jablow (1976) address some of these issues in small-scale kin-based societies and imply that it may be easier for elderly women to maintain productive work in the domestic sphere than it is for elderly men to work in the public sphere. While women may not expend as many calories per minute as men, their work in many societies begins at a younger age and lasts well into old age. Women's economic life centers on the household and is intimately bound up with the work of other women. Only extreme disability or death ends a woman's working life.

> An industrious and clever girl is undoubtedly a credit to her own kinsfolk, especially her mother, and she will be an asset to her husband. In her own household she will go on using those skills she learned as a girl. With the passage of time she may delegate some of the tasks to growing daughters and daughters-in-law, and eventually even to granddaughters. As an older woman she may thus be relieved of the more arduous work, but she is never completely idle. Whatever work the old woman does is important to her self-esteem. Her self-image demands that she continue as a productive member of the community as long as she can.   [Hammond and Jablow 1976:66–68]

This passage raises the issue of whether the inherent flexibility of work in the domestic sphere contributes to the longevity of women. With sedentary life comes a marked distinction between public and domestic domains in the lives of men and women.[1] Without making assumptions either about the exclusivity of these domains for the sexes or about the ranking of the domains on a single prestige scale, we can ponder the implications of the public/domestic dichotomy for the division of labor by age. Women begin their domestic work lives earlier and continue their productive tasks until their deaths. Does this arrangement contribute to the longevity of women, or does it shorten their lives? We need more research that examines changes in the productive roles of women and men when they are isolated from both older and younger generations, that is, when there is neither anyone from whom to learn nor anyone to whom tasks can be delegated.

The function of age as a variable in horticultural societies depends greatly on the unit or units of production. In egalitarian horticultural societies such as those in the Amazon basin, the household is the fundamental unit of production and consumption; households are composed of several extended families and are also primary units of distribution. Within households senior women coordinate the work of groups of female kin (Murphy and Murphy 1974:132). Young women, functioning primarily in the domestic sphere, begin to contribute to the economy much earlier than do boys. Seven-year-old girls will monitor one-year-old siblings. While similar patterns of older and younger sibling relationships are found among hunter-gatherers, it is difficult to conceive of a seven-year-old carrying a one-year-old for long gathering expeditions. Male Mundurucú children begin small-scale hunting around the age of 10. Adult hunting begins at age 14 (Murphy and Murphy 1974:75). The sedentary base seems to provide the young and the old much more opportunity to contribute to the economy. Perhaps this finding can be attributed to the population's short life span. Murphy and Murphy note that grandparents take care of children ''if they are still alive'' (1974:173).

Warfare may play a significant part in fixing the age ratios of a horticultural population. While Steven Polgar (1972:206) estimates that warfare seldom kills more than 10 percent of men of reproductive age, Napoleon Chagnon studied one Yanomamo village in which nearly 50 percent of the men were killed in war (Chagnon 1974). As populations

1. For a discussion of the domestic public dichotomy, see Rosaldo 1974 and Sanday 1974.

grow larger and denser, they become increasingly subject to infectious diseases, many of which, such as malaria and tuberculosis, may not in and of themselves be life-threatening, but which, when combined with other conditions such as malnutrition, can cause early death. All of these factors point to a shorter life span for many horticultural peoples than for hunter-gatherers, and thus perhaps the necessity of beginning one's economic life at an early age.

To summarize, the sedentary life of egalitarian horticulturalists has a greater effect on the division of labor by age than on the division of labor by sex. The sexual division of labor looks very much like that of hunter-gatherers, but the age division is quite different. People in sedentary economies begin work at a much earlier age and they remain working much longer.

Ranked Horticultural Societies

It is more difficult to generalize about age as a variable in the economies of larger, more complex, ranked horticultural societies such as the Trobriand Islanders and the Tikopia. Ethnographic emphasis on kinship has excluded age from consideration. African age systems are often described in terms of their contributions to ritual, not their role in subsistence activities (Gulliver 1965). This neglect raises an important issue for the study of primitive economies: the function of age in the relationship between ceremonial and ordinary exchange in societies at the tribal and chiefdom levels. By ceremonial exchange I mean exchanges that either take place in a religious context or function primarily to enhance power and prestige, not subsistence. By ordinary exchange I mean exchanges that occur outside of strictly ritual contexts and are oriented toward everyday subsistence needs. Obviously, in empirical reality, these two types of exchange overlap, and one is often accompanied by the other. Exchange of Kula valuables in the Trobriands, for example, is usually associated with the exchange of foodstuffs. The prominence of ceremonial exchange, especially in societies at the chiefdom level, suggests a rethinking of the function of age in the economy. How old does one have to be to function effectively as a big man, for example? Can a young chief marshal more resources by virtue of this kinship rank than a young big man whose kinship status may carry him less far toward his goals? Douglas Oliver says that Siuai men of Melanesia gain wealth and renown because of what they do beyond subsistence, not because of their vitality, economic solidity, general knowledge, or age (1955:73). Insofar as it may take time to marshal sufficient resources to engage in activities beyond subsistence, older men certainly have an advantage. Oliver describes a kind of reciprocity between young and old:

> While age by itself does not command great respect in Siuai, the offspring are usually tenderly affectionate toward aging parents, demonstrating by word and deed that they feel an obligation for their welfare. If the parents occupy the same hamlet or neighboring hamlets, the son or daughter will oft times perform much of the work of clearing and cultivating their parents' garden. Or, if they live too far apart for that, they usually take along baskets of food when they return for visits. As it is explained: "When we were children they fed and cared for us well; and now that they are aged we repay by giving food to them. For, if we did not, they would surely starve." [Oliver 1955:209]

Among the Siuai there is clearly a high correlation between age and high rank as an active feast giver and leader. Highest ranking leaders had been involved in competitive feasting for some 25 years previously (Oliver 1955:390). Young leaders start out with substantial support from kin.

A comparable ranked society is that of the Coast Salish of the Northwest Coast of the United States, and a similar pattern of kin support for leaders who grow powerful with age can be found. In the precontact period, all political and economic leadership was in the hands of the old. In order to become a powerful elder, however, a person had to have seniority in a large, wealthy family (Amoss 1981:33). Coast Salish adults were named teknonymously, suggesting that generational position defined the most important roles (Amoss 1981:230). Generational position combined with high kinship rank creates the prerequisites for leaders who can engage in the elaborate redistributive feasts (potlatches) for which many groups on the Northwest Coast are famous.

The Trobriand Islanders, with their highly elaborate kinship and exchange systems and their rich and mixed agricultural/maritime ecological base (see Malinowski 1978, Uberoi 1962, Weiner 1976), are a third case of ranked horticulturalists. Annette Weiner has written an entire book on the life cycle of the Trobriands from the point of view of ritual and exchange. Focusing on exchanges of male and female wealth within a life-course framework, she says that Trobriand exchange operates through transformations during specific phases in a life cycle (1976:19). For the Trobrianders, age also seems to be a variable that is embedded in the kinship structure. Malinowski maintains, for example, that "the structure of the sub-clan is also modified by the principle of seniority, that is age and superiority of generation give a man greater importance and a higher status within his sub-clan. . . . The various groups recognize with regard to each other a relative seniority. Thus, one of them is regarded as the eldest, that is, the most important" (1978:345–46). Age in the form of relative seniority serves to rank kinship groups and to determine the economic roles of people within the clans.

Trobriand women's economic roles take a somewhat different trajectory through the life course, and these roles are complicated by the matrilineal kinship system. Before marriage a girl works on her father's soil to produce goods for her parent's household and her father's sister's household. When she marries she will share her husband's garden and consume from her parents and her paternal aunt. Her own soil is held by her mother's brother; it will be inherited by her brother and he will provide for her as well.

The work tasks of Trobriand men also change through the life course, but again within the framework of kinship. While the gardening team retains a core of permanent workers, its composition changes over time. Young boys cultivate with the garden team for a period of time, but when they mature they return to their maternal communities. They are replaced by young men of the local descent group, who return from their villages of birth (father's villages) to join their maternal uncles and their subclan. The cycle continues as these men marry women from alien subclans (Malinowski 1978:357).

In sum, the function of age in ranked horticultural economies contrasts greatly with the patterns seen among egalitarian horticulturalists. Whereas age and kinship statuses complement one another in egalitarian societies, with age possibly superseding kinship, in ranked societies age is always in some way, if not subordinate to, embedded in the kinship system.

The question of the function of age as a variable in horticultural and pastoral societies with age-grade systems is one that is in great need of further study. Since age-grade systems and unilineal descent systems tend to exist simultaneously (Ritter 1980), we may inquire into the relative functions of age and kinship in the allocation of economic roles to individuals and to groups. Are age grades, for example, categories of producers, or categories of productive activities? Do the variables of age and kinship complement and crosscut one another? Or do age and kinship function in different domains of the culture? Which casts a wider net of relationships, age or kinship, and what bearing does the network have on economic life? Does one's kinship status function differently at different points of the life course?

Evans-Pritchard contends that age is expressed in a kinship idiom (1940:258). Gulliver says that among the Jie, "Although the age group is only a weak corporate group . . . nevertheless bonds of friendly equality between members of a group cut across the parochialism of clan and settlement to provide a wider network of personal links than kinship and neighborhood afford" (1965:186). The question is: How important are these age-based links for economic activity? Do they operate to facilitate productive activities, as through labor exchanges? Are age connections part of the structure of distribution networks? The relationship between labor division by age and that by sex in age-grade societies remains, to my knowledge, unexplored.

State Systems, Peasants, and Proletarians

At the state level, age functions very differently in economic organization than it does in kin-based egalitarian or ranked societies. With the development of class stratification systems based on private property, age becomes a dependent variable, subordinate to class in the structuring of economic processes. The higher a person's social class, the greater his or her longevity. In most instances longevity is inversely related to a person's actual contribution to subsistence. That is, the greater one's ability to extract a surplus from subordinates, the longer one lives. Class becomes the independent variable for dividing labor in state-level societies. Again, age affects production processes differentially, depending on the units of production and the political and economic contexts within which the units function.

If the household is the dominant unit of production and work is primarily organized by the household for the benefit of its members, the age composition of the household can greatly affect production processes. The Russian economist A. V. Chayanov, in his book *The Theory of Peasant Economy* (1966), addressed the problem of age as a variable in the household economy that he called the family farm, a subsistence unit without wage labor. For Chayanov household life cycles were critical determinants of production processes. The labor product, or amount produced, is not the same for all family economic units, but varies according to a number of factors, among them family size and composition. Age is an important variable because the number of workers in a household depends primarily on the ages and life-cycle stages of the family members. As the age ratios change in a family, so does the labor product: dependent children and elderly members contribute more and less, respectively, over time.

In what is probably one of the most sensitive descriptions of age as a variable in a rural agrarian economy, Conrad Arensberg, in *The Irish Countryman* (1968), reaffirms Chayanov's analysis of the family as a subsistence production unit. Both children and the elderly contribute to the subsistence base, the former as performers of small tasks such as errand running and child minding, the latter as managers and decision makers. Young and middle-aged adults perform the heavy physical work under the aegis of older men and women. As long as a married man's father is present in his household, that man is a "boy" who is economically subservient to his father. Thus even a 45-year-old married man may not be an economically viable adult in the Irish peasant social structure. Similarly, women in this patrilocal system are under the wing of a mother-in-law. This arrangement has its benefits for example, providing help with child care and relief from many responsibilities during pregnancy—but it also has its emotional costs. Theoretically, this is an interesting system. It provides a role for the elderly while at the same time providing much-needed help for young adults (see also Streib 1972).

The leisure time of hunter-gatherers is something peasants cannot afford. Rural agrarian economies in state systems are subject to many outside demands. The pressure to bring products to market on a certain day and the vagaries of the market-determined pricing system are only two such pressures. A great deal of labor is required to meet these demands, and it must be recruited from all available sources. It is not surprising that children are taken out of school to help with the harvest. Whereas hunter-gatherers can subsist without the labor of the very young and the very old, the primary peasant producers, young and middle-aged adults, need all the help they can get to produce their subsistence, distribute the products effectively, and reproduce the labor force. The help comes from children and the elderly. The Irish family farm is a well-functioning system that is a viable adaptation to the larger political and economic context in which it must operate.

Judith Friedlander's (1976) description of the multiple economic roles of a 65-year-old grandmother and head of a household in Hueyapan, Mexico, raises another set of questions regarding age and the division of labor in peasant households and villages. As a small landowner, subsistence agriculturalist, market woman, and *curandera*, Doña Zeferina plays a variety of social and economic roles. These roles are public but not political. Her work contrasts greatly with that of her 32-year-old daughter-in-law, whose work is entirely in the domestic sphere, that is, primarily child care and food preparation. How typical is Doña Zeferina, her household, and its division of labor by age? While large-scale statistical data are missing for this particular village, the Hueyapan case, in which childbearing women perform domestic work and older women play economic roles outside of the domestic domain, is not at all atypical.

Whether or not age ratios within households influence the conditions under which members of peasant households allocate work to domestic or public domains would be worthy of systematic research. The relationship between reproductive patterns and work outside the domestic sphere also merits further exploration. We know that many peasant women work in public spheres during their childbearing years, but the conditions under which they are able to do so are not known. Household life cycles and the needs of households at particular stages are likely to be significant determinants of how old the major producers or income earners will be.

Peasant villages have a great variety of mechanisms for providing for the economic viability of household consumption units. Dianne Kagan (1980:71) documents the "loaning" of grandchildren to their grandparents in a Colombian peasant village. By providing labor and social support for their households, the children keep the old people independent. The arrangement also provides subsistence relief for the grandchild's nuclear family. With one less mouth to feed, the other children will receive better nourishment. This arrangement presumes, however, that the labor of the child on loan is, at least temporarily, not needed in the nuclear household and acts to redistribute labor in the village. Neighborhood ties may also function to ensure the maintenance of the elderly as long as a reasonable exchange of services can be arranged. Such arrangements seem to be particularly common among women. Kagan describes a woman with four children in Bojacá who took an elderly neighbor, with whom no kin ties were shared, into her household to help her with her work (1980:71).

In virtually all rural agrarian villages in the Third World, households must have access to cash. In general, young men and women provide much of it, often having to leave the village and become wage laborers to do so. Older peasant women have few marketable skills, and when they are no longer strong enough to be traders or wage workers, they provide child-care services that enable their daughters to take paid employment. Interestingly though, it is not uncommon for older women to maintain their adult daughters when the daughters are periodically—often seasonally—unemployed. This is the case for Doña Zeferina, who, in addition to controlling land resources, has special marketable skills as a *curandera* (Friedlander 1976). Under certain conditions, older men may be able to maintain a cash income longer than their female counterparts, either by calling on the labor of younger clients who have become indebted to them or by calling on the support of peers. In the Caribbean, for example, men of all ages and classes tend to associate in peer groups, which by definition are composed of age mates. Caribbean crews arc both work groups and units of sociability (Wilson 1969, 1971). Peasant women, on the other hand, if they stay in their natal villages, may have greater access to subsistence goods through kin networks as well as to a sporadic cash income earned through wages or through the sale of small items in the village (Rothstein 1979:256).

In peasant economies in which the household is the smallest of several productive units and in which wage labor is predominant, age as a variable operates differently than it does in household-based subsistence economies. When young adults, particularly women, leave their extended family support systems behind in villages to seek work in towns and cities, their economic as well as their social viability may be compromised by the absence of younger or elderly women to provide child care. The dependent and often exploitive relationships created between spouses and the inaccessibility of the family farm, to use Chayanov's term, as a source of subsistence goods and reserve labor may also present severe hardships for recent migrants.

In somewhat extreme though not at all unrealistic or uncommon terms, Anna Rubbo (1975) describes the plight of poor women of childbearing age once they give up subsistence production in rural villages to become wage workers on commercial plantations in a Colombian frontier town. Among other things, Rubbo describes a society that has become age-segregated to meet the exigencies of agrarian capitalism. Since teenagers and elderly individuals are left behind in the rural villages, young adults must cope with small children in the towns without traditional economic and social supports. Concomitantly the village economy is undermined as more and more productive adults leave the rural areas.

Considerable research has been devoted in recent years to the peasant-to-worker transition in rural agrarian economies, and this research raises some interesting issues regarding age and economic change (Minge-Kalman 1978, Holmes 1982). Among these issues are those of work loads for older adults whose children have left the village for educational or economic reasons and are not available to work. John Cole and Phillip Katz (1973) have described a peasant-to-worker transition strategy based on child labor. When households are under economic stress, children are sent as migrant laborers. They describe groups of children from South Tyrol who appeared in the *Kindermarkt* of South Germany, where they were known to be auctioned off for a summer's work. Their earnings were negligible but their absence meant one less mouth to feed (1973: 50).

Processes of colonialism, modernization, development, and general incorporation into the world economy have many ramifications that differentially affect age groups. As manufactured goods begin to replace traditional craft items, for example, not only are whole occupations eliminated, but apprenticeship relationships that provide important roles for the elderly and that were common in precolonial periods also become extinct. In much of Africa and Latin America, traditional weaving is no longer done by either men or women. Among teenage Ben'ekie boys in Zaire, idleness and unemployment replace weaving apprenticeships (Fairley 1981). The occupational status of the older people to whom the young men traditionally would have been apprenticed is lowered. My own fieldwork in the West Indies shows a similar pattern. Few job opportunities exist, especially for male teenagers of the lower classes. While girls and women can usually work in the markets or in the domestic domain, teenage boys, since they have not attained full adult status but are no longer dependent children, have few economic opportunities. In Grenada, older teenage boys may be employed as shop tenders, but such jobs often require minimal literacy and transportation to the capital. Even if these conditions can be met, the jobs are extremely scarce. Expectations of upward mobility increase daily as radio communications and, in many parts of Latin America, television sets appear in barrio dwellings. As peasant villages come increasingly into contact with modern industrial societies and traditional age and sex statuses are undermined, male teenagers change from important subsistence producers into often frustrated consumers—frustrated because, unlike their female counterparts, they have few sources of income other than those that are illegal.

Patron-Client Relations

One of the institutions that most commonly organizes reciprocity within peasant societies is that of patronage or patron-client relations. While patronage and clientage are primarily based on differences of social class, one can also ask how, if at all, age functions as a factor in the development of patronage relations. Patron-client relations involve exchanges of goods and services between people whose roles represent fundamentally different class positions. By definition, a patron is someone of higher means if not higher social class than the client (Wolf 1966a, 1966b).

There is probably an age limit below which one cannot become an effective patron and above which one can no longer function as one. The determinants of the upper and lower age limits of patronage vary from culture to culture, depending on a whole series of variables, ranging from the amount of physical labor that is required to the amount of time it takes to acquire political and economic connections at the regional and state levels.

The dynamics of patron-client relations seem to be based on several factors, among them changes in the role of a patron during the patron's life span. Such changes may involve, for example, the accumulation of more and more clients or alterations in the patron's relationship to production processes. Over time patrons may accumulate such productive resources as land and increased means of communication and transportation, such as vehicles. As the patron controls more resources, he or she potentially can control more people. Does patronage depend on age? We know that there is a class component to patronage, but is there an age component? Are patrons always older than clients? Or always younger? Is there an age gap or differential?

In the West Indies as lower-class individuals grow older they do not accumulate productive resources of any significance; they do, however, accumulate clients in the form of loyal friends and followers who can be called upon to perform various tasks, and who in turn can receive credit from both male and female patrons. With age, female fish vendors, for example, expand their support systems from kin and peers to younger women in the community, who take turns marketing fish and sharing the profits with the older (head) vendor (Halperin 1972). Male patrons also gain clients as they age, but in different ways. Since their activities are concerned more with the public political sphere than with the domestic subsistence domain, they tend to collect clients for votes as well as for support at higher levels of state organization. This is true in Mexico as well (Halperin 1975). Some people move up the local or even the national stratification system with age.

Cargo Systems, Age, and Forms of Ceremonial Exchange in Peasant Villages

Cargos, civil-religious hierarchies common in Mesoamerican Indian societies, are organized in a ladder-like arrangement. A man first occupies a position low in the hierarchy and proceeds to move up to increasingly more expensive and more prestigious positions. The timing of a person's career is critical. As a man ages, his position in the hierarchy changes. Late entrance into the system can prevent mobility within it.

Probably one of the most complete descriptions of a *cargo* system, and one that includes age as a variable, is Frank Cancian's account of Zinacantan (1965), and I will draw upon it extensively here. Zinacantan is a township of 7,650 Tzotzil-speaking Maya Indians in the highlands of the state of Chiapas, in southeastern Mexico. Zinacantecos are primarily corn farmers who buy and sell corn as well as beans, chili peppers, flowers, and other cash crops in exchange for cotton for weaving clothes, metal tools, and other staples in the ladino city of San Cristóbal. The occupation of a religious office requires individuals to spend often large amounts of money to sponsor religious celebrations in honor of deities associated with Catholic saints. An incumbent receives no pay because his work is regarded as service to the community. The work of the civil government incumbents principally concerns such public works as the building and repair of roads and schools, the administration of justice, the settlement of disputes, and the management of relationships between the community and the larger outside world of the nation-state of Mexico.

Cancian states clearly that Zinacantan is not a typical civil-religious hierarchy in which an individual alternates between civil and religious offices, serving in one capacity or another for a year and then giving the office to another man. The *cargo* system is almost entirely religious; civil offices are filled by different recruitment mechanisms. There are 34 religious *cargos* at the lowest level, 12 offices at the second level, 6 at the third, and 2 on the fourth and final level of the religious hierarchy. Thus the system becomes increasingly selective at higher levels. The highest offices represent the apex of the social structure; only those who are rich can afford the most expensive *cargos*. In Zinacantan none of the civil offices counts for progress up the ladder of religious *cargos* (Cancian 1965:22). It is interesting also that a high civil office can be held by someone who is relatively young and unimportant. Cancian says that it is not uncommon to have a *presidente* in his late twenties; of the six *presidentes* who served between 1952 and 1963, four were younger than 30 when they entered office (1965:25). The system of recruitment for religious offices is entirely different and age is extremely important; men under 30 never hold high religious offices.

Cancian has performed some very interesting analyses of age and the *cargo* system, including the formulation of models that help to predict the age and conditions under which *cargos* are taken. In one model it is postulated that at least 90 percent of men take *cargos*. Since life expectancy in Zinacantan is relatively short and a person must take the *cargos* in hierarchial order, a delay of the first cargo until age 45, for example, will in all likelihood prevent a person from ever reaching the highest level (1965:168). A second model postulates a constant age at the first *cargo* and analyzes the results. Since the population of Zinacantan is increasing, under the second model's conditions the proportion of men who never take a first *cargo* will increase (1965:169). Cancian's analysis is one of the few to use age as a condition in a formal economic model. Cancian uses the model to compare postulated conditions with actual conditions, and his analysis is quite effective. Such formal models that include age as a component could add greatly to the precision as well as the time depth of economic analyses. The models would provide ways of systematizing the data by comparing expected conditions with observable facts.

Conclusion

Age has attracted little attention in the comparative study of economic processes. Aside from general assumptions about and references to age as one of the two basic principles (along with sex) that allocate labor in primitive societies, little systematic work has been done on age as a variable in economic analyses (Simmons 1945).

I have used an evolutionary framework to develop a consistent set of factors that can be used to define the political and demographic contexts for understanding age as a variable in the cross-cultural analysis of economic processes. I have emphasized production processes because, somewhat ironically, the ethnographic record seems to contain more data on the relationship between age and production processes than any other economic factor. The irony is that economic anthropology, as a whole, has until recently emphasized distribution processes to the exclusion of production. A focus on age draws from the ethnographic record data that have heretofore been ignored, and it has been possible to raise several theoretical issues concerning both production and distribution processes.

At the most general level, we can say that the relationship between age and economic processes is basically similar among all kin-based societies, both egalitarian and ranked. Property-based, stratified societies begin to manifest different patterns and relationships, depending on the context within which the units of production and consumption are found. Within these general evolutionary types some further distinctions can be made. Insofar as egalitarian societies encompass a variety of technologies and therefore various modes of adapting to their environments, age affects economic processes differently for egalitarian hunter-gatherers than it does for egalitarian horticulturalists. Among hunter-gatherers, abundant environments seem to exempt both the very young and the very old from productive activities and seem to permit a considerable amount of leisure time for people of all ages. Thus Marshall Sahlins' notion of "the original affluent society" (1972). It should be clear, however, that "affluence" as it is manifested by leisure is a result of several interrelated variables: abundant environments, egalitarian social organization, flexible divison of labor by sex, and simple technology. None of these variables, singly or even in pairs, would bring about affluence or leisure. In harsher environments, such as those inhabited by the polar Eskimo, the luxury of idelness is much less affordable and the elderly not only must be able to move with the group, a *sine qua non* in all hunting-gathering societies, they also must not be a burden to those younger. Thus the !Kung and the Tiwi can afford to support elders who are blind or crippled, but the Eskimo cannot. In the Tiwi case the marriage system and the division of labor by sex affects the division of labor by age by allowing both elderly and young men to be idle. At the hunter-gatherer level, some sex-role reversal also occurs with age, as in the case of elderly !Kung men who take on the female tasks of gathering.

Members of both egalitarian and ranked horticultural societies begin working at a much earlier age than hunter-gatherers and maintain production for most of their lives. This is particularly true of women. Girls in a sedentary society can care for young children without having to carry them on long gathering expeditions. As weaning foods are plentiful, children nurse for shorter periods of time and therefore also can be away from their mothers at a much younger age.

Aging seems to reverse the traditional sexual division of labor in a much more accentuated fashion in horticultural societies than at the hunter-gatherer level. In such societies both men and women can take on the productive and the distributive roles of the opposite sex. Judith Brown (1982) has argued that, cross-culturally, middle age lifts restrictions from women and confers on them the right to exert authority over certain kinsmen. She also notes the importance of older women in food distribution and in the supervision of food preparation (1982:154).

Brown's last point about food distribution raises an interesting theoretical issue for cultural economics. If productive processes are affected by age in a manner that includes sex-role reversal, are distribution processes so affected? In horticultural societies in which men are the primary distributors and women are the primary producers of both ritual and subsistence goods, for example, do older women become distributors? The work of Andrew Strathern (1971) and Marilyn Strathern (1972) on Melanesian exchange immediately comes to mind. The potlatch is another example. I hypothesize that sex-role reversal with age is much more flexible and possible in production processes than in distribution processes, especially at the chiefdom level. Since kinship principles are so prominent in these societies, such variables as the form of lineality might be worth testing with respect to the flexibility of the age and sex division of labor. Iroquois women tend to be powerful in all economic processes at all ages (Brown 1975). Within specific domains the same can be said of the Trobrianders (Weiner 1976).

In kin-based societies the lack of specialization in the divison of labor overall seems to enable people of all ages to match their skills and abilities with the various necessary tasks involved in the annual round. All men and all women are food producers and, to varying degrees, food distributors. Interestingly, the separation of producers from distributors occurs earlier in human cultural evolution than does the separation of producers and nonproducers. Age and sex statuses act to create these differences before class distinctions ever develop. The skills a young boy performs before puberty may be the very ones he needs in old age. Work groups in kin-based societies are often heterogeneous in age. Older and younger men and women commonly work together. Mat weaving, for example, in Samoa involves women of all ages; fishing brings together old and young men (Holmes 1972:75). Fishing brings together the old and young Eskimo of both sexes. Such arrangements in preindustrial societies make it possible to learn new skills and to change qualitatively the nature of one's work as one proceeds through the life course. In highly specialized postindustrial societies such qualitative changes cannot be accomplished easily. Once a person is unable to work at a specialized task, work must cease altogether. This is one of the many reasons that the elderly become isolated from production processes in industrial societies.[2] It is important to recognize, however, that the elderly in preindustrial societies are not more respected because of their revered position in the extended family. Rather, the basic interdependent and flexible nature of the division of labor, what Durkheim called organic solidarity, makes it possible for both young and old to function in the economies of preindustrial societies.

State-level societies present different issues surrounding age and economic organization. Probably the two most critical, and often related, factors impinging on age and economic organization are the class position of the individual and the unit of production within which individuals work. Modernization processes have greatly affected the economic activities of people of all ages, some positively, many negatively (Cowgill and Holmes, eds., 1972). Indigenous peasant agriculturalists in closed-corporate peasant communities (Wolf 1966b) operate in ways that are similar to those of horticulturalists in stateless kin-based societies. Links to larger political and economic entities through relations of patronage and brokerage create different economic functions for old and young. Once young men from tribal and peasant societies leave their indigenous groups and acquire wealth by using channels outside the traditional system, patterns of kin-based seniority become undermined and in some cases destroyed. We know that the shift from subsistence production to wage labor creates many stresses for children, young adults, and elderly members of extended families. For the elderly, subsistence patterns become diluted by the removal of young adult laborers. For children and

2. There is now a substantial literature on the economics of aging by economists. While the analyses are very interesting, they do not consider a great many variables; instead they focus on such conventional economic categories as labor supply, savings, investment, and income distribution. This literature also is restricted almost exclusively to industrial societies on the macro level, with brief mention of the underdeveloped world (Olson et al. 1981, Clark and Spengler 1980).

young adults, the absence of extended-family members when they move to areas where wage labor is available creates serious shortages of child carers and general social and economic support.

Some very basic questions are raised by an examination of age and economic organization, including the nature of reciprocity as a principle organizing production and exchange. Economic anthropologists generally agree that reciprocity is a dominant principle in nonmarket economies. If reciprocal exchange relationships, including trading partnerships, are defined as relationships between two equals, however, we can certainly inquire into the impact of age on reciprocal economic relationships. Can two individuals of radically different ages engage in reciprocal exchange, and if so, how equal is the exhange? What happens to the nature of reciprocity as the parties age? How does the age of the reciprocal relationship itself affect the kinds of transactions involved? Most of the exchange theorists are silent on this issue (Mauss 1966, Sahlins 1972, Dupré and Rey 1973, Polanyi 1957). Obviously individuals often act as representatives of groups, and in such cases perhaps the ages of the individuals make little difference.

The issue of intergenerational economic relationships must be examined cross-culturally. While an ideology of reciprocity probably always prevails to some extent between generations, the facts of reciprocity may be quite different. In state-level societies with private property, the dynamics of intergenerational exchange (Salamon and Lockhart 1980) will be different from exchange processes in prestate societies, in which the elderly control knowledge but not privately held resources. While intergenerational exchanges of goods and services are important in all societies, once societies develop private property and resources are no longer controlled by kin groups, the importance of intergenerational exchange is altered.

There seems to be little question that in societies in which kin are the basic means of economic support, insurance in old age, and buffers against starvation and destitution, exchanges of goods and services among people of varying ages and life-cycle stages are absolutely essential for the viability of the group. Such societies encompass a range of evolutionary types. The importance of intergenerational exchanges as the key survival strategy is also heightened when the group is near the bottom of a class stratification system. A striking example is Carol Stack's (1974) description of reciprocal exchange networks among poor urban blacks. Old women in particular are critical to the maintenance of the network because they care for children and allow younger women to work. An interesting point here is that women seem to provide the core of the network. Men operate in peer groups (Liebow 1967) in which certain kinds of reciprocal exchanges take place, but because men and women have different ways of articulating with the larger society, their patterns of exchange are very different.

Patterns of adaptation tend to repeat themselves in different cultural contexts. That patterns of production and reciprocal exchange in urban ghettos operate according to principles of generalized reciprocity should not be surprising; neither should the key child-care roles played by older siblings and older women. Kin-based economies still function within industrial societies, and there is increasing evidence that a hidden economy based on nonmarket principles is on the increase. The giving of food to elderly people by senior citizens' centers is only one example (Myerhoff 1978). Teenagers will need to create new survival strategies in our own culture as unemployment rises. Elderly people on fixed incomes also will need new strategies—mutual aid systems, perhaps, or reciprocal exchange systems of social and economic support which provide needed goods and services. The role that governmentally organized redistributive systems play in industrial societies in providing needed goods and services to age groups that are economically marginal remains to be fully explored.

To summarize, we can see numerous modes of livelihood in stratified state-level economies, and consequently various patterns of age and economic organization. If family production and consumption units are subsistence-based, without wage labor, children and the elderly are viable, indeed essential, contributors to the livelihood of the unit. The similarities between precapitalist formations in state systems and kin-based economies before the development of the state are substantial with respect to patterns of age and economic organization. It is important to note the difference between the introduction of wages and the introduction of a capitalist mode of production into processes of livelihood and into a state system as a whole. Once individuals become wage laborers and work in capitalist units of production, most of the social, economic, and political supports available in a noncapitalist economy disappear and the economic roles of people at all ages change dramatically.

REFERENCES

Amoss, Pamela T.
  1981   Coast Salish elders. *In* Other Ways of Growing Old, ed. Amoss and
          Stevan Harrell, pp. 227–48. Stanford: Stanford University Press.
Arensberg, Conrad
  1968   The Irish Countryman: An Anthropological Study. New York: Peter
          Smith. (First published 1937.)
Biesele, M., and Nancy Howell
  1981   "The old people give you life": Aging among !Kung hunter-gatherers.
          In Other Ways of Growing Old, ed. Pamela T. Amoss and Stevan
          Harrell, pp. 77–98. Stanford; Stanford University Press.
Brown, Judith K.
  1975   Iroquois women: An ethnohistoric note. *In* Toward an Anthropology of
          Women, ed. Rayna Reiter, pp. 235–51. New York: Monthly Review
          Press.
  1982   Cross-cultural perspectives on middle-aged women. Current An-
          thropology 23:143–56.
Cancian, Frank
  1965   Economics and Prestige in a Maya Community: The Religious Cargo
          System in Zinacantan. Stanford: Stanford University Press.
Chagnon, Napoleon
  1974   Studying the Yanomano. New York: Holt, Rinehart & Winston.
Chayanov, A. V.
  1966   A. V. Chayanov on the Theory of Peasant Economy, ed. David Thorn-
          er, Basil Kerblay, and R. E. F. Smith. Homewood, Ill.: Richard D.
          Irwin for the American Economic Association. (First published 1925.)
Clark, Robert L., and Joseph J. Spengler
  1980   The Economics of Individual and Population Aging. Cambridge:
          Cambridge University Press.
Cockburn, T. Aidan
  1971   Infectious diseases in ancient populations. Current Anthropology
          12:45–62.
Cole, John W., and Phillip S. Katz
  1973   Knecht to Arbiter: The proletarianization process in South Tyrol. Stud-
          ies in European Society 1:39–66.
Cowgill, Donald O.
  1972   A theory of aging in cross-cultural perspective. *In* Aging and Moderni-
          zation, ed. Donald O. Cowgill and Lowell D. Holmes, pp. 1–14. New
          York: Meredith.
Cowgill, Donald O., and Lowell D. Holmes, eds.
  1972   Aging and Modernization. New York: Meredith.

Draper, Patricia
  1975   !Kung women: Contrasts in sexual egalitarianism in foraging and sedentary contexts. *In* Toward an Anthropology of Women, ed. Rayna Reiter, pp. 77–109. New York: Monthly Review Press.
  1976   Social and economic constraints on child life. *In* Kalahari hunter-gatherers, ed. Richard B. Lee and Irven De Vore. Cambridge: Harvard University Press.
Dunn, Frederick L.
  1968   Epidemiological factors: Health and disease in hunter-gatherers. *In* Man the Hunter, ed. Richard B. Lee and Irven De Vore. Chicago: Aldine.
Dupré, Georges, and Pierre-Philippe Rey
  1973   Reflections on the pertinence of a theory of the history of exchange. Economy and society 2:131–63.
Durkheim, Emile
  1964   Division of Labor in Society. Glencoe, Ill.: Free Press.
Evans-Pritchard, E. E.
  1940   The Nuer. Oxford: Oxford University Press.
Fairley, Nancy
  1981   The economic roles of male teenagers: The case of Zaire. Paper presented to the Central States Anthropological Society, Cincinnati.
Fried, Morton
  1967   The Evolution of Political Society. New York: Random House.
Friedlander, Judith
  1976   Being Indian in Hueyapan. New York: St. Martin's Press.
Fries, James F.
  1980   Aging, natural death, and the compression of morbidity. New England Journal of Medicine 303:130–35.
Goodale, Jane C.
  1971   Tiwi wives. Seattle: University of Washington Press.
Gulliver, Philip H.
  1965   The Jie of Uganda. *In* Peoples of Africa, ed. James L. Gibbs. New York: Holt, Rinehart & Winston.
Halperin, Rhoda H.
  1972   Duality reconsidered: Some measures of womanhood in the Caribbean. Paper presented to the Northeastern Anthropological Association, Albany, N.Y.
  1975   Administración agraria y trabajo: Un caso de la economía política mexicana. Mexico City: Instituto Nacional Indigenista.
  1980   Ecology and mode of production: Seasonal variation and the divison of labor by sex among hunter-gatherers. Journal of Anthropological Research 36:379–99.

1982   New and old in economic anthropology. American Anthropologist 84:339–49.

Hammond, Dorothy, and Alta Jablow
1976   Women in Cultures of the World. Reading, Mass.: Cummings.

Hart, C. W. M., and Arnold R. Pilling
1960   The Tiwi of North Australia. New York: Holt, Rinehart & Winston.

Hoebel, E. Adamson
1954   The Law of Primitive Man. Cambridge: Harvard University Press.

Holmes, Douglas R.
1982   A peasant-worker model in a northern Italian context. Unpublished manuscript.

Holmes, Lowell D.
1972   The role and status of the aged in a changing Samoa. *In* Aging and Modernization, ed. Donald O. Cowgill and Lowell D. Holmes, pp. 73–90. New York: Meredith.

Howell, Nancy
1979   Demography of the Dobe !Kung. New York: Academic Press.

Johnson, Orna R., and Allen Johnson
1975   Male/female relations and the organization of work in a Machiguenga community. American Ethnologist 2:634–48.

Kagan, Dianne
1980   Activity and aging in a Colombian peasant village. *In* Aging in Culture and Society, ed. Christine L. Fry, pp. 65–79. New York: Praeger.

Kensinger, Kennteh M., Phyllis Rabineau, Helen Tanner, Susan G. Ferguson, and Alice Dawson
1975   The Cashinahua of Eastern Peru. Brown University Studies in Anthropology and Material Culture, vol. 1. Providence: Brown University Press.

Kolata, Gina B.
1974   !Kung hunter-gatherers: Feminism, diet, and birth control. Science 85:932–34.

Leacock, Eleanor
1978   Women's status in egalitarian society: Implications for social evolution. Current Anthropology 19:247–75.

Lee, Richard B.
1968   What hunters do for a living, or How to make out on scarce resources. *In* Man the Hunter, ed. Lee and Irven De Vore, pp. 30–48. Chicago: Aldine.
1979   The !Kung San: Men, Women, and Work in a Foraging Society. Cambridge: Cambridge University Press.

Liebow, Eliot
1967   Tally's Corner. Boston: Little, Brown.

Malinowski, Bronislaw
1978　Coral Gardens and Their Magic. New York: Dover. (First published New York: American Book Col. 1935.)

Mauss, Marcel
1966　Essai sur le don: Forme et raison de l'exchange dans les sociétés archaiques. In Sociologie et anthropologie. Paris: Presses Universitaires de France. (First published in L'Année Sociologique, 1923–24.)

Minge-Kalman, W.
1978　Houshold economy during the peasant-to-worker transition in the Swiss Alps. Ethnology 17:183.

Murphy, Yolanda, and Robert F. Murphy
1974　Women of the Forest. New York: Columbia University Press.

Myerhoff, Barbara
1978　Number Our Days. New York: Simon & Schuster.

Nag, Moni.
1973　Anthropology and population: Problems and perspectives. Population Studies 27:59–68.
1976　The economic view of children in agricultural societies: A review and a proposal. In Culture, Natality, and Family Planning, ed. John F. Marshall and Steven Polgar. Chapel Hill: University of North Carolina Press.

Netting, Robert M.
1977　Cultural Ecology. Menlo Park, Calif.: Benjamin/Cummings.

Oliver, Douglas
1955　A Solomon Island Society. Boston: Beacon Press.

Olson, Lawrence, Christopher Caton, and Martin Duffy
1981　The Elderly and the Future Economy. Lexington, Mass.: Lexington Books.

Polanyi, Karl
1957　The economy as instituted process. In Trade and Market in the Early Empires, ed. Karl Polanyi, Conrad Arensberg, and Harry W. Pearson New York: Free Press.

Polgar, Steven
1972　Population history and population policies from an anthropological perspective. Current Anthropology 13:203–11.

Ritter, Madeline Lattman
1980　The conditions favoring age-set organization. Journal of Anthropological Research 36:87–104.

Rosaldo, Michelle Z.
1974　Women, culture, and society: A theoretical overview. In Women, Culture, and Society, ed. Rosaldo and Louise Lamphere. Stanford: Stanford University Press.

Rose, F. G. G.
1960   Classification of Kin, Age Structure, and Marriage amongst the Groote Eylandt Aborigines: A Study in Method and a Theory of Australian Kinship. Oxford: Pergamon Press.

Rosman, Abraham, and Paula Rubel
1970   Potlatch and Sagali: The Structure of Exchange in Haida and Trobriand Societies. Transactions of the New York Academy of Sciences 32:732–42.
1978   Exchange as structure, or Why doesn't everyone eat his own pigs? *In* Research in Economic Anthropology, ed. George Dalton. Greenwich, Conn.: JAI Press.

Rothstein, Frances
1979   Two different worlds: Gender and industrialization in rural Mexico. *In* New Directions in Political Economy: An Approach from Anthropology, ed. Madeline Barbara Leons and Rothstein. Westport, Conn.: Greenwood Press.

Rubbo, Anna
1975   The spread of capitalism in rural Colombia. *In* Toward an Anthropology of Women, ed. Rayna Reiter. New York: Monthly Review Press.

Sahlins, Marshall
1972   Stone Age Economics. Chicago: Aldine.

Salamon, S., and V. Lockhart
1980   Land ownership and the position of elderly in farm families. Human Organization 39:324–31.

Sanday, Peggy R.
1974   Female status in the public domain. *In* Women, Culture, and Society, ed. M. Z. Rosaldo and Louise Lamphere. Stanford: Stanford University Press.

Simmons, Leo W.
1945   The Role of the Aged in Primitive Society. New Haven: Yale University Press.

Stack, Carol
1974   All Our Kin. New York: Harper & Row.

Strathern, Andrew
1971   The Rope of Moka: Big-Men and Ceremonial exchange in Mount Hagen. Cambridge: Cambridge University Press.

Strathern, Marilyn
1972   Women in Between. New York: Seminar Press.

Streib, Gordon G.
1972   Old age in Ireland: Demographic and sociological aspects. *In* Aging and Modernization, ed. Donald O. Cowgill and Lowell D. Holmes. New York: Meredith.

Uberoi, J. P. Singh
1962   The Politics of the Kula Ring: An Analysis of the Findings of Bronislaw Malinowski. Manchester: Manchester University Press.
Weiner, Annette
1976   Women of Value, Men of Renown. Austin: University of Texas Press.
Wilson, Peter J.
1969   Reputation and respectability: A suggestion for Caribbean ethnology. Man n.s. 4:70–84.
1971   Caribbean crews: Peer groups and male society. Caribbean Studies 10:18–34.
Wolf, Eric
1966a Kinship, friendship, and patron-client relations in complex societies. In The Social Anthropology of Complex Societies, ed. Michael Banton. ASA Monographs. London: Tavistock.
1966b Peasants. Englewood Cliffs, N.J.: Prentice-Hall.
Wolfe, Alvin
1977   The supranational organization of production: An evolutionary perspective. Current Anthropology 18:615–36.

7

Age and Social Change

Nancy Foner

The study of age is a neglected area in anthropology. Although anthropologists have long been aware that age is an important factor in social life, they have yet to explore systematically how the analysis of the social aspects of age can contribute to our understanding of the structure and dynamics of society. This chapter is an attempt to begin to fill in this gap by focusing on age and social change. What does the study of age have to tell us about patterns of change in nonindustrial societies?[1]

For one thing, this chapter shows how the study of age further specifies some limitations of a widely used model of change: the modernization model. Many anthropologists, of course, have challenged the common assumption in modernization studies that nonwestern societies will replicate changes Western countries experienced as they industrialized. They have shown that such institutions as the family do not automatically become "modernized" in the Western image as nonindustrial societies come into contact with industrial powers. Questions about modernization concepts, however, are generally put aside when it comes to dealing with the social position of various age groupings. The prediction of the mod-

---

1. Following Jack Goody (1976:117), I use "nonindustrial societies" to refer to societies in which the economy is based on hunting and gathering, pastoralism, or agriculture, including the nonindustrial sectors of industrial societies.

ernization model that the status of the old will inevitably deteriorate as urbanization and industrialization proceed is too often uncritically accepted. Anthropologists who study changing age patterns tend either to endorse the modernization model openly or implicitly to follow its premises. Available evidence on age and change, however, makes clear that the impact of change on the status of the old is not so simple as the modernization model would have us believe.

By raising additional questions about the inevitability and universality of modernization processes, the study of age as a social phenomenon contributes to the anthropological critique of modernization theory. And the study of age illuminates the processes of change in nonindustrial societies in yet another way. A theoretical perspective developed in the sociology of age—the age-stratification perspective—can shed light on the sources as well as the effects of change in the nonindustrial world.

To date, the age-stratification perspective has gone unnoticed by anthropologists who study change. This neglect undoubtedly stems from the fact that the model was developed by sociologists primarily with reference to our own society. Moreover, anthropologists concerned with change have generally paid little attention to age and so have hardly been searching for a theory of aging to inform their work. The age-stratification perspective provides insights into the processes of change in nonindustrial societies by showing how forces for change are related to age systems. One of the unfortunate consequences of modernization concepts is that they lead to an image of "traditional" (as opposed to "modern") society as unchanging. In contrast to the modernization model, the age-stratification approach does not simply point to changes that ensue as a result of contact with Western countries. The age-stratification perspective bids us to consider social changes in precolonial and precontact days as well as those in more recent times.

The key concept developed by age-stratification theorists to analyze change is the succession of cohorts. Examination of the process of cohort succession reveals how one cohort (individuals who were born in the same time period and age together) follows another, each influenced by the social and historical context in which its members grew up and matured. The characteristics of each cohort are thus a product of the changing social environment its members experience over the life course. And the very fact that cohorts have different characteristics—size and composition, for example—can provide a further impetus to social change.

The Modernization Model Reconsidered

The view that the "passing of traditional society" ushers in a decline in the overall status of the old—what has been called the modernization model—has explicitly or implicitly guided much of what has been written about changing age relations in nonindustrial societies. According to Donald Cowgill and Lowell Holmes (1972), well-known proponents of the modernization model in anthropology-and-aging circles, modernization inevitably worsens the prestige and power of the old. In a revision of the model, Cowgill (1974) specifies how urbanization, the spread of literacy and mass education, and the introduction of scientific and health technology undermine old people's status. The elderly, the argument goes, were respected for their experience and expertise in premodern societies, where they controlled property and played important roles in the extended family. Their situation, however, is much worse in the modern world. The aged not only multiply in numbers. They are relegated to less prestigious jobs or are forced to retire altogether, while the young acquire the knowledge to equip them for specialized and more lucrative jobs. No longer is there a mystique of age or a reverence for the old on the basis of their superior knowledge and wisdom. Indeed, old people's wisdom becomes obsolete.

When we reexamine the way social changes associated with modernization affect the status of the old in nonindustrial societies, however, we find that this outcome is not inevitable. Not only does historical research on our own preindustrial past show that the modernization model distorts and simplifies changes in age relations in England and America; ethnographic evidence on other nonindustrial societies also cautions that changes in the status of the old are more complex and varied than the modernization model suggests.

The Historical Critique

The central question in most historical writings on old age, David Hackett Fischer (1978:268) writes, is the validity of the modernization model. Lately historians of aging have marshaled considerable evidence to show how limited the model is in light of the history of Western industrial countries—the base that modernization theorists use for their assumptions about the direction of change in present-day nonindustrial societies.

Of course, historians do not agree on all the particulars. They differ, for example, on the extent to which the aged were respected in early modern England and America, and on the timing of and reasons for changes in the position of the elderly through the years.[2] Yet certain common themes emerge in historians' general criticisms of the modernization model.

In the first place, historians of aging challenge the premise that certain changes in age relations followed on the heels of industrialization. Peter Laslett (1977) shows that extensive shifts in the proportion of the aged in the English population did not occur until a century or more after the onset of industrialization. And the dramatic undermining of the authority of age in America, according to Fischer (1978:102), came before industrialization, urbanization, and mass education had any effect.[3]

Quite apart from matters of causation, historians of aging have criticized the modernization model's before-and-after approach: the notion of a uniformly better "before" for the aged in traditional times, followed by a worse "after" in modern days. The model fits what Laslett (1976:91) calls the "world we have lost syndrome," or the tendency to hold up today's problems against the backdrop of an idealized past. According to Laslett (1976:89–91), "existent informal dogmatic theory" assumes that "before" the aged were respected, held useful and valued roles, and found a secure place in the family; "after," they have been brutally deprived. Historical evidence shows, however, that such a view romanticizes the past.

The situation of the elderly in preindustrial Europe and America, it is noted, was no paradise on earth. In Andrew Achenbaum and Peter Stearns's words (1978:309), "it mixed official respect, some real power, considerable economic and physical degradation, and cultural derision, and therefore almost inevitably improved in some respects as it deteriorated in others with the onset of modernization."

Nor can we assume, as the modernization model implies, that the position of old people in preindustrial Western societies was uniform.

---

2. A useful guide to some of these disagreements can be found in Fischer's (1978) bibliographic essay reviewing the contributions various historians have made to the "modernization and age" question.

3. Why old people's position changed in certain ways in Western Europe and America is subject to debate. Fischer (1978), for one, places strong emphasis on the role of ideas of liberty and equality in effecting changes in age relations in the United States.

Their condition varied not only among these societies (Laslett 1976:113–15) but within them—according to class, sex, and racial group, for example (Fischer 1978).

There are also many continuities between past and present. We cannot confidently say, Laslett argues (1977:176–77), that the elderly were better provided for in preindustrial England than they are now. According to Laslett, there is no reason to suppose that in the traditional era "deliberate provision was made for the physical, emotional or economic needs of aged persons, aged relations or aged parents in a way which was in any sense superior to the provision now being made by the children, the relatives and the friends of aged persons in our own day, not to speak of the elaborate machinery of an anxiously protective welfare state." Across the Atlantic, Fischer (1978:230) points out that ambivalent attitudes and conduct toward the old have characterized every period of American history.

Obviously, there have been many changes in the past few centuries. And many of these changes have led to declines in old people's authority and prestige. But to view shifts in old people's situation as a "fall from grace or manifest destiny from a remote point" is, Achenbaum says (1978:166–67), risky and naive. The history of growing old in America, he notes, has been filled with "too many surprises, ironies, and exceptions" to say that changes in old people's situation were ever one-directional, uniform, or inevitable. And Fischer observes (1978:230) that it is impossible to say that the condition of the aged in America became worse—or better—with the passage of time. "It became better in some ways," he says, "and worse in others."

Far from steadily deteriorating, old people's situation has, in recent decades, improved in many ways—the modernization model running in reverse, as Fischer puts it (1978:267). Thus, although serious difficulties still beset the elderly in this country, increased government health and welfare measures (including the wider availability and size of retirement benefits) have provided crucial services for and improved the condition of the elderly in many ways (see Achenbaum 1978:143–57).

The Anthropological Record

Historians of aging point out the need to look at the modernization model with a critical eye. They have shown that the model does not accurately describe changes in age relations that occurred as Western societies industrialized. What about changes in the nonwestern, nonindustrial world?[4]

In evaluating the model's relevance for studying old age in nonwestern societies, I adopt a narrower focus than that of historians of aging, who range over such diverse topics as the care the aged received in the family, old people's longevity and health, the political and economic influence of the old, and general cultural attitudes toward the aged. The concern here is with the status of the old—that is, with the share of social benefits and rewards that the old obtain through access to various social roles. Is the modernization model right to predict that the status of the old inevitably declines as nonindustrial societies come under the influence of Western industrial countries?

The answer, I argue, is no—not because such declines never happen, but because they are not inevitable. Far from leading to declines in old people's status, contact with the industrial world has, in some societies, strengthened or reinforced old people's status in many ways. And where anthropologists have charted changes in the status of the old over the years, a bumpy up-and-down path is often revealed, with the authority or prestige of the old declining at one point in time, for example, but improving at a later stage.

Support for the Modernization Model. Although the modernization model overemphasizes the negative impact of the industrial world on the old in nonindustrial societies, it is not always wide of the mark. Let us first consider some of the evidence that supports the model's pessimistic predictions about the status of the old before we look at the brighter side of the picture. Numerous anthropological accounts do report that in many societies the imposition of colonial rule, the introduction of wage labor and Christianity, and other related changes have undermined the position of old people in a variety of ways.

How do such declines come about? Several analytically separate but empirically connected processes are involved. For one thing, the way rewards and valued roles are allocated among age strata may change so

---

4. Whereas the validity of the modernization model is a central question in historical writings on old age, the same cannot be said of the writings of anthropologists of aging. Indeed, the latter have tended not to evaluate the modernization model critically in the light of ethnographic data. One exception is Pamela Amoss (1981). In addition, a few anthropologists (e.g., Keith 1980, Simic 1978) have, in passing, noted some of the problems with the modernization model. A chapter in my own comparative study of old age (N. Foner 1984) pulls together ethnographic data to evaluate the model critically.

that the old hold fewer of them. Roles the old fill that were once highly valued may no longer bring so much esteem, influence, or wealth. These roles can even disappear altogether. And new roles may emerge in which younger people predominate.

In many societies the advent of wage labor and a money economy has lessened old people's economic dominance because young people have greater access to a wider variety of relatively lucrative economic roles than in the past. Among the Kpelle of Liberia, for example, in order to obtain wives, young men used to have to indebt themselves to older men. New wage-earning opportunities, however, have meant that young men can avoid relying on their fathers for bridewealth payments. They can even avoid brideservice by giving money payments to in-laws (Bledsoe 1980:118–20). In the case of the Giriama of Kenya, the switch to a cash-crop economy has reduced old men's control over crucial productive resources in the community while some younger men have much greater scope to acquire wealth than before (Parkin 1972).

The highly valued political roles old men once filled sometimes fade in importance, and new skills often qualify younger men for new political positions. This is what happened among the Asmat hunters and gatherers of New Guinea. As recently as 1930, old Asmat men who were local influentials—*tesmaypits*—arranged raiding, rituals, trade, and the periodic relocation of villages. With the imposition of Indonesian rule, the suppression of headhunting and related rituals, and the establishment of relatively permanent coastal villages, former *tesmaypits* became relatively powerless old men in their communities. Their ritual, political, and headhunting skills, once a source of power and glory, were meaningless in the new situation. Now men under 40, who read, write, and speak Indonesian, are chosen for local government offices (Van Arsdale 1981).

In the Asmat case, old men's ritual dominance was also threatened as younger men became leaders of new religions. In other societies, too, ritual powers of elders are less valued as new faiths take hold. And the advent of national courts in a number of societies has reduced old men's sway over the wheels of justice because they cannot dominate these new bodies.

Another process that undermines the status of the old is frequently at work. Old people's authority decreases as sanctions at their command (religious or economic sanctions, for example) lose force. Where traditional religous beliefs disappear or decline, mystical sanctions the old once wielded are often less effective—perhaps no longer thought to operate at all. And young people are sometimes less cowed by their elders' threats to withhold various kinds of economic benefits when the young can go off to earn good wages on their own.

Finally, the legitimacy of old people's prestige and power may come under fire. The very fact that they occupy fewer rewarded roles calls into question their right to respect and influence. Even when the old still have considerable political and economic power, new values and ideas may raise doubts about their right to wield it. These new ideas and values, which are disseminated through such agencies as schools, courts, churches, and political parties, frequently give legitimacy to, and sometimes actually spur, young people's challenges to the dominance of the old (see, for example, Schapera 1971:242, Wilson 1977:19).

Limitations of the Modernization Model. This account of old people's declines is only part of the story. We cannot assume that the powers and prestige of the old invariably deteriorate in changing nonindustrial societies. In some societies, the elderly continue to fill valued roles and to command deference from the young. Sometimes their influence and prestige actually increase with change. Far from being conservative upholders of the status quo, the old may react to certain changes in new ways that preserve or fortify their position (see, for example, Fowler 1982 on the Arapahoes).

In several African societies, for instance, the power of influential old men was increased under British colonial rule. In the Nyakyusa case, the British maintained elderly chiefs in office much longer than would have been possible in precolonial days (Wilson 1977). Among the Afikpo Igbo of Nigeria, the powers of elders—which in the nineteenth century had been circumscribed by men in certain non-Afikpo lineages—generally were expanded under British rule (Ottenberg 1971).

In many societies, old men's control of land has ensured (perhaps in some cases increased) their economic authority. What has happened in these societies is that new occupational opportunities for young people have been very limited. Jobs for most young people have been mainly unskilled and poorly paid, when they are available at all. Wage earnings often have limited buying power as well. Meanwhile, with dramatic population increases and the introduction of cash crops and new farming techniques, land has become an ever more scarce resource. And a valued one. For land provides subsistence as well as cash crops and a source of social security. In this situation, the old are clearly in an advantageous position when seniority or age gives them control over land.

An entirely new benefit has improved the economic position of the old in several North American groups: old-age pensions (see Goodwin 1942, on the Western Apache; Hughes 1961, on the St. Lawrence Island Eskimos; Williams 1980, on nonreservation Indians in Oklahoma). In poor communities where cash is hard to come by, old-age pensioners provide a steady source of income for their households, and in several Native American communities these contributions have been a definite gain, particularly for the disabled old. Thus, before the advent of pensions among the Western Apache, the very old were poor and economically dependent on the young. When Grenville Goodwin (1942:517) lived among them in the 1930s, however, old people who received monthly army pensions were often the wealthiest members of their families, and younger relatives came to them for money. The very frail old also usually received better care than before. Younger people, Goodwin says, had an interest in keeping old relatives alive: when they died, the pensions ceased.

Finally, a report on the Coast Salish of Washington State and British Columbia shows that the elderly recently gained prestige as ritual experts and sources of information about indigeneous ways as part of a religious revival movement (Amoss 1981). Old people dominated revived traditional-style rituals because they knew the ropes. They were the ones who remembered how these rituals were practiced—how speeches should be made, for instance, and the family regalia displayed.

Note that these examples refer to certain aspects of old people's status. This observation leads to a crucial point. Since the overall status of the elderly is multidimensional, it is too simple to say that change leads to improvements or declines in their status. Rather, we must specify (as I have done in the preceding examples) which dimensions of the status of the old we are talking about: which social rewards and valued roles they lose or gain. With change, all components of old people's status rarely vary in exactly the same way. In other words, the elderly may lose some rewards and valued roles at the same time that they keep or expand the scope of others. Giriama elders in the 1960s, for example, were losing economic ground in the community as many sold land and palms to enterprising younger men. But elders continued to be recognized as ritual experts and to be sought as witnesses in cases involving claims to land and palms (Parkin 1972).

Nor is the direction of change in particular aspects of old people's status—say, their religious authority—necessarily consistent over time.

In the early period of contact with industrial powers, for example, old people's ritual authority may have declined, but with later developments it may increase. Such was the case among the Coast Salish. Contact with the white world was initially devastating for the Coast Salish aged. Among other things, they lost their central place in the religious life of the people. The rituals they dominated were either suppressed by missionaries and Indian agents or "abandoned as useless by a progressively demoralized people" (Amoss 1981:235). Meanwhile, young men assumed leadership positions in new faiths. In the past few decades, however, the old once more have become valued for their ritual knowledge, and they run the revived Indian religious ceremonies.

Alternately, an increase in rewards for the elderly may be followed by later declines. Thus British rule enabled Nyakyusa chiefs to hang onto power much longer than was possible before conquest. With Tanzania's independence, however, old chiefs were losing their authority while some young men gained leadership positions in the ruling political party (Wilson 1977:98, 187).

To sum up so far, a model that proposes that it's downhill all the way for the aged in changing nonindustrial societies is seriously flawed. This critique has, I suggest, relevance for the general anthropological study of change. It emphasizes that changes in the past hundred years or so in nonwestern societies—such as the imposition of colonial rule, integration into a world economic system, the introduction of new religions, the spread of Western education, and the emergence of newly independent governments—have not swept through with uniform effect. It is not just that these societies do not imitate Western patterns of change. There are also significant differences among nonindustrial societies. Thus in trying to understand how contact with the industrial world has affected the old, as well as other age strata, in these societies, we must consider a variety of factors that vary from place to place. These factors include the particular external forces of change, such as the nature of colonial rule and subsequent political and economic developments in national centers since independence; the peculiar social, economic, and political conditions as well as cultural beliefs and values in each local setting; and the often unanticipated actions and decisions of individuals in these settings as they respond to, and can thereby influence, the course of change. And finally, it should be borne in mind that all of these particular external forces of change, local conditions, and individual responses vary not only from place to place but, within a society, from one time period to another.

Insights from the Sociology of Age:
The Age Stratification Model

The review of the modernization model has emphasized the negative: the limitations of the model. On the positive side, a theoretical perspective in the sociology of age—the age-stratification model—provides a useful analytic framework for interpreting the relationship between age-related phenomena and social change (for an elaboration of the age-stratification model, see Riley et al. 1972). While modernization theory tends to contrast modern societies with a model of a static "traditional" past, the age-stratification perspective reminds us that there is a potential for change in all societies—in nonindustrial societies, before as well as after contact with the West. Then, too, by stressing that individuals are not only influenced by but also help to shape social change, the age-stratification perspective gets us away from notions about the inevitability of change. Thus, while the age-stratification model was developed with Western industrial societies in mind, it raises important questions about the effects and sources of change that are relevant to anthropological studies.

The Succession of Cohorts: Effects of Change

The concepts of cohort analysis and cohort succession seldom crop up in social and cultural anthropology. It is true, of course, that although they do not use the term "cohort,"[5] many anthropologists discuss how individuals born about the same period differ in attitudes and behavior from those born later or earlier. But there has been no systematic theoretical analysis in the anthropological literature of the ways birth cohorts differ from each other and of how cohort differences not only reflect but can also lead to social change.

The principal contribution of the age-stratification model to the study of social change is to elaborate these points. What is key here is that social changes do not, in general, affect all cohorts the same way.[6] This

5. Sometimes the term "generation" is used. I prefer to use the term "cohort" to refer to people born at the same time, as to use "generation" in this way, as David Kertzer (1982) points out, leads to conceptual confusion. "Generation," as Kertzer argues, should be used in its genealogical, kinship-related sense.

6. There are methodological problems in determining to what extent differences among age strata at any given time are due to cohort membership, to the process of aging (the fact that members of a cohort are at a particular life stage), or to the circumstances in the particular period under study (see Riley et al. 1972:27–90, 583–618).

variation comes about, first of all, because as one cohort succeeds another, each cohort has lived through a different segment of history.[7] Members of a given cohort are born and come of age in a particular historical environment and together they experience later historical events and changes as they pass through subsequent life stages. Thus each cohort has a unique historical past and "bears the stamp of the historical context through which it flows" (A. Foner 1978:S343); and each cohort is unique in the age at which its members experience important historical events and other social changes. The members of only one cohort in the United States, for example, faced World War II in their twenties, and only one cohort retired in the early years after the establishment of the social security system (A. Foner 1982:224). Or to use an example from nonwestern societies, only one cohort experienced the onset of colonial rule or struggles for independence during youth. Still another important point is that social changes can affect such crucial features of cohorts as their size, sex composition, and the capacities of their members. In turn, the size and composition of cohorts and the abilities of the cohort members can influence the lives of individuals in a cohort and, as I discuss later, can bring about further social changes.

Because of social change, then, each cohort has unique life-course experiences that mark it off from cohorts that have preceded and come after it.[8] No two cohorts experience youth, adulthood, and old age under exactly the same historical circumstances. Thus, when we study the effects of social change on "the old" (or "the young") in a society, it is essential to know which cohort of old (or young) people is being considered—with all its unique characteristics.

Age-stratification theorists illustrate these points with examples from modern American society, where we know that continual and far-reach-

7. The concept of a cohort, I should stress, is a construct of the outside observer. Members of a cohort need not have an awareness of a common cohort identity. The age boundaries of a cohort, moreover, are quite arbitrary, chosen by the observer for particular purposes of study, so that a cohort can include individuals born within a span of, say, as short as five years or as long as thirty years. Here I focus on the factors that cohort members have in common. But there are crucial differences among cohort members that can shape their life experiences—sex, wealth, and race differences, to name but a few.

8. The Ilongots of northern Luzon, Philippines, actually had a sense that each successive cohort "followed its own path." From the beginning of this century, Renato Rosaldo writes (1980:112), "the Ilongot population has experienced such shifting historical conditions that a sense has emerged that each generation [cohort] grows up in a world unlike that of its predecessors." Whether individuals in other societies have a similar sense is a subject well worth investigating.

ing changes have given each cohort a unique stamp. But are there cohort differences in nonindustrial societies? Unfortunately, there are few available detailed anthropological or historical reports on the same society for an extended time period that provide systematic information on how changes in nonindustrial societies lead to differing cohort experiences. Yet it seems likely that in nonindustrial societies, as in industrial America, gradual and hardly perceptible changes, as well as sudden and dramatic shifts, mean that successive cohorts differ from each other in a variety of ways. Even before Western industrial influence, such events as epidemics, natural disasters, and contact with other social groups could have altered "the collective lives of successive cohorts" (Riley 1978:45). It is possible, for example, that in some societies in certain precontact periods, the ranks of one cohort were decimated by disease, famine, or war. The relatively small size of this cohort could have influenced the attitudes and behavior of its members, a point I will consider in the next section. In addition, coming of age during a time of famine, war, or disease may have had a lasting influence on members of this cohort, perhaps giving them an outlook on life and perhaps also behavior patterns that differed form those of people who grew up in less troubled days.

Or consider how contact with the industrial world may have left its mark on different cohorts in nonwestern societies. The political attitudes, work histories, and family lives, for example, of the cohort that came of age during the first years of colonial rule could have differed markedly from those of cohorts who came of age earlier. When members of this cohort reached old age, surely they had a different backlog of experiences and perhaps different expectations than previous cohorts of old people. They probably differed also from later cohorts of old people who experienced further social, economic, and political changes throughout their lives.

That individuals in some cohorts confront particularly dramatic historical circumstances—wars or depressions, for example—in their youth may partly explain why members of these cohorts have a strong sense of their cohort identity. The experience of sharing traumatic or momentous events when they came of age—and the effect of these events on their life-course patterns and their attitudes and values—can give them a sense of "we-ness" that continues as they age. Or the common memory of catastrophic events may reinforce or enhance their sense of a collective identity. This is what seems to have happened among the one marital cohort (individuals who got married in the same period) that Renato

Rosaldo describes in his study of the headhunting Ilongots of northern Luzon, Philippines. According to Rosaldo (1980:113), the twenty people in this marital cohort "acquired a self-conscious, though loosely bound, sense of their collective identity through a series of intermarriages in 1955– 58." Their collective consciousness was strengthened in subsequent years as they "held one another's hands" through coordinated residential moves, so that the people who married at the same time also grew old together (Rosaldo 1980:120). Their collective consciousness was also solidified by their shared remembrances of the traumatic events that occurred when they were young, that is, remembrance of the "time of the Japanese" in 1945, when about one-third of the local population was lost through disease, starvation, or bullets as a result of the massive influx of retreating Japanese troops. The sense of collective identity among the ten men in the marital cohort was further deepened by the fact that before they married they had taken heads in quick succession and had gone on raids together.

Whether other marital cohorts among the Ilongots had as strong a sense of collective consciousness as the one Rosaldo analyzes is an open question. But among the Ilongots, as in other societies, social change over the years means that the process of growing up and growing older is at least somewhat different for members of successive cohorts.

The Succession of Cohorts: Sources of Change

More than just reflecting change, cohort differences, according to age-stratification theorists, can also exert pressure toward change.[9] Of course, political, economic, social, or demographic trends external to the age system (or to the society)—such as colonial rule or natural disasters—influence the social environment to which cohorts must adjust. But cohorts are not only acted upon; they also react. By the way they respond to their social environment, members of a given cohort can help to redefine patterns of behavior, reshape social institutions, and alter attitudes and values. What needs stressing is that neither the responses of given cohorts to their changing environment nor the consequences of these responses for behavior patterns, social institutions, or cultural values are always predictable or inevitable.

Members of particular cohorts can help to mold social or cultural changes at all life stages. Cohorts just assuming adult roles, Anne Foner suggests (1982:224), have a special effect on age patterns of behavior.

9. See A. Foner 1982, Riley et al. 1972:515–82, Riley 1978, and Waring 1975 on how cohort differences can contribute to change in our own society.

Because they have not had time to internalize established ways firmly, they may be especially receptive to new ideas and behavior and thus play an active role in contributing to change.

But while we often think of young people as innovators, members of particular cohorts can also contribute to change in middle or old age. Take the reaction to Christian influence of old men in the ritual elder age grade among the Tiriki of Kenya (Sangree 1966). Ritual elders seemed to have hastened the demise of the ancestor cult over which they traditionally presided. To be sure, challenges from Christian missionaries and converts might have led to the decline of the cult no matter what the elders did. In addition to being ignored in their ritual capacity, ritual elders found that their ritual functions were ridiculed by Christian converts and missionaries, even condemned as causes of social and individual distress. Given these circumstances, the ritual elders might have tried to hold onto their ritual roles in the ancestor cult until the bitter end. They chose not to do so, however. Instead, they gave up most of their ritual duties. "Rather than continue to administer a cult which has lost its general social significance, and in so doing expose themselves to charges of being responsible for contemporary social woes," Walter Sangree writes (1966:167), "the Tiriki elders have abdicated their principal ritual roles." This abdication of ritual functions may in fact have played a role in maintaining the ritual elders' credibility and prestige. Ritual elders continued to be leaders of initiation ceremonies, and they were still respected and feared by juniors for their sorcery powers and for their potent curses.

Members of cohorts, then, can help to shape the course of change as they experience and respond to events and new circumstances at particular life stages. The fact that successive cohorts are of varying sizes and compositions can also contribute to change. A few examples help to illustrate this point.

The Samburu of Kenya are an age-set society in which young men in the *moran* age grade were, in Paul Spencer's words (1965:100), "odd men out," unable to control family and settlement affairs until they became elders. When an unusually large age set occupied the *moran* grade, there were, for various reasons, pressures to delay the promotion of members of this set to elderhood as well as to delay the initiation of the subsequent set.[10] Thus there was a change in the timing of the transition to age-graded roles.

10. Although Paul Spencer (1965:167–72) notes that political and economic developments as well as such factors as epidemics can affect the size of sets, he suggests that the

Among the Arapahoes of the Northern Plains, a change in the composition of the cohort of old men at the end of the nineteenth century provided an impetus to further changes in the society. Hardships both before and as a result of reservation settlement severely reduced the number of elders, including many priests who died without having properly trained their successors. In the absence of ritual experts, crucial aspects of religious rituals were altered or reinterpreted to accommodate the level of training and ability of the old men picked to fill ritual leadership roles. Indeed, the very structure of ritual leadership changed (Fowler 1982).

There is another development in some societies. When new economic opportunities or such events as famines, crop failures, and wars lead to the temporary or permanent emigration (or removal) of large numbers of younger men, old people and women who stay behind assume some of the roles that younger men formerly filled. In one Ilongot local cluster (of thirty-five people) in 1940, lowland troops arrested seven local men, thereby removing *every* able-bodied adult man from the group. Throughout the 1940s, the women in that local cluster took on the traditional male tasks of hunting and butchering in addition to their regular home and garden chores. "This shift in the sexual divison of labor," Rosaldo says (1980:72), "was so deeply formative for that cohort of . . . women that they alone among the Ilongots still hunt side by side with their men. In 1974 I participated in hunts in which these women, then over 40 years of age, led barking dogs through the prickly underbrush in flushing out the game." (Among the Bashu of eastern Zaire, women's assumption of male responsibilities as a result of male emigration for wage labor had far-reaching consequences for the society; see Packard 1980.)

Still another example shows that the absence of large numbers of younger men in a cohort can lead to changes in age norms. Among the Afikpo Igbo of Nigeria, the absence of many young men from their villages for extended periods of time led to shifts in the rules regarding initiation into an age set. Formerly, a man who was away from his village when his agemates were joining an age set could not join this set. Instead, he had to join a junior set that was open to recruitment when he returned. Later, however, with so many young men away at work for years at a time, men were allowed to join an age set *in absentia* (Ottenberg, cited in A. Foner and Kertzer 1979:129–30).

Samburu attitude toward their age-set system—which influenced elders' preferences as to when their sons should be initiated—may partly explain the pattern of alternately large and small sets that he documented.

The analysis of the way cohort differences can shape the direction of change brings us back to the modernization model. The analysis points out that changes in age patterns of behavior are not, as is implied by the modernization model, automatic responses to such processes as urbanization, industrialization, and the growth of bureaucratic organizations. Rather, cultural and social patterns can shift, often in quite surprising ways, as members of cohorts of varying sizes, compositions, and histories react to modernizing processes in the world around them.

Conclusion

The investigation of age has, I have tried to show, important lessons for the anthropological study of change. It emphasizes the need to revise one model of change and the virtues of applying another. It shows, too, that by looking beyond the boundaries of anthropology—in this case, to history and sociology—we can gain fresh insights into the processes of social change. Crucial questions still need to be explored. The analysis in this chapter suggests several lines of inquiry that deserve further examination.

I have made clear that the modernization model is too simple in predicting how the status of the old changes as nonindustrial societies come under Western influence. An alternative approach, which captures the complexities involved, should consider what kinds of changes worsen or improve various aspects of the status of the old in particular social and cultural settings. And of course the old are not the only ones affected by contact with the industrial world. Individuals in other age strata (socially recognized divisons based on age)[11] are also influenced by these changes. Thus the study of change—before as well as after contact with the West— should look at the way change affects all age strata in a society and not simply the old.

Although change affects all age strata in a society, it often affects each one differently. It is possible, for example, that individuals in only one age stratum—the old, for example—will benefit from a particular type of change. Indeed, the gains of one age stratum frequently take place at the expense of another. Several cases cited in this chapter have shown how changes that widened young people's economic and political oppor-

11. An age stratum is not necessarily a social group. Nor do people in an age stratum usually have "stratum awareness"—that is, awareness that they have common interests.

tunities spelled declines in old people's economic and political power. There is also another possibility. Rather than hit various age strata differently, certain changes can have the same impact on all age strata in a society. What are gains for one age stratum, then, are gains for all—a situation that could happen, for instance, if economic changes raised everyone's standard of living.

The very fact that some age strata enjoy gains or suffer losses as a result of change has implications for social relations. This area too needs to be explored. How do changes affect relations among age strata? Do these relations become more relaxed or do they become more tension-ridden? This question is especially pertinent in cases where members of one age stratum increase their prestige, authority, or wealth while members of another age stratum experience social losses. And how do changes affect relations *within* an age stratum? After all, gains or losses are seldom evenly distributed among individuals in an age stratum. Do tensions or conflicts develop or increase between people of similar age when one becomes more successful and another less successful as a result of change?

Another question worth pursuing is how age norms in a society influence the course of change. Age norms are social rules about what people in each age stratum ought to do. Members of each age stratum are expected to fill certain roles and to act in a manner that is appropriate to their age and age-related roles. As I showed in discussing the modernization model, age norms often shift as a society undergoes social, political, and economic changes. In many societies, notions of what roles were fitting for the aged and whether respect and influence were due them changed as their economic, political, and ritual authority was undercut and as new ideas and values spread. But while age norms frequently bend with the times, they sometimes remain relatively unaffected by change, and they can even retard the pace of change. Cultural traditions, we know, often die hard, and age norms are no exception. The idea that old age deserves respect and deference, for example, is strongly rooted in some places, especially when seniors are still believed to have moral and mystical power over their descendants (see Wilson 1977:105). Despite blows to the economic and political authority of older people, members of a society may still feel that younger people should defer to the elderly.

When we analyze change it is also crucial to consider that age systems are systems of structured inequality, and that the way individuals in a society respond to various events and changes may depend on their location in the system of age inequality.[12] Age strata in a society have un-equal access to highly valued roles and social rewards. Those on top of the age hierarchy want to safeguard their privileges, while subordinate age strata often want a larger share of the social goods of their society.

Introducing the notion of age inequality—or age stratification—raises important questions about the processes of change that require further investigation. How does position in an age hierarchy influence reactions to political, social, and economic pressures and trends? And how can these reactions further affect the course of change? Members of advan-taged or disadvantaged age strata often "seize the time," responding to new values, opportunities, and allies so as to preserve or improve their position. Sometimes, for example, the elderly champion customary ways—such as rituals or political arrangements—that ensure their domi-nance and privileges. In other cases, the old, as well as younger people, support and actively promote changes—the introduction of Christianity, for example, or the creation of new political roles—that enable them to hold onto or expand their influence and prestige. They may even intro-duce innovations for this purpose. Whether or not efforts to bolster the traditional order or bring about innovations are successful obviously de-pends on a wide variety of factors. What is significant is that such attempts are made and that they can help to mold social, political, and economic developments in a society.

Finally, there is the importance of cohort succession. I have already discussed at length how cohort differences can both reflect and lead to change. Closer attention to the processes of cohort succession will, I believe, significantly broaden the anthropological study of change. We need more systematic and finely drawn studies, with considerable time depth, that detail how various cohorts have been affected by the social changes they experienced as they grew up and matured. Of special in-terest is how social changes can shape the size and composition of cohorts and the abilities of cohort members. We need to know more, as well, about how the size and composition of cohorts and the capacities of cohort members can go on to bring pressure for further change.

In these concluding remarks, I have raised a number of questions about change that follow from a study of age and age-related processes. As anthropologists explore the theoretical significance of age for our under-standing of social change, they will undoubtedly pose additional ques-

12. For a general theoretical discussion of age inequality, see A. Foner 1975, 1979. See N. Foner 1982 and 1984 for an analysis of age inequalities in nonindustrial societies.

tions about change that can enrich the work of their own as well as other disciplines.

REFERENCES

Achenbaum, W. Andrew
1978   Old Age in the New Land: The American Experience since 1790. Baltimore: Johns Hopkins University Press.
Achenbaum, W. Andrew, and Peter Stearns
1978   Old age and modernization. Gerontologist 18:307–12.
Amoss, Pamela
1981   Coast Salish elders. *In* Other Ways of Growing Old, ed. Amoss and Stevan Harrell, pp. 227–47. Stanford: Stanford University Press.
Bledsoe, Caroline H.
1980   Women and Marriage in Kpelle Society. Stanford: Stanford University Press.
Cowgill, Donald O.
1974   Aging and modernization: A revision of the theory. *In* Communities and Environmental Policy, ed. Jaber F. Gubrium, pp. 124–46. Springfield, Ill.: Charles C. Thomas.
Cowgill, Donald O., and Lowell Holmes
1972   Summary and conclusions: The theory in review. *In* Aging and Modernization, ed. Cowgill and Holmes, pp. 305–23. New York: Appleton-Century-Crofts.
Fischer, David Hackett
1978   Growing Old in America. Expanded ed. New York: Oxford University Press.
Foner, Anne
1975   Age in society: Structure and change. American Behavioral Scientist 19:144–66.
1978   Age stratification and the changing family. American Journal of Sociology 84 (suppl.): S340–65.
1979   Ascribed and achieved bases of stratification. Annual Review of Sociology 5:219–42.
1982   Perspectives on changing age systems. *In* Aging from Birth to Death, vol. 2: Sociotemporal Perspectives, ed. Matilda White Riley, Ronald Abeles, and Michael Teitelbaum, pp. 217–28. Boulder: Westview Press.
Foner, Anne, and David Kertzer
1979   Intrinsic and extrinsic sources of change in life-course transitions. *In* Aging from Birth to Death: Interdisciplinary Perspectives, ed. Matilda White Riley, pp. 121–36. Boulder: Westview Press.

Foner, Nancy
  1982   Some consequences of age inequality in nonindustrial societies. *In* Aging from Birth to Death, vol. 2: Sociotemporal Perspectives, ed. Matilda White Riley, Ronald Abeles, and Michael Teitelbaum, pp. 71–85. Boulder: Westview Press.
  1984   Ages in Conflict: A Cross-Cultural Perspective on Inequality between Old and Young. New York: Columbia University Press.
Fowler, Loretta
  1982   Arapahoe Politics, 1851–1978: Symbols in Crises of Authority. Lincoln: University of Nebraska Press.
Goodwin, Grenville
  1942   The Social Organization of the Western Apache. Chicago: University of Chicago Press.
Goody, Jack
  1976   Aging in nonindustrial societies. *In* Handbook of Aging and the Social Sciences, ed. Robert H. Binstock and Ethel Shanas, pp. 117–29. New York: Van Nostrand Reinhold.
Hughes, Charles
  1961   The concept and use of time in the middle years: The St. Lawrence Island Eskimos. *In* Aging and Leisure, ed. R. W. Kleemeier, pp. 91–95. New York: Oxford University Press.
Keith, Jennie
  1980   "The best is yet to be": Toward an anthropology of age. Annual Review of Anthropology 9:339–64.
Kertzer, David I.
  1982   Generation and age in cross-cultural perspective. *In* Aging from Birth to Death, vol. 2: Sociotemporal Perspectives, ed. Matilda White Riley, Ronald Abeles, and Michael Teitelbaum, pp. 27–50. Boulder: Westview Press.
Laslett, Peter
  1976   Societal development and aging. *In* Handbook of Aging and the Social Sciences, ed. Robert H. Binstock and Ethel Shanas, pp. 87–116. New York: Van Nostrand Reinhold.
  1977   Family Life and Illicit Love in Earlier Generations. Cambridge: Cambridge University Press.
Ottenberg, Simon
  1971   Leadership and Authority in an African Society. Seattle: University of Washington Press.
Packard, Randall M.
  1980   Social change and the history of misfortune among the Bashu of eastern Zaire. *In* Explorations in African Systems of Thought, ed. Ivan Karp and Charles S. Bird, pp. 237–67. Bloomington: Indiana University Press.

Parkin, David J.
  1972   Palms, Wines, and Witnesses. San Francisco: Chandler.
Riley, Matilda White
  1978   Aging, social change, and the power of ideas. Daedalus 107:39–52.
Riley, Matilda White, Marilyn Johnson, and Anne Foner
  1972   Aging and Society: A Sociology of Age Stratification. New York:
         Russell Sage Foundation.
Rosaldo, Renato
  1980   Ilongot Headhunting, 1883–1974: A Study in Society and History.
         Stanford: Stanford University Press.
Sangree, Walter H.
  1966   Age, Prayer, and Politics in Tiriki, Kenya. Oxford: Oxford University
         Press.
Schapera, Isaac
  1971   Married Life in an African Tribe. Harmondsworth: Penguin. First pub-
         lished 1940.
Simic, Andrei
  1978   Introduction: Aging and the aged in cultural perspective. In Life's
         Career—Aging, ed. Barbara Myerhoff and Simic, pp. 9–22. Beverly
         Hills, Calif.: Sage.
Spencer, Paul
  1965   The Samburu: A Study of Gerontocracy in a Nomadic Tribe. London:
         Routledge & Kegan Paul.
Van Arsdale, Peter W.
  1981   The elderly Asmat of New Guinea. In Other Ways of Growing Old,
         ed. Pamela Amoss and Stevan Harrell, pp. 111–24. Stanford: Stanford
         University Press.
Waring, Joan
  1975   Social replenishment and social change: The problem of disordered
         cohort flow. American Behavioral Scientist 9:237–56.
Williams, Gerry C.
  1980   Warriors no more: A study of the American Indian elderly. In Aging in
         Culture and Society, ed. Christine L. Fry, pp. 101–11. New York: J.
         F. Bergin.
Wilson, Monica
  1977   For Men and Elders. London: International African Institute.

Part Three / Age and Culture

8

Age and Linguistic Change

Penelope Eckert

Aging and age differences are important in a variety of areas of linguistic study, but linguists have yet to develop an explicit and coherent picture of linguistic behavior through the life span. Although knowledge of linguistic phenomena specific to particular age groups abounds, this knowledge has not been integrated into a lifelong developmental scheme. Such an integration will require the systematic study of a wider range of age groups and a social theory of aging to provide context and explanation for the linguistic findings. Among the subfields of linguistics, sociolinguistics stands to gain perhaps the most from such a theory, since age is one of the most important independent variables in the study of sociolinguistic variation. Ambiguities that arise in any study that relates behavior differences to age differences therefore surface regularly in the study of sociolinguistic variation. This discussion will focus on the sociolinguistic study of linguistic change—particularly sound change—as an area of linguistics that stands particularly to benefit from increased anthropological understanding of aging.

The Ambiguity of Age Differences

The problem of the status of age as an independent variable arises in any study that relates behavior differences to age differences. Age dif-

219

ferences have the dynamic and ambiguous possibility of representing at once different developmental stages, age-dependent differences in orientation to social and linguistic phenomena (age grading), changes in cognitive style and in cognitive and motor capacity, and historical change in apparent time. These factors, furthermore, are not mutually exclusive. While some historical changes may affect the speech only of those whose linguistic system is in the early stages of development, other changes could conceivably influence the speech of a larger segment of the community. And although these factors can be isolated in theory, they cannot always be observed separately in the speech of the individual or the community, for some features may be attributable to more than one of these factors simultaneously. Baby talk, for example, can be not only a stage in the acquisition of language but a register, and children moving out of the baby-talk stage have been observed to shift between baby talk and more adult talk, perhaps as a way of negotiating the change in life stage. This is an example not only of the influence of the speaker's age (or life stage) on speech, but also of that of the addressee, for speakers frequently adjust their speech according to expectations about appropriate behavior toward members of different age groups. Post-baby-talk children (Gleason 1973) and adults (Ferguson 1964) frequently use baby talk to children, and people of most ages tend to speak in a more conservative or formal style to the aged (for a summary of speech differences according to the age of both speaker and addressee, see Helfrich 1979). They may also use baby talk to mitigate their change in life stage. The actual tracing of individual linguistic development, therefore, will involve the interaction of all factors.

This interaction is of pressing importance to the sociolinguistic theory of linguistic change, especially since the relation between social variation and historical change is of major concern to this field. The absence of a strong theory of linguistic aging currently limits researchers to a fragmented view of age differences in language.

The Social Motivations of Sound Change

The community studies that comprised the early phase of work on sociolinguistic variation showed that selected features of linguistic form covary not only with region but with certain broad categories, particularly age, sex, ethnicity, and socioeconomic class. In recent years sociolinguists have focused particular attention on the fact that much of this variation is not only an expression of social differences but the manifestation of linguistic change in progress.

Since historically significant linguistic changes travel great distances over fairly long periods of time, for the purposes of this discussion it is useful to think in terms of a given linguistic change traveling through communities of speakers and across geographic space. When I speak of change I am referring here to the propagation rather than the initiation of change. Ideally, a linguistic change can be traced as it spreads through social and geographic space, and the correlation of innovative form with social categories and groups within that space will indicate the relative chronology of the adoption of the change by different segments of society. The salience of social categories in linguistic change is at least twofold: a person's place in a social matrix through which linguistic change is spreading is determined by that individual's social contacts, and by the particular social networks in which he or she participates. Individuals will be actually exposed to a change with sufficient intensity and intimacy at different times, depending on when it travels to their location in the social matrix. In addition, as a change spreads through social networks, it becomes popularly associated with the social categories that have adopted it. Therefore, the individual's reaction to a given change will be colored by (1) the social connotations that particular change has acquired during its recent travels and (2) the recipient's own social identity and resulting reactions to the connotations of the change.

Adoption of a linguistic change is an expression of affiliation in the social category (or categories) associated with that change. To the extent that our social networks are heterogeneous, our use of a new form will be more conservative than that of some people we interact with, and less conservative than that of others. Insofar as our social orientations shift when we interact with various people and in various situations, our use of innovative variables will shift. Much of what we recognize as shifting between formal and familiar speech styles involves a movement back and forth in linguistic time: formal speech tends to shift to historically conservative forms. Each individual's speech, therefore, represents a tiny piece of history, contextualized within the larger but still tiny piece of history represented by the speech of the various social categories that make up the community. The correlation of patterns of linguistic variation with the individual's place in the social structure allows us to examine social forces in change, and the accumulation of such correlations is allowing us to move from description into the development of social theories of the spread of sound change. Social categories presumably function in the spread of change as determinants both of the frequency and intensity of the contact required for transmission of change and of those aspects of social identity that lead speakers to be variously influenced by the speech of those with whom they come into contact.

Social Categories and Sound Change

The social categories that have been found so far to correlate fairly consistently with linguistic variation are socioeconomic class, ethnicity, sex, and age. These factors combine with linguistic variants to form a cross-cutting system of social markers. These markers are organized into a kind of cognitive social map of the flow of linguistic change. The relations among these markers can be relatively complex, since they can all interact differently with linguistic form.

Socioeconomic class defines the general grid through which sound change travels. Degree of innovation generally correlates inversely with socioeconomic level, indicating that most sound change spreads upward through the socioeconomic hierarchy. The picture of sound change that prevails in sociolinguistic thought is that regular changes ("natural" changes, according to Kroch 1978) enter communities through the upper working class and move upward through the socioeconomic hierarchy. These changes remain relatively unconscious to the speakers until they reach the lower middle class, by which time they have become stigmatized through their association with working-class speech. At that point they can become relatively conscious social markers and spread with somewhat more difficulty, at times even becoming reversed (Labov 1972b). Changes that respond to prestige norms (and that are frequently reactions to changes moving upward) tend to originate in the lower middle and middle classes and move downward (Labov 1972a). Such changes tend to rely more on conscious effort, and although it is assumed that natural changes can begin in the middle class, observations so far indicate that they rarely do so. As a result, linguistic variation is overwhelmingly associated with socioeconomic class, and stylistic variation is undoubtedly associated in the speakers' minds above all with socioeconomic mobility.

Because ethnicity plays a more varied role from community to community and from ethnic group to ethnic group than the more crosscutting category of socioeconomic class, it plays a wider variety of roles in sociolinguistic variation. Ethnicity can play a great or a negligible role in variation; it can speed up or slow down the propagation of a change (as illustrated by Irish and Jewish speakers' reactions to vocalic variables in New York City [Labov 1966]), or it can foster the development of altogether different dialect features, as in the case of American Black English.

Sex shows what appears at the moment to be a fairly consistent influence: women in general show more advanced linguistic patterns than men of comparable social categories. Women, however, also show greater style shifting toward the conservative end of the spectrum in formal speech. In other words, women show a broader stylistic range than men, a range that makes them historically both more innovative and more conservative.

Age differences, inasmuch as they crosscut synchrony and diachrony, hold a key to and a particularly problematic position in the study of linguistic change in progress. Correlations of linguistic variation with age categories are ambiguously a result of age as a reflection of apparent time and of age as a social category. To date, only the former has been systematically treated in linguistic studies. Data on variation do in fact generally indicate a regular inverse correlation between age and linguistic innovation. Thus, by and large, sociolinguists have been encouraged to think of age differences in speech as representing above all change in apparent time. An understanding of age as a social category, however, plays an implicit role in theories of the social constraints on linguistic change, particularly inasmuch as sociolinguists have spent time considering the age categories in which linguistic change takes place. Such considerations are part of a general interest nowadays in explaining the relation between social categories and linguistic change.

In the early stages of sociolinguistics, the attempt to view language in a dynamic framework led to a static treatment of the social categories—a treatment that is now becoming more informed as we understand more and more the interactions between linguistic and social dynamics. Most work in recent years has been aimed at breaking down the broad social categories to identify the specific social processes that affect linguistic behavior. Most of this effort so far has concentrated on the components of socioeconomic class and the social relations that enter into that larger grid. Linguists have also become increasingly sensitive to interactions among the categories of social influence on language change. Lesley Milroy and Sue Margrain (1978), for instance, have found that certain sex differences in dialectal features of English spoken in Ireland can be explained independently of sex, in terms of differences in men's and women's local social networks. The biggest problem is perhaps the separation of these social factors from each other, and the isolation within each broad category of the actual social influences that make that category linguistically salient.

The biological categories of sex and age have been the least creatively treated in sociolinguistics, perhaps because their biological basis allows researchers to assume that they accurately classify individuals, whereas nonascriptive categories present a categorization problem from the start. The acceptance of biological categories as sufficiently representing social categories creates increasing problems as researchers give increasing consideration to the reasons that such categories make people behave linguistically as they do. Various linguists have explained sex differences in speech, for example, on the basis of differences in aspirations, roles, and orientation to society. Clearly, social gender is the category in question, rather than biological sex. Insofar as individuals' linguistic behavior is part of a strategy associated with social roles, it is the roles that each individual plays that correlate with linguistic variation, and sex, like socioeconomic class, is only a rough predictor of the roles the individual will be playing.

Age presents a set of problems almost identical to those associated with sex, and clearly a coherent theory of the relation between age and social categories will lead to a more comprehensive understanding of the interaction between individuals' age and linguistic behavior. Since linguistic change serves to mark social category affiliation, the study of aging in relation to linguistic change is not separate from the study of aging in relation to other forms of social behavior.

Linguistics, like most fields, has focused on particular life stages as other interests have dictated. Although linguists thus have not consciously sketched a coherent picture of lifelong linguistic development, an implicit set of assumptions has emerged through this spotty attention to different age groups. Clearly, one problem at this stage is to disentangle myths about aging from conclusions based solidly on linguistic evidence. Another problem is to reexamine our interpretation of correlations between age and linguistic variation in the light of independent analyses of age as a social category. Finally, we can consider our conclusions about the role of aging in universal linguistic processes (such as change) on the basis of a cross-cultural aging framework. Any elucidation of the relation between life stages and social orientation will move sociolinguistics closer to an explanatory science of linguistic change.

Linguistic Change in a Life-Course Perspective

The individual learns the basic structure of his or her native language during the first few years of life, and then begins what may well be a lifelong process of elaboration. Some of this elaboration is clearly the result of a continuing acquisition process: certain parts of the linguistic system continue to develop throughout life as the individual accumulates experience with language and its use. Other parts of language may simply change along with the individual's communicative needs at various stages of life, but not necessarily as a result of any increase in skill.

After the initial acquisition of the basic system, beyond the age of about 6, the only further development required for grammatically acceptable adult speech is the ironing out of such morphological patterns as those of the English strong verbs (which have anomalous past tenses and participles, e.g., *run*) and subject-verb agreement. At the same time, the speaker increases his or her repertoire through the elaboration of basic syntactic and discourse structures. the combination of syntactic constructions, for instance, that may have been used only separately before.

One of the most important assumptions in regard to aging in linguistics has been that there is a critical age for learning language. The process of language acquisition begins the individual's linguistic life with a frenzy of activity that appears to slow down quickly after the major grammatical structures have been learned. Precious little is known about what happens to the individual's linguistic capacity or linguistic behavior after this time, but a kind of necessity seems to be built into linguists' view of the life span: everything that requires any great learning ability must happen at an early age. If it is true that the bulk of one's native language is acquired very young and that foreign languages are more easily learned during childhood, it does not necessarily follow that language development ends with childhood. It will be necessary at some point to disentangle empirical observations of linguistic behavior from the popular notion that the mind decays beyond middle age—a notion that is particularly accelerated in linguistics because of the dramatic development of the early years. David Sankoff and Rejean Lessard (1975) have shown that enrichment of vocabulary continues at least to the age of 50, and while grammatical development is most noticeable during childhood, there is no evidence that it does not continue well beyond. Studies on syntactic development beyond youth have been few and inconclusive (see Helfrich 1979), but it is nonetheless probable that speakers increase their skill in manipulating complex syntactic and discourse patterns well into adulthood.

Certainly the basic means of referential communication are acquired in the early years of childhood, and the receptivity of young children to additional languages is striking. It is possible, though, that the loss of facility in learning a second language in adulthood is the result not of a loss of some underlying language-learning ability, but simply of the differences in the social context in which children and adults learn second languages (Burling 1981).

Another kind of elaboration that follows closely on the acquisition of basic linguistic structure is the development of stylistic range, which is linked to the development of local social dialect features. While the basic linguistic skills are learned primarily from adults, the child's peers are the main force in dialect formation. Children acquire the dialect of their community, whatever their parents' dialect may be, and within the range of dialects in the community, the child's dialect comes to resemble most closely that of his or her peer group (Labov 1974, Wolfram 1969). Peer influence during dialect development seems to be strongest during pre-adolescence. It is this age group, furthermore, that shows the highest incidence of stigmatized linguistic features within their socioeconomic group (Wolfram 1969), and while some stigmatized features are stable social markers, others are innovations—changes in progress. It appears that the main impetus of sound change is focused in this group. One explanation for this observation is that the eagerness of the preadolescent society to distinguish itself from adults—and of groups of preadolescents to emphasize their own separate identity within the peer society—leads to the exaggeration of certain sound patterns (Eckert 1981). Because of the path of spread of linguistic change, any change away from adult speech will be in the direction of the lower end of the socioeconomic hierarchy. Eugene Hammel suggested at the NIA workshop that the desire for independence from adults translates into emulation of peers in lower socioeconomic strata, where children are generally more independent of parents. My own work with suburban adolescents has certainly shown it to be the case that middle-class adolescents regard working-class adolescents as free of parental domination.

An obvious conclusion is that the overwhelming innovativeness of preadolescent and adolescent speech is a result of the place of that age set in the age hierarchy. Solidarity within the age set results from its particularly powerless position in a society dominated by the middle-aged, and causes its members to develop symbolic (linguistic) means to set themselves apart as a solidary category from this power structure. If such innovation is purely a result of powerlessness, one might look to the aged in our society for parallel developments, as suggested by Keith and Kertzer's observation in the introduction to this volume that adolescence and early old age are both "periods of transition, of powerlessness, and of possible identity confusion." But other factors lead one to believe that it is the particular combination of age and powerlessness that lead to innovative linguistic strategies. The most important of these factors is that adolescents are not only trying to set themselves off from adults, they are also developing the linguistic means to set themselves off from others in their age set. It is the intensity of the more general socialization process, not just their relative powerlessness in society, that lends force to preadolescents' and adolescents' linguistic innovation. The question one might ask, though, is whether linguistic change is slower in societies where the young are less excluded from adult power. To go further, within our own society, one might consider the possibility that the observed greater receptivity of working-class speakers to linguistic change is a result of greater peer solidarity than exists among middle-class adolescents; and if so, whether peer solidarity is a result of greater accentuation in working-class families of the hierarchical aspect of age that Basil Bernstein has so heavily emphasized (1971).

There lingers, after all the social motivations for linguistic innovation among preadolescents and adolescents, the possibility that this kind of linguistic elaboration follows so closely on the initial acquisition of language as part of the necessary flow of linguistic development. If social motivations for linguistic innovations are indeed identical in old age and adolescence, it still remains an empirical question whether the kinds of systematic and motor controls required to develop the complex phonological patterns characteristic of linguistic variation can be developed at any age, or whether they are significantly greater in youth.

During and after adolescence, the extreme pattern of innovation is gradually tempered as speakers encounter a wider range of speech styles. Exposure to people from a wider social range seems to introduce the second (and longer) phase of dialect acquisition—the adjustment of speech patterns to the norms of the wider community.

The continual question of language-learning ability translates most clearly into innovation-learning ability at the point where speakers begin to outgrow their innovative patterns, for all of this adjustment is regarded as a reversal of linguistic patterns that have become natural during the crucial dialect-learning period of preadolescence. This reversal is considered to rely on somewhat conscious effort, and while a small amount of work indicates that this is so (Mahl 1972, cited in Kroch 1978), our understanding of dialect-formation processes beyond preadolescence is weak. Not only is there no conclusive evidence of this phase of linguistic development, there is nothing to substantiate the generally accepted claim that this linguistic retrenchment is less systematic than the period of innovation that precedes it.

It is generally accepted that speech becomes more conservative as people enter the work force and seek to raise their employment and social status. This alteration of dialect represents an increased repertoire: the addition of a wider variety of styles in the ranges of careful speech to serve the demands of an increasing range of social contacts. And while most of this alteration seems to be aimed at the conservative end of the speech continuum, there is also no doubt an important development of style toward the innovative end. To the extent that the amount of correction corresponds to the individual's or the cohort's entry into an upwardly mobile lifestyle, the onset of this period of correction will depend on how and when such entry begins. It should be emphasized that while linguistic correction associated with upward mobility is aimed at an external norm, there is no reason to assume that—at least for many people—the conservative linguistic behavior is not as much a peer-group phenomenon as it is aimed at the normative group.

It is assumed that middle-class speakers (who acquire in preadolescence a form of speech that is historically advanced for their middle-class community) begin to correct their speech earlier than working-class speakers, because there is more correction and influence from prestigious speech in their homes and neighborhoods. And it has been postulated (Wolfram and Fasold 1974) that upper-middle-class speakers tend to reduce their style shifting toward the end of college, at which time they have had maximum exposure to the patterns of style shifting to the extent that upward mobility continues to necessitate linguistic adjustment. The chronological boundaries of linguistic age cohorts may differ from one social class to another because of the differential entry times into different sectors. Thus entrance into the relative power structure of the middle-aged life stage may bring increasing conservatism—that is, decreasing localism—in one's speech. David Sankoff and Suzanne Laberge (1978) have examined the relation between patterns of sociolinguistic variation and degree of involvement in the standard language marketplace, an important step toward the recognition that broad social categories such as age and socioeconomic class interact over more basic issues of linguistic needs.

This notion of linguistic marketplace takes on added interest when one considers the implications of retirement for linguistic development. Relatively little has been written about dialect development beyond the corrective phase in early adulthood. But insofar as linguistic correction is spurred by participation in normative social roles, one might expect the changing social role participation associated with retirement and old age to be accompanied by changes in linguistic orientation. William Labov has observed (1972a) that older men's linguistic behavior seems to relax along with their concern for power relationships. Some of the data in community studies do suggest that older speakers relax in their speech, but since most of these studies group together all speakers over the age of 50 or 60, it is impossible to see potential differences between those who are still functioning fully in their middle-aged roles and those who are in complete or partial retirement, and between those who have acquired new roles in old age and those who have not.

The elderly, being the farthest from the experience of young and middle-aged researchers, comprise the age group that is most subject to stereotyping in linguistic as well as in other research. Linguistic evidence is thin for this age group, and so is serious speculation, although there are a number of intriguing possibilities to consider. For instance, it is possible that the age solidarity that has been observed in retirement communities may encourage substantial changes in linguistic patterns. There is no particular reason for these changes to be historically innovative, but they may nonetheless be innovative for the speakers themselves. Insofar as increased age brings people closer to being the conservative norm setters of the language, the oldest age groups in a community will be native speakers of the most conservative local dialects in their particular socioeconomic strata. Certain of these conservative patterns may become intensified as an expression of age-set solidarity.

Conclusion

I have referred to the particular life stages of childhood, preadolescence, adolescence, early adulthood, middle age, old age. In the final analysis, these and related stages may not be clearly associated with linguistic differences, and linguists will eventually have to shift their perspective to the roles and linguistic needs associated with life stages. No one should be more sensitive to the fluidity of the boundaries between life stages than the sociolinguist, who is a major adovocate of attention to fluidity within the subject matter of linguistics. Each individual enters each stage of life at his or her own time, rather than at a given age, and gradually, role by role. Thus linguistic behavior may depend not only on one's age or apparent stage of life, but on one's relation to a variety of roles associated with given life stages. One may be adult in the domestic but not the external domain, or vice versa; one may play some adult roles in a given domain but not in others. And certainly the gradual progress from one life stage to the next will be different for members of different social categories, and the implications of each stage for these categories may differ radically.

Not only the boundaries of life stages are gradual; so are the boundaries of age cohorts. And inasmuch as the cohort accelerates linguistic change at least partially as an expression of age solidarity, this can be a very suggestive fact for linguists. The description of the cohort will vary not only according to historical time and place but according to the cohort unit. My work in the Detroit suburbs has already suggested that working-class adolescents function in age-heterogeneous networks, whereas middle-class adolescents restrict their associations more to people of precisely their own age. The implications of this difference in social networks for linguistic change are complex, for while on the one hand one may speculate that a large cohort would make for increased linguistic conservatism, on the other hand this large cohort will give working-class speakers a stronger sense of cohort strength and allow them to innovate with greater confidence. Relations between generations, furthermore, are not the same in all social categories, so not all cohort units will involve themselves equally eagerly in linguistic change. Important external events that bind together large age ranges into a cohort, furthermore, over time will change the configuration of age groups that respond linguistically to these events.

Two areas of study would best respond to the most immediate needs for understanding the role of aging in linguistic change: (1) the lack of information about the language of older speakers must be corrected, and (2) the social correlates of aging in linguistic variation must be explored directly, with careful attention to the difficulties involved in equating biological and social categories.

One reason for the lack of information about patterns of variation of older speakers has been the difficulty of gathering a sample of older speakers equivalent to that of younger speakers within a community, particularly because of the sociolinguistic requirement that speakers be natives of the community under study. To solve this problem of numbers, sociolinguists commonly group older speakers in larger age chunks, and therefore virtually nothing is known of linguistic differences among older age groups. Another serious obstacle to the study of the speech of the elderly has been the implicit assumption that the elderly lack the physiological and/or mental capacity to modify their dialects significantly. It is probably safe to say that less is known about developments in linguistic capacity than about the other aspects of language and aging, and the reasons that linguists do not study the language of the elderly today are probably not significantly different from the reasons that they did not study the language of minorities a generation ago.

Insofar as sociolinguists takes as a first principle that speakers linguistically respond to and manipulate their social status, it is obvious that they should be looking to the elderly in our society for verification of some of their fundamental assumptions. It is generally acknowledged nowadays that retirement is one of the most problematic life events, and among the most shocking changes in social status. If changes in speech are thought to accompany changes in status, retirement should be of primary interest to the sociolinguist. A study of linguistic variation as a function of retirement would provide information not only about retirement itself as a linguistically significant state but about the significance of the workplace as a linguistic influence for all age groups. The full force of the role of aging in linguistic change, of course, cannot be evaluated until our models transcend the institutions of our own society. Still a new field, the study of sociolinguistic variation has not yet developed a significant cross-cultural perspective. The study of linguistic variation in cultures with different age-grading systems would shed a good deal of light on the role of aging in linguistic change.

It is actually difficult to separate the needs of understanding the relation between language and aging from the general needs of sociolinguistics. Age cannot be isolated from other social variables that constrain sociolinguistic variation. The salience of socioeconomic class varies with time of life; the salience of age varies with socioeconomic milieu. The same applies to sex and ethnicity. The clearest need in sociolinguistics is to clarify the relation between biological age and social age. So long as linguists appeal to age grading to explain age differences in linguistic patterns, they need a clearer understanding of the social significance of age groups in our culture. Such understanding requires careful study of the linguistic requirements of the varying life stages in all segments of society. The interactions of age with other parameters that affect linguistic variation are clearly endless. Increasing sophistication about the specific content of each of these parameters will eventually lead sociolinguistics to more precise and explanatory formulations of the social motivations of linguistic change. It is apparent that the framework offered by an anthropology of aging will provide a very crucial—and to date a largely ignored—component of the social explanation of linguistic change.

REFERENCES

Bernstein, Basil
    1971   Class, Codes, and Control, vol. 1: Theoretical Studies toward a Sociology of Language. London: Routledge & Kegan Paul.
Burling, Robbins
    1981   The social constraints on adult language learning. Annals of the New York Academy of Sciences 379:279–90.
Eckert, Penelope
    1981   Language development and linguistic change. Paper delivered at the Tenth Annual Conference on New Ways of Analyzing Variation in English, Philadelphia.
Ferguson, Charles
    1964   Baby talk in six languages. American Anthropologist 66:103.
Gleason, Jean Berko
    1973   The acquisition of code-switching ability. In Cognitive Problems and the Acquisition of Language, ed. T. E. Moore, pp.159–67. New York: Academic Press.
Helfrich, Hede
    1979   Age markers in speech. In Social Markers in Speech, ed. Klaus R. Scherer and Howard Giles, pp. 63–108. Cambridge: Cambridge University Press.
Kroch, Anthony
    1978   Toward a theory of social dialect variation. Language in Society 7:17–36.
Labov, William
    1966   The Social Stratification of English in New York City. Washington, D.C.: Center for Applied Linguistics.
    1972a   Hypercorrection by the lower middle class as a factor in linguistic

change. *In* Sociolinguistic Patterns, ed. Labov, pp. 122–42. Philadelphia: University of Pennsylvania Press.

1972b On the Mechanism of Linguistic Change. *In* Sociolinguistic Patterns, ed. Labov, pp. 160–82. Philadelphia: University of Pennsylvania Press.

1974 Language change as a form of communication. *In* Human Communication: Theoretical Explorations, ed. M. Silverstein. Hillsdale, N.J.: Lawrence Erlbaum.

Mahl, G.
1972 People talking when they can't hear their voices. *In* Studies in Dyadic Communication, ed. P. Siegman and B. Pope. New York: Pergamon Press.

Milroy, Lesley
1980 Language and Social Networks. London: Blackwell.

Milroy, Lesley, and Sue Margrain
1978 Vernacular language loyalty and social network. Language in Society 9 (1):43.

Sankoff, David, and Suzanne Laberge
1978 The linguistic market and the statistical explanation of variability. *In* Linguistic Variation: Models and Methods, ed. Sankoff, pp. 239–50.

Sankoff, David, and Rejean Lessard
1975 Vocabulary richness: A sociolinguistic analysis. Science 190:680.

Wolfram, Walt
1969 A Sociolinguistic Description of Detroit Negro Speech. Washington: Center for Applied Linguistics.

Wolfram, Walt, and Ralph Fasold
1974 The Study of Social Dialects in American English. Englewood Cliffs, N.J.: Prentice-Hall.

9

Age and Culture as Theory

Ronald Cohen

Although anthropologists have long elaborated theories about culture, they have not adequately considered culture as theory or policy. Viewed this way, culture offers moral understandings and explanations of human experience (R. Cohen 1981:206–8). These theories cum policies are found in the literary traditions, myths, legends, and folklore of a community and both influence and are affected by physical and social experience. The plot, the characters, and the outcomes provide the expressive mode for declaring the policy. The elements are not precise; the meanings can shift and change as required. In this sense, the social theory carried in traditions is a living, evolving corpus of guidelines, lessons, or moral precepts, guiding and responding to the community's encounters with varying conditions over time.

Greater attention to age in anthropological research leads to fuller understanding of culture as theory and policy in several ways. First, the variation in norms and explanations about aging and the position of the aged highlights diversity in cultural theories; and examination of the relationship between norms and behaviors, or theory and practice, reveals conditions under which cultural policies are implemented in varying degrees. Second, aging is an ideal focus for the broadest questions about culture as theory or policy for action because it is both universal and

234

elemental. There are three ways in which aging and age can be examined from the perspective of culture as policy: age roles and norms; phenomenology of aging; and aging as an independent variable to whose physical effects cultural theories respond.[1] In traditional anthropological style, I shall approach these three issues from the perspective of my own fieldwork in West Africa.

Roles of the Aged and Norms for Their Treatment

Data from West Africa indicate that, as conventional wisdom in gerontology states, the status of many of the aged does tend to decline with urbanization and modernization. Housing shortages, high divorce rates, and physical mobility are leading old people into destitution and abandonments, in some cases for the first time. This is especially true for older women, divorced after or around menopause, whose children may have moved to another town. The impersonality and growing heterogeneity of such towns is associated with widespread destitution (Hardiman n.d.). The problem is exacerbated by the fact that community leaders deny its existence, claiming that African extended families have always cared for and respected their older members. Only in alienated "white" society, they say, is old age a problem. No matter how urban or Westernized people are, however, cults of the dead tend to protect and enhance the status of the aged. In Freetown (A. Cohen 1980) old Creole family houses cannot be sold without the consent of the dead who reside there, and who must be persuaded to move. As a result of this custom, many old houses remain in the central city, and older people have an important role to play as intermediaries between the living and the dead. Belief in the power of the dead to do great harm should they be angered, thwarted, or disobeyed is very strong. This belief produces important functions and powers for the aged people in each household, making them central to economic planning.

In Buraland in northeastern Nigeria, where I carried out intensive fieldwork (1972–74) among a people partly centralized and Muslim, partly uncentralized, both groups perceive close links between the living and the dead, especially the recently deceased older generation. Their

---

1. By restricting myself to sociocultural materials, I purposely exclude biological, demographic, and macroeconomic aspects of aging. Although essential to its understanding, these fields are peripheral to my competence.

advice, blessings, and wishes are constantly sought in a compound shrine tended by the eldest or most senior male member. The immanence of the dead is a clear and powerfully felt force in everyday life. Manipulation of their alleged wishes is part of the politics of everyday life, and interpretation of the will of the dead is a language for personal and factional conflict and competition.

The Bura have very widely ramifying exogamy rules, forbidding marriage within one's lineage and clan segment. The elders of each lineage carry the genealogical knowledge necessary to sanction or prohibit marriages. In the 1970s, university-trained young people attempted unsuccessfully to abrogate the wider exogamy relations, thus narrowing the number of forbidden mates. The elders realized the reform was a threat to their power, fought it bitterly, and won. Even today, therefore, a Bura couple must check with home-based elders who can assess the legitimacy of the union if they wish to have their marriage sanctioned and blessed in Buraland.

Such situations are not new. My own data corroborate previous findings that in many traditional societies, older people, especially men in lineage-based systems, generally increase their status with age. The idealized norm, however, is not universally achieved. Even in these simple and so-called homogeneous societies, some men and women fail in life, and live out their days with few supporters and an insecure subsistence. Extreme poverty has been rare, but not every man becomes an "elder" in his own lineage. A few people do not accumulate enough supporters, enough of a reputation for wise choices, or enough experience to provide a storehouse of information on options when decisions are in order. Such men and women do not benefit from the norms of increased status associated with age.

Most people, however, men especially, do gain the benefits of old age, for several reasons. First there is the pride each corporate lineage takes in itself vis-à-vis other lineages. To honor its older members, to give them respect, and to demand respect from others are part of their corporate identity. In a lineage-based society respect for the older members of one's own group is thus part of pride and loyalty to one's own self-identification with the society's basic age policy. In effect, aging (before senility or other major age-related disabilities) is associated with eldership—increased leadership, respect, wisdom, experience, and supernatural powers stemming from proximity to the recent dead.

Among the Bura this entire complex of aging, respect, and increased status for older people is enhanced by the dramaturgy of funerals. Thirty days after a person's death a special ceremony is held to celebrate the end of mourning, to settle the estate, including the negotiation of leviratic unions, and to pay last respects to the dead. Lineage mates and joking relations (a special form of affinal and matrifilial kin) enact scenes from the life of the deceased. His exploits in hunting, warfare, decision making, and wife capture are recalled by actors who use his weapons and even dress or walk as he did. Joking relations also recall more shameful or humorous events and go about saying that all should be forgotten, that the deceased was not that important anyway and will not be missed. Should these insults become too difficult to swallow, violence may break out.[2] People say that these enactments help as well to introduce the deceased to his new community among the dead.

The important point is one that is universal, although the Bura seem to have elaborated it enormously. The culture produces a spur to each person to play the game of life as well and as close to the cultural ideal as possible. As people age in Bura, they become increasingly aware, even concerned, about the *kuri twa* (life drama) to be portrayed during their own oncoming funerals. At that time a ridiculous, weak, poorly performed old age will undoubtedly be remembered, commented on, even exemplified in theatrical form before the entire community.

Although such concerns are less important to young people, especially Western-educated ones, many contemporary old people feel very strongly that the traditional (pre-Islamic, pre-Christian) funeral must be performed in their own case. In one instance a man demanded such a funeral as his dying wish. His Christian family decided against it. Within the next four months, seventeen grass-roofed huts caught fire among the members of this particular lineage. The various diagnoses and countermoves showed that the man who had held the dying relative—the one who had listened and agreed to the request—had a spirit familiar. The spirit was carrying out the vengeance of the dead man against his lineage mates for not performing a traditional funeral. Vengeance was required particularly for failure to perform the ritualized dramaturgy of the deceased's life accomplishments, which he had specially requested.

I interpret this episode to mean that the more funeral practices dramatize a person's successes and failures, the more aging will be associated

2. Thoughtful Bura say that these shameful statements help people get over their grief. They may also make explicit secret ambivalence felt by the survivors about the death of their relative.

with attempts to achieve culturally idealized norms of behavior. Funerary practices can help to maintain the individual within community norms, counteracting disengagement from the expectations of his or her age-related roles. Postmortal judgments of all kinds do the same thing to a community of believers.

The general theoretical point being illustrated is a comparative one. We have still to examine carefully what modes of behavior and ideology human groups have evolved to constrain age-related roles. The example of a theatricalized funeral service used to spur people on to a conforming old age indicates that we still have things to learn about the variance of adjustments already made in various communities.

Age as Inner Experience

The experience of old age is a function of the specific context in which the person finds herself or himself, the kinds of decisions each must make, and the particular theory a person develops and accepts about how the later phases of life should be carried on. L. Auerbach (1981) puts it very well:

> In their typification of the appropriateness of life events, individuals are guided by practical theories about living. Through such theories people make sense of their experience, discover continuities or discontinuities between past and present, and predict how these will affect future events. Making such theories of life change requires constant interpretation and re-interpretation of past, present, and future events so that these events will be seen as a developmental process. While this process is subjective, individuals do not act alone but are joined in constructing such theories by others in their social environment.

The difficulty is to tap this inner experience in order to understand how, why, and when decisions and theories are applied, and why they change. Below I have transcribed material from Bura life histories taken in 1973 from village men and women, all of whom were over 70 at the time. At or near the end of their accounts many were stimulated to comment on their present lives. They did so honestly and thoughtfully, often using events to make a more general point.[3]

3. I have altered the language toward standard English in order to catch the emotional connotations of the original interviews.

A Village Woman Adjusts to a New Age Status

When my husband died [1968] his patrilineal kin decided that I should *not* be inherited [by his brother] because I was too old and should go instead to live with my oldest son, Yamta [in the same village]. I moved there and was treated well.

Yamta's wives would not allow me to cook and provided me with food. All I could do was to thread cotton part of the time. I wasn't allowed to help on the household farm plots, or to have my own farm. Soon I got fed up and asked for more work, because I was used to it, but my son said no.

My son also ordered me to urinate and defecate in a pit latrine *inside the compound.* I said I could not mix my stools with those of other people—I must go alone to the bush to excrete. I then left that town to go to my son Garga's compound, fifteen miles away, where life is more as it used to be. But it was very difficult. Garga had three wives. On the surface, they were friendly, but they were never open or intimate. I kept losing my temper at everything they did—because old people behave like children again. This angered them and so we quarreled often. Last year [1972] I moved back to Yamta's, where I have been ever since.

Everything is going very well. I enjoy it here now—except that my eyes are getting dim and I must walk with a stick. But people here are kind and I will stay.

The message is clear. Shocked by her husband's death, she received an even worse blow: she could not remain in his lineage as a wife to one of his heirs. Even older widows are normally kept on, but for some reason she was rejected and told to live with her son by a previous marriage (he was not, that is, a member of the rejecting lineage). Her self-respect received another blow when her son ordained that his mother was to be nurtured rather than permitted to contribute normal adult energy and skills to his compound. Finally, times have changed, and her deeply rooted sense of morally appropriate personal hygiene and vulnerability has been assaulted by novel notions of toiletry practiced in her son's household. But at her other son's home there was hostility diaphanously clothed in politeness. Her ugly outbursts of temper made her realize that her own reactions to people's behavior was that of an old person. And so four years after her husband's death she accepted her new role in life, chose the best context, and settled for what she could get, a decent, kind enviornment among loved ones, while she resigned herself to the limitations of old age.

A Contented Man

I now do nothing but farm. [He had been a teacher in a primary school but had retired nearly ten years earlier.] I am healthy and strong; my [farm] plots are big; I am content. What I hate most and always avoid is trouble with others, or to be looked down on by others.

I like most to plant fruit trees for my grandchildren to use later on [when I am gone].

My desire now is that my son should finish his schooling [in England] successfully and come home to a good job while I'm still alive. It would be good if all my children got holidays at the same time so they could come home and I would see them all, and they could see each other and be together.

My sons have bought me a bicycle. I am pleased. I have wanted one for a long time but was afraid to buy it because people would gossip and ask why my sons had not bought one for me. Now all is well.

This man's health allows him an active productive role in the community. He worries only about his reputation and the continuity of his family, their ties to one another, to him, and to their birthplace. Significantly, this former schoolteacher does not mention cultural change as a problem, but the proliferation of his seed may not result in as large and powerful a group as would have been the case in days gone by. And that bothers him. Still he is indeed doing quite well.

The Man Who Learned by Making Mistakes

I was not so old [late fifties], so I married a young rebellious girl. She always insulted me. I beat her, but she abused me even more. I once became so angry that I took a knife to kill her. But I realized that I was still not old enough to be considered not responsible for my actions. Therefore, the village would punish me if I harmed her. After a while she ran away with a younger man.

Now I was old. I decided to throw out my *haptu* [ancestor shrine] and join the church where my children all go to pray. But every time I went I had terrible nightmares—lions, snakes, hyenas, and other wild beasts would come and eat me. Other times I would be on fire, consumed in flames, or under deep black waters choking to death.

I went to the bush where I had thrown the *haptu* and put it back in my compound so it would leave me alone. And there were no more terrible dreams.

Church is nice. I don't believe all those things [Christian beliefs] but it's a nice place. My children do not use the *haptu* at all. It will be buried with me or taken back to its original village, from which my lineage originally came.

Old age for this man was first rejected. He married a young girl to show himself and the world that he was still young. She was probably forced into the marriage (that point is not clear); in any case, she reacted to him as to an old and undesirable mate. The failure of the union was his lesson in accepting his new age status. His vigor meant that he must still abide by the rules, even though he could not at his age seek all the rewards of youth and maturity. Acceptance meant a new desire to conform and be with his children. But rejection of his religion led him into depths of psychological torment.

So age for him meant giving up some things, holding on to others. Only by trying and learning what works could he come to some theory of old age that applied to himself.

Old Age Is Hell

The Old Diviner Woman

> This world belongs to you, not me.
> Before it belonged to the old.
> The running of family and village affairs—
> everything came from the old people.
> People sought their advice; even poor old
> people were respected, obeyed.
> Old people were the most intelligent, most
> understanding.
> They knew more.
> Now the old have no place, they are left alone,
> neglected, uncared for, not respected.
> The new ways are good for health, bad for families,
> bad for the old.[4]

This woman inherited a *jisku* or magical divination stone from her mother. This is a ouija-like metate stone that passes from a female specialist to one of her daughters for diagnoses and divination concerning family matters—sickness, fertility, and most especially naming. The *jisku* is given a long list of names. When the new infant's "real" name is mentioned by the diviner, the stone cannot be lifted off the ground. Wrong naming is believed to result in sickness and poor growth for the

---

4. This woman's words were so poetic that I have written them in free verse format (I define poetry as an experience looking for an image or a means of verbal expression).

neonate. Such conditions therefore lead to a search for a new name, and the process is repeated.

This woman has lived her entire life in the expectation that her old age would bring respect and a steady income once she inherited the *jisku*. But the village is now largely Christian. People baptize and name babies in church; they deal with health matters in a well-run and well-equipped mission hospital. The old diagnostic procedures and naming practices are dying out. And with them has gone the old woman's entire vision of a decent and dignified old age. Her plans, well grounded in her culture, have become obsolete. She is frustrated, angry, resigned. She understands, but her theory cannot solve the problem. One is reminded of the Rawlsian conception of happiness as the capacity to make plans and carry them out.

The Lonely Old Farmer

I was poisoned six years ago. It left me with constant stomach pains and weakness. Now I am like a cripple. Ever since that terrible time I do not farm. Someone did this to me, someone who does not want me to be successful. I don't know who. I have never clashed with other men over women, nor have I ever done anything that could lead to such enmity. It was not in my food. It was thrown on a path, intended for me alone—my name was used when it [the sorcery stuff or "medicine"] was made.

At first I could not bend down to urinate and defecate. After some treatment in the mission hospital it got better. But it is still there and I cannot farm anymore. My wives farm and so we get some food. And my children, all of whom have moved away from the village, send me money regularly.

But I am very sad. My children are either working elsewhere or in school away from here. It never seems to end; they go from one school on to another one, and when they finally finish they get jobs and work in other places.

I am lonely and old. I want my children and grandchildren around me. This always makes me sad. But I do a lot of weaving and ropemaking.

Old age and infirmity hit this man suddenly; so precipitous was the change in his capacity to work that he cannot believe it was a natural set of events. Culture supplies a theory for him, but still he is troubled. Most enmity between men that can lead to sorcery involves women. Elopements are common among the Bura: men persuade women to run off with them, then arrange for a violent pseudocapture. Such activity plus homicides are the reasons most frequently given for feuds between lineages, often lasting for generations. Our farmer has avoided such hostilities—or won't admit to them. His infirmity is real; some form of illness has left him in a weakened condition. His response has been to become old and inactive.

Now he is self-consciously old and sad because his expectations of a venerable old age surrounded by descendants is an impossibility. His children have prospered; they send him money. But his expectations, normal for his culture, like those of the diviner woman, have been cut off by a new kind of scope offered to his children by a changing world. Weaving and ropemaking are activities of the disabled and the old who cannot carry out the normal productive work of adults.

The cases indicate dramatically that culture may offer channels for choice, but it does not in any meaningful way actually direct or channel the course of any particular old age. In each case there is disengagement, integration, and activity. One of these things does not exclude the others. Each context forces its participants to ask questions about what has happened, and the participants find some solution or theory to explain their predicament. When social change is severe, cutting off the past from the present, older expectations simply do not apply; the really incisive intelligent response—that of the diviner woman, for example—leads to a realization that there is no solution. She played the game according to one set of rules; history has changed the rules and she must lose out. When a theory is available that explains what has happened—it was the result of someone's evil intentions—it is actually more satisfying than a more rational response, albeit less valid empirically. Still it gives meaning to the meaningless and is therefore less frustrating. And all of these cases, the happy contented adaptations, the sad and angry old people, all of them took place in one tiny society with what anthropologists usually call a homogeneous culture. Old age is never stereotyped by culture, only guided by it. Culture is policy, not behavior (R. Cohen 1981).

Aging as an Independent Variable

In comparative theoretical terms more work needs to be done on aging as an independent variable (see Keith 1980). Gerontologists are bound to continue probing into every corner to find out what affects the aging process, what it is, and how many of its negative features can be understood and alleviated. Operationally, however, the social-anthropological task must include comparison of the observable effects of aging in different cultures and their development over time.

Some comparisons are already well developed. All societies, for example, cut the life course into grades that are determined partly by physiological aging. However culture and context may vary, basic similarities in the life cycle are a constant stimulus that makes for similar grades across societies. Infancy in one society is more like infancy in another than either is to puberty. Even though Boran boys in Ethiopia and Kenya can be initiated into old age sets, with consequent effects on their social relations, everyone still understands their chronological age and its impact on their culturally ordained age role (Legesse 1973).

Closely related to age grading is the notion of seniority or status ascribed by birth order. Grading and age sets relate cohorts by seniority, but birth order also relates individuals with families, or even with particular grade. Combined with lineages or some form of communal organization based on age, these aging effects are associated with the sociopolitical ideology of eldership. This latter concept is widespread in West Africa, China, and the Near East. Wherever it is found, it is characterized by gerontocratic principles of leadership, and all old people are highly respected. Some whose experience and success throughout life accrue extra prestige become true ''elders''—people whose advice is sought by the entire community. They give counsel to the community leadership, or become part of the leadership, and often such societies develop beliefs in which the old stand as active intermediaries between the recently deceased and the living.

Underlying these aging effects is another less well-researched factor, that of experience. The attribution of positive value to older people who are still active or capable of being active is a community's way of using an important resource. In this context, experience is the application to contemporary problems of previous solutions or modes of solution. The greater the similarity of present conditions to past ones, the greater the potential value of successful experience. Where younger, more inexperienced members must reason through each step of a decision and its possible outcomes, more experienced members know unthinkingly which outcomes are the best for the group, which will lead to disaster, and which are a waste of time and effort. Research on experience indicates that even though young people's brains work more rapidly in organic terms, older people solve problems of great complexity within their competences because of large numbers of stored outcomes already available to them through experience. Farmers or traders, for example, who must calculate profits at different market prices under differing conditions of transportation, storage, and other costs, can be divided into more and less experienced decision makers. Less experienced ones actually compute differing profit outcomes; more experienced ones do not. They have done so under so many differing conditions for so long that they know the answers without doing the actual computations (C. Gladwin, personal communication). Experienced people, therefore, do not calculate outcomes; they know from the values of inputs that they have seen many times before that outcomes are available to them without working through problems. Experience is thus a shortcut to problem solving, therefore a community resource.

These linked conceptions of seniority, eldership, and experience add depth to Simone de Beauvoir's suggestion (1972:78) that ethnologically old age is worse for nomadic than for sedentary groups. Without denying this treatment of aging as a factor dependent on ecological adaptation, I suggest that aging is tied to higher status for reasons of seniority and experience whenever continuities of adaptation are available.

The two factors that run counter to this generalization are, first, that change is always present, and second, that the old who are very infirm must be cared for and nurtured as dependent members of a community, just like children. Yesterday's adaptation may be tomorrow's maladaptation. Under conditions of rapid change, the value of experience as a communal resource is reduced. When and exactly how this decline occurs is unclear. Clearly in times of rapid economic and political change it is not always advisable to use older solutions to problems without careful consideration of their suitability. But where does such caution stop? How widely does it apply? Should a mother's advice on child training be considered out of date in a differently organized macroeconomy? Should an elder's advice on wise political behavior be ignored because the groups competing for scarce rewards differ as do the rewards themselves? Or are some forms of experience transferable across changing conditons? The durability of the Bible, the Koran, and other holy writings suggest that *plus ça change, plus c'est la même chose.* But again, how much? and why?

Even when they are valued and elaborated, seniority, eldership, and experience must sometimes bow to infirmity and the loss of skills necessary to permit the aged to participate actively in communal life. Some old people, indeed many, do not want to participate, and pull away from active interest in local affairs. Quite possibly some form of disengagement may be physiologically based, albeit variable, for old people as a group. Whatever its etiology, infirmity means that higher status given to old people can dwindle for basic physiological reasons. Within this obvious limitation, however, cultures vary enormously from murder or abandonment to a ritualized respect that maintains the higher status of old people simply because they are old. Thus Kanuri old people are revered and respected (R. Cohen 1967). They bless people by the laying on of hands; they have a special status at weddings, where their presence is believed to bring long life to the young couple. They are told of all decisions, and younger people interpret their responses as both agreement and a blessing on the enterprise. They are thus included as participants until death even when they cannot actually participate actively.

This last point brings up the problem of competence and role change. Every society must cope with the fact that persons and roles age at different rates. Some roles and organizations have short lives, so that their incumbents must be transferred to other roles. The more ubiquitous, more profound problem is that of retirement and replacement of people in roles that outlast individual life spans.

Given the universality of the problem, it is not surprising that societies develop their own theoretical explanations. These are not abstract statements of cause-and-effect relationships. Instead they involve real-life dramas of gods and goddesses, kings and princes, spirits and anthropomorphized animals. The plot, the characters, and the events and outcomes proclaim social theory and social policy. One brief example from my field data will illustrate the point.

Among the Pabir of northeastern Nigeria, just south of Borno emirate, the royal origin myth includes a well-known section on the death of the founder of the dynasty. In it the original king calls his sons together to discuss succession to the throne. He asks them to boil stones into grain balls. The youngest son achieves this impossible feat, then invites his father to come and join him. The father now knows which son will succeed him. With the help of the other sons, the king tricks his youngest into going under the straw roof of a hut under construction and burns him up after he is caught in this trap. But the son miraculously escapes and waits in a tree for people going to his funeral. He then orders them to tell the king that he is alive and well, and that he invites the king to come and eat. On hearing the news, the king disappears into his house, sits on his stool, and starts to sink into the ground. A daughter discovers this magical burial and tells her mother, the queen, who does not believe the story. After a number of tries, the daughter finally convinces the mother, but they are too late, and are able to save only a topknot of the king's hair.

This story is repeated publicly much more often than many other episodes of the royal origin myth. It is replete with the Pabir theory of recruitment and retirement. No person likes to be replaced. The job the king is doing is too difficult for the inexperienced young. But replacement will occur, and who is the most likely person to get the job? The best of those qualified, whether he is young or old, though normally the eldest should be the first in line. But, like all of us, the father really does not want to be replaced. His search for a successor is in effect a conspiracy to do away with a would-be rival. The youngest son is declared the most likely candidate because of his power—he boils stones into grain balls—and because of the invitation he sends to his father. Seniors invite subordinates; juniors go to superiors; therefore, the son's invitation is open rebellion, open declaration that he wishes it publicly understood that he can supersede his father. And so the monarch tries to kill his successor. His meeting over succession was actually a plot to discover who was his most dangerous opposition. But the son escapes miraculously from the burning roof (the traditional mode of execution for witches and sorcerers, indicating the son's rising power and the father's decline). His defiance over the funeral is the climax. The father cannot stand this second demonstration of his own lack of power and dies by burying himself alive magically.

The mother-daughter section reemphasizes the same theme in regard to women. The daughter has true understanding. The mother rejects it by denying her daughter the maturity to play a full role. This denial destroys the mother's capacity to aid her husband. Daughters, too, must replace their mothers. Mothers, too, fail to appreciate that the young grow up. Sexual status is irrelevant to the role replacement demanded by the human life cycle.

Conclusions and Implications

The discussion above indicates that the understanding of aging requires that we look at the process in at least three ways: as a dependent variable, as an inner experience, and as a causal force that shapes the society, its institutions, and social history. The experience of aging may be similar across cultures or different. How? Why? At this point more quantification and hypothesis testing can begin. The few reports of people's own experience of old age, for example, suggest that several years are required before they settle into oldness as an identity feature. How widespread is this experience? Where and why does it take more and less time to make the transition? First, however, we must know more about the experience of oldness from the point of view of old people themselves. Here is a classic anthropological task and one that needs doing.

The impact of aging on society is clearly a difficult question and should be examined quantitatively, since the effects of aging must be compared with those of other factors before we can assess its potency as a determinant in social evolution. At the same time, as a society develops, it sifts and winnows values and guidelines—policies, if you will (R. Cohen 1981)—about aging that amount to its own social theory, that is, its moral understanding and explanation of this and all other important life-cycle experiences. I accept the notion that a people's traditions express its own insights into how people *ought* to behave, ought to age, ought to retire, ought to treat one another and nature if they are to survive. These moral precepts are social theories—explanations of human experience in terms of what is morally obligatory.[5] In this view, the comparative understanding of aging requires that we look at the full range of explanations available in the human records, ask how and why they differ, and then ask whether our own social theories, our own attempts to shape policy haven't omitted or included features that may defeat our best intentions. In the process, this intensified attention to aging and age will illuminate the notion of culture as theory and policy by examining it in terms of an aspect of human experience both elemental and universal.

REFERENCES

Auerbach, L.
    1981   An overview of major theoretical issues in social gerontology. Photocopied manuscript.
Beauvoir, Simone de
    1972   The Coming of Age. Trans. P. O'Brian. New York: Putnam.
Cohen, Abner
    1980   The Politics of Elite Culture. Berkeley: University of California Press.

5. I distinguish social theory from social science theory. The latter explains but does not evaluate or recommend; the former takes on this additional policy feature, making it less "valid" but more useful.

Cohen, Ronald
  1967 The Kanuri of Bornu. New York: Holt, Rinehart & Winston.
  1981 Evolutionary epistemology and human values. Current Anthropology
        22(3):201–18.
Foner, Anne, and David I. Kertzer
  1978 Transitions over the life-course: Lessons from age-set societies. Amer-
        ican Journal of Sociology 83:1081–1104.
Hardiman, M.
  n.d. Report on a social survey of Maiduguri. Mimeo.
Keith, Jennie
  1980 The best is yet to be: Toward an anthropology of age. Annual Review
        of Anthropology 9:339–64.
Legesse, Asmarom
  1973 Gada. New York: Free Press.

10

"It's Just Old Age": Old Age as a Diagnosis in American and Chinese Medicine

Andrea Sankar

During the first weeks of my fieldwork among elderly Buddhist nuns in Hong Kong (Sankar 1978, 1981) we played a game that took me quite a while to understand, so different and unexpected were the cultural values it assumed from those with which I was raised. Soon after being introduced to various nuns, I would inevitably be asked to guess their age. With tact so exaggerated that I hoped it would be considered humorous, I guessed at least ten years less than I estimated their ages to be. Far from being flattered, the women laughed at my lack of perceptiveness and proudly informed me of their real ages, usually older than my real estimates. The older they were, the prouder they were of their age. In part I was slow to understand the game because of the strange culture and language, but I now realize that in large part I simply could not accept the

Work for this paper was supported by NIA grant #1F32AG05176-01. I am grateful to the Medical Anthropology Program of the University of California–San Francisco for use of its facilities and access to its resources during the course of my grant tenure. I have sought the criticism and advice of many friends and colleagues in the preparation of this work. Although they are not responsible for the final product, I thank especially Michael Taussig, Frithjof Bergmann, Jessica Muller, Deborah Gordon, Margaret Locke, Charlotte Ikels, Eugene Anderson, and Emily Ahern.

notion that this group of old women could be proud of growing old. Old age was, they informed me over and over again and in many ways, potentially the best time of life. It was a time when one deserved and received the respect of others, when one could spoil oneself and indulge in little luxuries and favorite pastimes, a time when one could relax and enjoy the fruits of a life in which hard work and drudgery had been dominant.

Traditional Chinese healers—physicians, shamans, herbalists, fortunetellers—do not move readily to the diagnosis "It's just old age." Such a diagnosis is unlikely within the theory of Chinese medicine. Sickness is caused by imbalance; health is balance,and this is the expected state of being at all times during the life cycle. One does of course hear the explanation "It's just old age" (*Lauh le*),[1] usually in regard to nonacute problems. A gradual slowing down and limitation on activity are acknowledged to be related to age. Of course elderly Chinese have health problems similar to those found among elderly Americans—failing hearing and eyesight, chronic degenerative diseases—but among the Chinese the symptoms are interpreted differently. Part of the explanation lies in the nature of clinical interaction in traditional Chinese medicine, part in the elderly themselves and their attitude toward health and illness, and part in the role of the elderly in Chinese society.

These initial impressions conformed to some extent to the stereotype revealed by a Harris poll on aging (Harris et al. 1976), which indicated that Americans believe that the main causes of the disabilities associated with old age is age itself. For Americans old age is seen as a kind of disease, a terminal illness that uniformly begins in the sixties. This stereotype persists despite data indicating the relatively low incidence of institutionalization among people 65 and older (Hickey 1980).

In the United States the cultural meaning of old age as a time of sickness is shared and further elaborated by the medical profession. Whether old age is the cause of disease or its characteristics are caused by disease is a question that still eludes definitive resolution, despite debate and research. This theoretical ambivalence beomes concrete when a physician, unable to diagnose the nature of an elderly patient's complaint, retreats from the standards of scientific medicine to the cultural justification for the limits of his diagnostic powers by stating, "It's just old age."

---

1. This is Cantonese, the language in which the research was conducted.

To understand the radical differences in these two cultures' approaches to old age, one would have to examine both the concepts of health and disease and the role of old age within American and Chinese cultures. Yet because such a project is clearly beyond the scope of this chapter, I have chosen to address each of these issues only in part, as they bear on the larger question of old age as a medical concept within each culture.[2] What is the role of old age in diagnosis both from the perspective of medical epistemology and within a specific clinical context? What is the meaning of old age as a diagnosis, and how does it function for the individual involved and for the old person's family?

I have chosen to examine the medical concept of old age for several reasons: (1) such a discussion addresses the stereotype of aging in the United States directly; (2) it contributes to the cross-cultural analysis of the distinction between illness and disease by questioning the concept of disease in this particular case; (3) it illustrates the practical implications of a diagnosis of old age; (4) it addresses the nonbiological rationale behind such a diagnosis.

Old Age in the United States

In the Western medical tradition, old age is a gray area where purely quantifiable technological diagnoses are often imprecise and must give way to or incorporate the subjective judgments of health-care providers.

2. Data for the discussion of Chinese medicine are drawn mainly from fieldwork conducted in Hong Kong in 1975 and 1976. To supplement my observations I have drawn on the published works of other sinologists (Ahern 1975a, 1975b; Anderson and Anderson 1977; Bowers, ed., 1974; Chang 1977; Gould-Martin 1975; Harrell 1981; Hsu and Hsu 1977; Ikels 1979; Kleinman 1980; Topley 1975, 1976; Whyte and Parish 1978) and have communicated with several of them. Unfortunately, little, if any, work has focused directly on the question of health and old age, or on the distinction between old age and disease in Chinese medicine and in Chinese culture in general. When Chinese medicine is discussed, the reference is to the practices of Taiwan and Hong Kong.

Data for American case study were collected at a major West Coast teaching hospital in 1980 and 1981. The research focused on a home-care program that was part of an ambulatory and community medicine rotation. During this eight-week rotation, fourth-year medical and pharmacy students had to visit two or three patients at home one afternoon a week. During each rotation four teams were observed on these visits and on any additional visits that proved necessary. A total of twenty-four medical and twenty pharmacy students underwent a total of 416 systematic observations. Almost all staff meetings and patient conferences were observed during this period. Sixteen patients and their families were closely followed and interviewed for periods ranging from one month to sixteen months.

Because of the ambiguous medical status of old age, examination of its role in diagnosis and treatment sheds light not only on the specific health concerns of the elderly patient but also on the nature of modern Western medicine. A case study of the elderly should illuminate the area where technique and technology, empirical method and medical practice, science and art, practical reason and cultural reason are blended by medical praxis.

The Disease

In nineteenth-century medical diagnosis, old age was synonymous with disease. Physicians used the diagnosis "old and infirm" to describe the no longer young who were irreversibly ill (Pernick 1979). "Old" distinguished those who were about to die from the healthy elderly, who were "advanced in years." It does not appear to have been relevant at this time whether old age caused disease or its disabilities were caused by it, for old age was in fact synonymous with disease. As the century progressed, however, the direction of causality became a key research question. In the late nineteenth century, Western medicine underwent a revolution of sorts as it moved to establish itself as a rigorous scientific discipline governed by stringent rules of evidence, predictability, and replication. The notion of specific etiology which has since been characterized as the "germ theory" or "golden bullet approach" was introduced by Rudolf Virchow in the latter third of the nineteenth century. This theory established the premise that a single specific agent could be identified as the cause of each specific disease. Inspired by success in developing treatments for infectious disease based on this theory, researchers sought to identify the cause of the disease of old age and thereby to cure it.

To this end considerable research was carried out (see Stearns 1976). One of the more notable efforts was undertaken by Ilya Ilich Metchnikoff (1906), who in 1908 was awarded the Nobel Prize for physiology and medicine—notable because of his articulation of the connection between old age and disease. In 1911 Metchnikoff proposed that the disabilities associated with old age were caused by one of three factors: syphilis, alchoholism, or a poison produced by the bacteria of the large intestine. These factors, he proposed, caused arteriosclerosis, which in turn caused the disabilities of old age. Metchnikoff saw old age as a pathological condition, a chronic malady for which there was no cure, except possibly removal of the large intestine. Such early research efforts were an important step in the medicalization of old age. No lasting direct link between old age and disease was established as a result of these researches, but the endeavor served to strengthen the tie between old age and disease (Achenbaum 1978).

Despite the lack of success in research directed specifically toward the question of old age, the domain of old age as a diagnosis has been steadily shrinking as medical research informed by the doctrine of specific etiology has continued to seek out and identify causes of the various conditions that we commonly associate with old age. Thus more and more of the conditions previously attributed to old age are now classified as individual diseases. Most notable is arteriosclerosis and the numerous conditons that derive from it. The key here is the fact that medical research and understanding have made great progress in dissecting and illuminating the general syndrome of old age; yet, despite the fact that the sphere of problems attributed to old age grows smaller and that the numbers of specific identifiable degenerative diseases increase, old age remains as a powerful diagnostic concept within medicine and the related health disciplines

Laboratory research, which has contributed to the circumscription of old age as an explanatory principle, does not appear likely to provide us with a definitive solution to this dilemma. The most widely accepted theory of biological aging is that proposed by biologist Leonard Hayflick. Hayflick (1977) has argued that the cells of each individual of a species are capable of doubling only a limited number of times during its life span. Until that number is reached, cells double in a normal, active way. After that they fail to grow and then they die. This process is thought to account for the organ insufficiency that is seen as antecedent to degenerative disease. Critics of this view argue that there is no proof that this pheonomenon can explain human aging (Manton 1982). Some suggest that specific pathological states cause the aging process. They argue that if the chronic illnesses can be eliminated, the life span can be greatly extended (Walford 1969, Verbrugge 1983).

We are left, then, without a clear-cut medical definition of old age. Its causal relationship to the degenerative conditions associated with advanced years has not been determined. Absolute identification of the aging mechanisms is not likely to resolve the problem. For in fact the problem may ultimately be one of interpretation; that is, the biological process and its causal role in disease may depend on the perspective of a particular branch of medicine. Thus what immunologists take to be the precursors of disease are cited by geriatricians as the signs of age (Fries 1980). To examine the present role of old age within medical practice, we must then go beyond advances in medical understanding and turn to the contexts in which the diagnosis is generated and applied.

The Physician

In connection with writing a yearly report, the medical team with which I worked in San Francisco was assigning patients to diagnostic categories. I noticed that two patients had been assigned the major diagnosis of old age. When this diagnosis was questioned, the following conversation ensued:

Medical director: We decided to list everyone over ninety-five as suffering old age.

Pharmacist: But we are treating Mrs. E. for a heart condition.

Medical director: Yes, but I can't say her main diagnosis is heart disease; she's ninety-nine and walks around the block. Just compare her to Mr. C., who can't walk across the living room without pain. I can't put her in that category.

Pharmacist: Yes, I see that, but then why are we treating her?

Medical director: Because she's getting old and a lot of things are starting to go wrong. We decided a while ago that by the time someone is that old, what's wrong with them is probably due to their age.

Pharmacist: Probably, but what about people that old who have nothing wrong with them?

Medical director: Then what should I say is wrong with her?

This debate was not resolved, nor was it considered to be terribly important. Many of the problems from which the patient suffered, which could have been affected by old age, had been identified as specific diseases or disabilities, and she continued to receive treatment for them. The physician continued to treat what he could treat and left unresolved the complex problem of etiology.

Because there was something to treat and the patient was satisfied with that treatment, the dilemma did not have to be confronted. Yet such is not always the case. Mrs. E., the patient discussed by the medical director and the pharmacist, was a 99-year-old former nurse of German origin. She suffered from arthritis, cataracts, and heart disease. Her health problems seemed cyclical, with periods of stability and periods of great fragility and weakness. She lived alone in a senior center, and her great fear was that she might have to move into a nursing home if she lost further function. Most physicians I observed remarked that they enjoyed dealing with her because she was so articulate and knowledgeable. One physician who encountered Mrs. E. during one of her relatively healthy stages, however, expressed frustration and sometimes anger at having to treat Mrs. E. until she discovered a pulled muscle, missed by other physicians in exams. She analyzed her experience this way:

> I had a lot of trouble with Mrs. E. to begin with. I mean she just did not seem to need me, not like Mr. B. I used to get angry and impatient with her complaints. I thought, "You're so healthy comparatively, you should be grateful instead of complaining." I really felt it was a bad use of my time. And then, remember, I discovered that pulled muscle, I recognized it when other people hadn't. It used to happen to me so I knew how painful it could be. Then I understood about the pain in her chest and the trouble with her arm and her complaints that the doctors had missed something. After that I didn't mind so much working with her. But she still needs me less than Mr. B.

It is possible to resolve the gray areas of medicine that are embodied in old age if treatment is possible. When treatment is not possible, as we shall soon see, then the lack of resolution or certainty confronts the physician. When praxis fails, the diagnosticians' retreat is into irrationalism embodied in the notion of nature. A health problem is redefined as something beyond the scope of medicine and attributable to old age, to nature.

> Mr. X., 78, formerly a successful and energetic businessman, has been deteriorating in the past few years. He lives alone and is very proud of his independence. Recently he underwent a hospitalization for congestive heart failure. While recovering in a convalescent home, he was not able to walk after a fall, and his leg, which had been injured in an automobile accident twenty years previously, gave him serious trouble. Because he had been unable to walk for a few weeks, they grew weak and unsteady. Physical therapy helped to restore function to the legs but he remained unstable. At his insistence, he left the home earlier than planned and returned to his apartment, accompanied by his social worker. Once home

he had great difficulty using his walker, and continued to bump into things and generally created a great deal of anxiety on his behalf. He explained his unsteadiness as the cause of his accident and described the accident as if it had just happened. He expressed the hope that his doctors would be able to treat his problem and restore complete function to his legs. His care providers did not agree with his assessment of the situation. They thought his focus on the accident, so many years ago, was a form of denial that he was aging. "He doesn't want to admit he is getting old," said his nurse. "He focuses on the accident because that is something his doctors can fix."

The implication is straightforward. Old age is something doctors cannot fix; therefore, there is nothing they can do for it or for the patient. This was not a careful clinical judgment, yet it represents the quick and easy association between old age and disease characteristic of American culture. To say "It's just old age" is tantamount to admitting that one does not understand the problem. Again, the situation focuses itself when the patient is unsatisfied and pushes the physician or health-care provider beyond his limits.

Yet there are other instances when physicians do not resort to a diagnosis faulting nature when they fail to understand a complaint. The diagnosis "It's just old age" is not simply an excuse for ignorance; it portends a more complex significance. In many cases "It's just old age" embodies the message "I don't want to treat you." Here we travel well beyond the legitimate limits of medical knowledge and the individual physician's diagnositc abilities. Here we are within the subjective, cultural meanings attached to old age. Considerable research has been undertaken to identify and document physician antipathy to the elderly (Institute of Medicine 1978, Kutner 1978). Yet despite numerous programs designed to ameliorate the problem (Beeson 1979, Birenbaum et al. 1979), it persists. In part physicians simply reflect the society of which they are a part. Thus physician informants frequently remarked that although they did not mind treating the elderly, especially those with something interesting to say, they felt it was not a good use of their skill and expertise. This issue has ramifications beyond the specific clinical setting. Perhaps the best-known instance of this attitude concerns hemodialysis (Childress 1971). Here the case against the elderly was more explicit; elderly persons were denied access to hemodialysis on the basis of the supposition that they had fewer significant, socially useful years left to live. While denial of treatment is rare now because of special congressional mechanisms for payment, age is still a factor considered by physicians before they embark on treatment. Old age is a factor in less dramatic decisions as well. One of the patients with whom I worked, a 92-year-old man, was scheduled for bilateral hip replacement when Medicare refused to pay for the operation, saying he was too old. The decision was reversed and the patient, a highly motivated individual, regained use of both legs, moved back into the community, and became self-sufficient.

In part the physicians are responding to singular aspects of medical training in which elderly patients embody the negative values of that endeavor. Most diseases from which the hospitalized elderly suffer are long-term degenerative diseases. These diseases cannot be cured. The structure of medical education, which puts a premium on the unusual, exotic case presentation, has little time for a serious consideraton of advanced arthritis, diabetes, or arteriosclerosis (Kleinbach 1974). Not valued as people, the hospitalized elderly are also not valued as medical subjects.

But in large part physicians are also responding to a deep dilemma within modern medicine; namely, its faith in reason and science, which stands in direct opposition to its ultimate failure in the face of death. For many informants old age was a kind of terminal illness. Unlike cancer, it offered no hope for remission. The cost-benefit equation of resources to lives saved does not and cannot apply; ultimately no lives are saved. Physicians who are taught that correct diagnosis and cure are their main responsibility cannot help encountering elderly patients with some mixture of frustration, anger, and despair.[3]

The Patient

Not circumscribed by the rules of evidence that limit physicians' diagnoses and not conflicted about the object of their endeavors, my elderly

---

3. This association between old age and terminal illness is clearly articulated when the physician is actually dealing with terminal illness in the elderly and sometimes not so elderly. Here the label "old age" is used not to justify nontreatment but to describe advanced pathology. Physician informants often characterize the severe physical changes wrought by degenerative diseases as premature aging. The "rapid aging" associated with terminal cancer is said to be a quick indication of the progress of the disease. One way of describing a patient's decline is to say that he or she seems to have aged. Although most physicians would not maintain that this physical deterioration was actually old age, their quick association of pathological process and natural aging reflects the stereotypes popular among the lay public. It may also indicate that, the fashionable "no one ever died of old age" philosophy to the contrary, American medicine does perceive old age as a pathological process.

informants were mainly concerned with maintaining their health and could be clear and concise concerning the distinction between their complaints due to old age and those due to illness.

According to Mrs. E., she suffered from the following problems:

Well, the medical problems I have have been mostly orthopedics—arthritis and orthopedics. It started when I had injured my arm and arthritis set in, so I came here for treatment of that. I was working too then, you see, and just gradually over the years it got worse. . . . I know that it was arthritis but I had to have treatment for it, I couldn't treat it alone according to my knowledge, I thought I need more. That's why I started to come up here and they gave me Cortisone. I had tissue therapy. So I know almost every medical department other than arthritis and orthopedics—I have gone through the mill.

These are all distinct problems, which she described as having specific beginnings and which got worse or improved over time. She expected her physicians should be able to help her with these problems. To assist them she diligently read newspapers and journals for the latest medical information that might enhance her care and carefully passed on this information to her physicians.

She made a clear distinction between these problems and her great age. About her age she commented:

In the elevator ten days ago, the door hit me and I lost my glasses, so you see I have to watch it. Any unevenness in elevation or . . . So it's—it's hard to remember what to do and what not to do. So I feel a little bit discouraged. . . . My back has been giving me trouble and it's getting hard for me to get up and lift myself and it's getting worse all the time. Seems like my upper part is too heavy for my bone structure, that's why I've been a little discouraged lately because it's been more and more difficult for me at times. So I realize that my time is not very long but I am not afraid, you understand.

Mrs. E. was not seeking treatment for these conditions. The problems that she identified as disease, however, those she recognized as acute episodes or marked departures from a previously stable condition, she believed her physician should be able to treat so as to return her to her previous functional status or something close to it.

Not all patients were as articulate or thoughful as Mrs. E. Some, tending toward hypochondriasis, did report every little pain, the sort of thing Mrs. E. would have classified as "aging." But those who were unanxious, thoughtful observers of their own physical conditon could be surprisingly clear, in the face of medical confusion, as to which problems were due to aging and which to disease. Said another 99-year-old woman: "This is my body and I don't want any medical student probing around where they're not suppose to. Some of these aches and pains have just grown with me and I want them left alone. Let the doctors fix what needs to be fixed and don't touch the rest."

This clarity is notably absent in the terminally ill. Such patients appear to attach a meaning to old age which is in flat contradiction to that casually articulated by physicians, namely, that terminal illness produces premature aging. Although I have no systematic evidence to substantiate this observation, my impression from my own research and from discussions with people in the field is that when faced with the prospect of imminent death, individuals more readily attribute their problems to old age. True, old age is also seen as a terminal disease, but it is one with an unpredictable trajectory and indeterminate time of death.

One informant, a 78-year-old former foundry worker, was suffering from end-stage chronic obstructive pulmonary disease. Among other things, he was on twenty-four-hour oxygen therapy, requiring him to wear a nose tube at all times; he continually suffered from the sensation that he was suffocating; and he was confined to bed and had great difficulty eating because to do so expended the precious little reserves of breath he had. When asked about his health problems, he replied:

> That's the sixty-four-thousand-dollar question. Going back thirty years, I worked in smoke and dust and dirt. I used to have a doctor who wrote in the paper who said that emphysema was caused by having a cold all of your life. So I don't know what to lay it on. . . . Hell, there's nothing wrong with me. I just got bum lungs. The rest, it's just—it's just old age.

This was the case with a friend's 78-year-old mother, who was confronted with a diagnosis of widespread bone cancer. This formerly active woman suddenly began to act, as she said, "old." Having previously rejected the label—along with some of the benefits that go with it, such as senior discounts—she suddenly decided to sell her home, move into a senior citizens' complex, and begin "acting her age." Simone de Beauvior (1964) related a similar reaction in her mother. Shortly after her mother's admission to a hospital for treatment of widespread cancer, she announced that she had decided to "act her age" and accept the fact that she really was old. She talked about slowing down and taking better care of herself after she was discharged. As Beauvior points out, this was a marked change in her mother, who previously would not allow the subject of age to be mentioned in her presence.

The Family

Elderly patients who seek assistance for complaints they have identified as disease not only face possible rejection from their physician; they may also encounter resistance within their own family. As individuals age they pass into a space where those younger than they lack the empathy to follow. What do middle-aged people know of cold extremities, brittle bones, forgetfulness, weakness? In attempting to interpret or understand elderly relatives, individuals may turn to the common knowledge available within our culture, which casts the elderly in the role of perpetual patients. According to a Harris poll (1976), even the elderly see themselves in this role. Some research has begun to address this phenomenon of nonagreement between generations and its possible consequences for care of the elderly (see Hickey and Rakowski 1980 for a psychological examination of the problem).

Historical processes have contributed to the shaping of this stereotype in America. The status of elders in our culture had become associated with the meaning "about to die." When the term "old" was used exclusively to designate one who was "old and infirm," suffering from irreversible pathology, this was an appropriate meaning for the word. The criteria for the use of the label have changed, and now a chronological marker of 65 triggers its application for most people. In part this change grew out of political and labor struggles to establish a fair retirement age and a just pension system. Unions wanted a functional definition and management a chronological one (see Roebuck 1979 for a detailed account of this process in England; see Achenbaum 1978 for an account of the process in the United States). The passage of social security legislation fixed a chronological definition to old age in the United States. Although most men and women of 65 were functionally capable, their age became the marker for the onset of old age. The rationale behind assignment of the label has changed, but the meaning has not. Thus attainment of age 65, relatively young in terms of our rates of mortality, now consigns numerous healthy, fully functioning individuals to the status "about to die" (Clark 1972, 1973).

American Perceptions of Old Age

The actual number of pathological complaints and disabilities that are attributed to old age by the medical profession has been drastically reduced in the last century. Such specific conditions as arteriosclerosis have been identified, along with their side effects, and now receive treatment. Yet as we have seen, old age continues to occupy an important place within the diagnostic schema of the physicians studied. Because the aging process has a biological basis but one imperfectly understood, it provides fertile ground for cultural interpretation. Advances in medical understanding which provide both the theoretical basis and the technological means for individual interventions have limited the contexts in which physicians encounter the gray area of old age. Yet when they do, the diagnosis reflects primarily two conflicts within modern medical science. The first meaning can be translated, ''I don't know.'' Such an admission in the age of rapid advances in technological interventions and ever-increasing precision in diagnosis is threatening to the physician's faith in his own diagnostic abilities as well as to both the patient's and the physician's investment in the infallibility of Western scientific medicine. The second problem may be translated, ''I don't want to treat you.'' Such a subjective dismissal is antithetical both to the objective scientific standards the medical profession seeks to maintain and to the fundamental humanitarianism of the Hippocratic oath.

Within the family the mitigating act of medical intervention, which helps keep ambiguity and prejudice at a distance, is absent. For a family member who has limited access to advances in medical knowledge and whose understanding of old age is colored by the historically evolved association between old age and the status ''about to die,'' the sphere of old age as a diagnosis is much larger than it is for the medical profession. When one directly encounters visible physical and sometimes mental changes in a family member and lacks the experiences that would enable one to empathize and understand, one's own anxieties about the inevitability of death are associated with old age as a disease—a disease whose only outcome is ultimately death.

From the patient's singular perspective, the gray area of old age is narrowly circumscribed by personal history, function, and feeling. The patient knows when a new pain or a sudden decrease in function occurs. My informants defined such deficits as medically curable. The slow, gradual change, the diminishment in function, the increase in pain, is usually separated off and defined as age. The patient's perception is not always accurate. Beauvoir's mother preferred to account for her increasing pain as age rather than face the diagnosis of cancer. One patient informant whose joints had gradually frozen over the years from ankylosina spondylitis, so that he was confined to an apartment, able only to stargaze through a mirror propped on his chin, felt the gradual onset to be old age and ruled out any effective intervention. An operation and subsequent physical therapy returned him to a level of functioning he had not experienced in ten years. Not all problems a patient defines as disease-based can be addressed by medical intervention. The body's ability to recover from trauma or disease is age-related. The older patient may never regain his or her previous functional status. For the physician and the family, the subjective element in the diagnosis of old age is large and serves to articulate fear, anxiety, prejudice, and frustration. For many patients, however, the self-assessment reflects in many cases an accurate determination based on empirical observation into which few cultural interpretations intrude.

Old Age and Death in Chinese Society

Comparisons between such separate entities as the Chinese and American medical systems are at best hazardous, even when they are limited to a specific question such as the role of old age in diagnosis. One faces problems in establishing equivalents both for terminology and for concepts. The differences between the two sets of meanings are large indeed. It is precisely within the scope of the different meanings that the significance of the latter half of this essay lies. I shall extend this examination only a minimal distance into an analysis of the structure of Chinese medicine, only so far as to give coherence and background to the meanings discussed. I shall circumscribe the account so as to establish a contrast to the medical interpretation of old age in American culture.

The principles and concepts of Chinese medicine reflect the theories and systems that govern the cosmological and social aspects of Chinese life. Central to the whole structure is a system of balances. Imbalance and disharmony cause disease. Imbalance and disharmony can arise from a wide variety of causes, some of which are recognized by Western medicine, many of which are not. Yin and yang are the basic forces governing the universe and all things within it. Yin represents the dark, wet, cold, female, the negative. Yang is its opposite, light, warm, dry, male, the positive. Within the universe the two forces are in balance; and if they are not, great calamities result. The individual is also composed of yin and yang forces. Emily Ahern (1975a) describes these forces as two separate selves: the yin self, which lives in the world of ghosts, is exactly analogous to the yang self, which exists in the world of the living. Sometimes the concept of two distinct worlds is collapsed into the single human body, which is portrayed as having both a yin and a yang part, each part embodying aspects of the world from which it comes.[4]

The cosmological forces that govern the universe need to be in balance for a harmonious society, and within society forces represented by various individuals or occasions, such as weddings and deaths, need to be balanced for harmonious social relationships to exist. So too in the body, health is associated with harmony and balance. Yin and yang operate almost every level of existence. Thus imbalances between yin and yang within the cosmos have their counterparts in society and in the body. Problems between adults, for example, can affect the health of those involved and the health of their children.

Within the body concepts of hot and cold and to a lesser extent clean and poison are considered more immediate and therefore weighty in their effect on health than yin and yang. Physical health depends on a delicate balance of hot and cold at all times. Once again balance and harmony are considered to be the way of nature, but they can be endangered by time of year, personal disposition and constitution, and age. Balance between hot and cold is maintained by the ingestion of foods that are believed to contain the qualities of hot and cold. When my informants had eaten too much deep-fried food, which was considered hot, the head nun fixed us a cool soup of apples, fungus, and nuts. An imbalance can also be caused by an exterior problem, such as a birth, a death, a wedding, or anything that produces an excess of one element over the other. Thus when a woman loses a considerable amount of blood in giving birth, she is said to be cold and is given a "hot" soup of chicken, wine, and sesame oil to "heat her up."

Disease that results from imbalance can have both internal and external causes. Internal causes include those most frequently recognized by Western medicine, such as physical and psychological problems, and those not often recognized, such as social problems. External causes have

4. As anthropologist Emily Ahern (1975a) has indicated, significant incongruities do exist, and these discrepancies may themselves provide the basis for healing powers.

to do with the realm of the supernatural. According to Ahern (1975a), there is a third source of causality, which also arises from within the body. It explains colds, menstrual cramps, and other "naturally" occurring problems that seem to afflict everyone at one time or another. Such problems are considered so trivial as not to require treatment.

Many problems that arise in the course of living and that are treated medically in China are not labeled as medical problems in Western medicine: such things as business problems, disagreements between children and parents, and inability to find a husband. Their inclusion within the medical sphere is accomplished by more than a simple fiat of cultural labeling. Physician and anthropologist Arthur Kleinman (1980) has written at length on the Chinese tendency to somatize, that is, to give physical expression to psychological distress. Symptoms of the anxiety produced by a business failure, a difficult infant, or impending spinsterhood are defined as health problems and treated medically.

Medical care in Chinese society can be obtained from a variety of sources. In Hong Kong, Taiwan, and some overseas Chinese communities one can visit Chinese-trained doctors, herbalists, bone setters, shamans, or *tang kis* (fortunetellers). All except the latter two are to be found in the People's Republic of China. The patient also has the option of visiting a Western-trained physician. Physicians of Chinese medicine are trained in the principles of Chinese medical knowledge and theory that have been in use for almost two thousand years. Although their training is not uniform or necessarily consistent with this body of knowledge, it is a clear articulation of general diagnostic principles. Diagnosis is made by observation, palpation, and pulse taking, the latter being preferred by many physicians. Unlike Western physicians, Chinese doctors do not consider knowledge of the anatomy important. The diagnostic logic is inductive rather than deductive. The aim of the diagnosis is to identify changes in function rather than to locate underlying pathology.

When faced with a self- or family-diagnosed illness, the patient can make a choice among these kinds of practitioners. Each offers a different kind of care and a different approach to a specific problem. Choice of a healer is in large part determined by the suspected etiology of a complaint. Certain categories of affliction are seen as best treated by specific types of healers. Something with an internal etiology and experienced as acutely disabling, such as appendicitis, is best treated by a Western-trained physician. For less dramatic but still serious problems involving a fever, Western-trained physicians are also sought out. Western medicine is not, however, perceived as the most efficacious treatment for many kinds of disease. Several recent studies (Kleinman 1980; Ahern 1975a, 1975b; Gould-Martin and Ngin 1981) indicate that many Chinese perceive Western medicine as effective in treating only symptoms, not the underlying disease, and express dissatisfaction with the treatment they have received. The strongest source of dissatisfaction arises from the unwillingness or inability of Western-trained physicians to explain the cause of illness. Because the different types of disease,internal and external, may have exactly the same symptoms, and because efficacious treatment depends on understanding the cause of the disease, Western medicine's failure to provide an explanation for an illness is troublesome for many patients. Among other problems, it leads to the belief that Western medicine is effective only in dealing with short-term acute problems, and that if the treatment if not immediately effective, it has failed.

Old Age

Within the Chinese medical system old age is thought to create a special susceptibility to disease. In this respect it is structurally similar to infancy and childhood. Both phases of the life cycle are characterized as having insufficient yang and by a soul that is not firmly attached to the body. In the elderly the yang, or life force, has been diminished and is gradually being surmounted by the ascension of yin, or negativity. Because of their unstable cosmological and elemental constitution, diseases in both the elderly and children are seen not as self-limiting but as being potential threats to life, and consequently as demanding immediate treatment. During the adult years, ranging from the late teens to late middle age, when the forces should have achieved a balance and harmony within the individual, minor disturbances and illnesses caused perhaps by excessive or careless eating can be corrected by the body's own balancing system; the same indulgences by the elderly lead to serious problems that call for specific correctives, usually diet therapy. Because of the delicate internal balance, both the elderly and children are also more susceptible to exterior (supernatural) causes of disease, and must take special care to guard against them.[5]

5. The ideas of why old age creates special vulnerability are fairly clear and accepted; my informants both within the nunnery and within the larger Hong Kong society held these notions. The treatment for this vulnerability, however, reflects the complex and often conflicting concepts involved in Chinese medicine. Marjorie Topley (1975, 1976) has analyzed Chinese medicine in terms of the amoral contributions of Chinese culture

To say that old age is not considered a disease does not mean that specific physiological changes are not attributed to advanced years. *"Lauh le,"* sighed an elderly nun in response to a question about why she had to leave so early for market. "I can no longer stand the heat of the day. I must leave early so I can get back before it's too hot." *"Lauh le"* was also the response I got when I inquired about the nuns' use of taped chants. "We used to be able to chant all night long for funerals and special festivals. Now our voices get tired quickly. We can't chant all night anymore, and when we do our voices are weak; so we use these tapes of ourselves to make our sound louder. It has to be loud enough for the Buddha to hear." *"Lauh le,"* groaned the aging boat builder in the village near the nunnery. He just couldn't work as hard as he used to, and his eyesight wasn't so good anymore.

All these complaints might come under Ahern's category of naturally occurring trivial problems of internal etiology (1975a). As in the cases of colds and menstrual cramps, there is little one can do about them. Yet for some people, at least, *lauh le* appears to have a more profound meaning. Although we cannot adequately understand its significance, it is worthwhile at least to mention it here. According to Charlotte Ikles (personal communication), *lauh le* can refer to serious debilitating physical problems. She quotes one informant, a woman in her seventies, who suffered from blindness in one eye, deafness in one ear, and loosening teeth yet declined to seek medical care, as saying that these conditions were inevitable in old age. "In old age all the diseases come out."

Her statement poses interesting questions. This conceptualization of

---

and of the moral and supernatural influences of Buddhism. Because the elderly suffer from an insufficient yang force, which is the precursor to disease, diet therapy to maintain a balance between hot and cold (and by analogy between yin and yang) often stresses supplements of hot foods, provided in special tonics or meats (Ahern, personal communication). Many elderly people, however, influenced by Buddhism, choose a *chai* or vegetarian diet, believed to be purifying and to consist mainly of cold foods, such as fungi. My informants were among the most strict in this respect, living in a *chai t'ang*, devoted to the practice of *chai* diet and meditation. But an informal survey of elderly people in secular Hong Kong revealed that many Buddhists take a vow to eat *chai* on the first and fifteenth of each month, and/or swear off red meat entirely after turning 60. People who follow the *chai* diet therefore are seriously increasing the natural imbalance in yin and yang brought on by increased age. There is the counterbalancing factor of Taoism, however, which holds that fungi are essential to longevity, and that a diet heavy in fungi will increase the life span. Thus one of the first things I was told in interviewing informants about their *chai* diet was that it was extremely healthy (for adults; very few felt it was healthy for children, who need hot foods to grow) and would lead to a long life, longer than the normal span.

lauh le does not seem to fit within the categories established by Ahern (1975a) and further articulated by Gould-Martin (1975). Although the physical condition is conceived of as naturally occurring and untreatable, it is by no means trivial. The notion that there is something within the body that must come out is strikingly similar to the case of measles analyzed by Marjorie Topley (1976). Topley describes the difficulty of persuading Hong Kong mothers to have their infants inoculated against measles, which was taking a high toll at the time. Through her research Topley discovered that mothers purposely withheld treatment, believing that the pustules that formed were the body's expulsion of womb poison. If the rash did not form, the child would maintain the poison within its body, where it would cause serious damage. Possibly some such notion of pollution and poison is operating in the old woman's conception of her illness, its natural etiology, and the ineffectualness of treatment.

Such an understanding is at variance with the responses of my informants as well as data gathered by Arthur Kleinman. Among my informants two nuns in their seventies suffering from dental problems elected the expensive solution of dentures rather than endure painful and prolonged treatment. Another informant treated her general weakness with deer tail, which she had to consume on the hill behind the nunnery so as not to break the prohibition against nonvegetarian food. Kleinman's (1980) study of illness experience in 115 households over a period of one month found that of 139 elderly (those over 60), who made up 19 percent of the sample, there were 112 reported sickness episodes, 27.2 percent of all reported episodes at a rate of 0.81 sickness episode per elderly person per month. All of these episodes received treatment of some sort.

From another perspective the distinction between what is treatable and what is not treatable, *lauh le,* carries far less weight than it would in the Western system of self-diagnosis. For the nuns' concern was less with disease and its implied cure than with maintaining health. The maintenance of a healthy body will affect the individual's well-being spiritually and socially as well as physically, for all these levels are connected. Scrupulous attention to and awareness of health in all matters and at all ages characterized my informants. Cognizance of the healthful or dangerous properties of food is part of this awareness (although this knowledge is slowly being lost by the younger generations in modern Hong Kong). So, too, is attention to physical fitness. Daily exercise was a rule for the nuns and lay informants in Hong Kong except the most feeble and bedbound. In the early morning one could see Western-attired businessmen in the parks and plazas of downtown Hong Kong, with their suit coats neatly folded on their breifcases, going through the ritual movements of *tai chi chuan.*

Every summer the Buddhist nunneries and monasteries in the Hong Kong area would join together on a nearby island to sponsor an "old people's festival" (*lauh yahn yuen*), which was attended by up to a thousand people and lasted almost a week. While much of the focus of the festival was on spiritual preparation for death, it was also devoted to health. People gathered together to eat vegetarian food and pray for health and long life. The real health benefit, according to my informants, came from the three-hour walk to the festival and back each day for a week. This exercise, they claimed, did as much good as all the sutras they had chanted. The old people's festival symbolized the attention to health rather than disease which characterized both my religious and lay informants.

The Physician

Old age does not provide a metaphor by which to articulate the gray areas of Chinese medicine. Nor is it used as a rationale for dismissing those elderly people whose health problems may create frustration and defy solution. In analyzing why this is the case, we need to turn to the individual practitioners and their relationship to and interaction with their elderly patients. Such an endeavor, however, is beyond the scope of the data I gathered and has not yet been systematically addressed in the literature. Because the examination of the interaction of physician and patient is an important part of the appreciation of both the health problems of the Chinese elderly and the role old age plays within the Chinese medical system, I wish to suggest the most salient areas where research might be undertaken and to discuss the possible implications and relevance of such research.

Despite attention to health, elderly Chinese are not quick to seek out a physician. Although concern about health was an important and sometimes major part of life for the elderly nuns and their lay associates, they rarely saw physicians, herbalists, or fortunetellers, preferring to treat their illnesses themselves with diet therapy. This pattern is substantiated by Kleinman (1980), who reports that 100% of all sickness episodes reported by his 139 elderly informants were first treated in the home. Of these cases, 86 percent received only family treatment. When the elderly sought care outside the home, they did so primarily for chronic illnesses;

two-thirds of the chronic illnesses identified in the study were experienced by the elderly. People suffering from illnesses labeled as severe by the research team received treatment from at least one practitioner outside of the home. Only 29 were treated by Western-trained doctors, 45 by Chinese-trained physicians, and 40 by folk healers. The low use of Western-trained physicians despite the perceived seriousness of the problem reflects the belief that Western medicine addresses only the symptoms and not the underlying causes of disease. The high use of folk healers represents a suspected external or supernatural etiology. Disorders that do not respond quickly to treatment or are not self-limiting are suspected to have at least in part an external etiology.

Encounters between elderly Chinese patients and their healers primarily concern the treatment of chronic illness, as they do in the United States. The physician's relationship to the patient is in part structured by the interpretation of chronicity within the medical system. Thus in seeking to understand the medical meaning of old age, we must analyze the place of chronicity within the structure of Chinese medicine. We need to know what the physician's expectations of his treatment outcomes are, how much responsibility he accepts for the treatment, and what the aims of an intervention are (i.e., cure or palliation). Research must also address the conceptual relationship between old age and disease. Topley (1976) speaks of geriatrics as one of the specialties in Chinese medicine. It would be useful to analyze the work of geriatricians in order to understand what the perceived relationship between old age and disease is and how this relationship in turn affects the kinds of medical interventions sought and the willingness of the physician to treat.

The effect of age on access to treatment is important in the understanding of health problems of elderly Chinese. Here three main questions might be addressed: (1) the effect of cultural orientation toward maintenance of health rather than toward treatment of disease; (2) willingness to treat the health problems of the elderly directly; (3) cultural attitudes and values concerning old age. My informants' orientation toward maintenance of health rather than treatment of disease meant that any perturbation received treatment in an attempt to maintain a balanced state of health. It also meant that a great range of preventive measures were taken to ensure against imbalance. Future research might examine whether such a cultural orientation facilitates access to health-care providers; in other words, can a person secure treatment without presenting any clear evidence of pathology? The aches and pains of growing old may receive attention and treatment as conditions that threaten the self-defined balance of the patient and thus could lead to disease.

When my informants experienced the gradual weakness they associated with *lauh le* they often took a strengthening tonic, something that restored the vitality that had gradually diminished with age. Often they took such tonics to prevent the imbalance that could lead to more serious illness. Sometimes those tonics were prescribed in combination with stronger medicines aimed at more serious health problems. Here the purpose was to treat the underlying imbalances as well as the more serious exacerbations. If the manifestations of old age can be addressed directly through treatment interventions, what effect does this have on access to treatment in general for the elderly?

Finally, what effect do cultural attitudes and values concerning old age have on the healers' willingness to treat? on the status of the elderly person as a patient? on the use of old age as a metaphor for imprecision and doubt in the system of medical care?

The Family

If one ever wishes to present an example of a culture where old age is venerated, it is probably China that first comes to mind. So strong was the explicit power of the elderly, underwritten by Confucian legal and moral traditions, that when the Communists first came to power, veneration of the elderly and acquiesence to their power was expressly forbidden (Davis-Friedman 1979). The origins of this power date back to the first century B.C. and the time of Kung Fu-tze, or Confucius. His articulation of the concept of filial piety helped to establish the moral and later the legal basis for a gerontocracy that was maintained culturally until the mid-twentieth century, and, some people argue, continues today. After the age of 60, each additional year of life was a blessing on the elder and his or her family. The sixtieth birthday marked the beginning of old age. It was celebrated as the ascent to a higher status.

In direct contradistinction to the American custom, advertisers in Hong Kong who wish to promote such luxury products as expensive brandy or watches often depict the birthday party of an elder as the appropriate occasion for such a gift. Ancient laws allocated special meat rations to those who had attained advanced ages. These allotments were similar to the status markers denoting the nobility (Chang, ed., 1977; Hsu and Hsu 1977).

The elderly in the People's Republic retain a high status position. The harsh decrees of the early days of the republic have been modified; children are now legally responsible for the care of their parents. The affection and respect accorded the elderly still remain, especially in rural areas. There the parents still maintain considerable control over the social and economic lives of their adult children (Davis-Friedman 1979, Whyte and Parish 1978). With social space allotted to them, the importance of the sick role to legitimize dependence is in effect negligible for the elderly. In fact, the opposite attitude very much obtains. Elderly people whose children are successful enough to care for them take great pride in the fact thaty they are able to rely on their children. (This is not always the case in Hong Kong, however; see Ikels 1979 for a detailed discussion.)

Very little research has been done on the interpretation of symptoms within the family. (Topley's [1970] study of mothers and children is a notable exception.) Kleinman's (1980) statistics on health-seeking behavior, however, seem to corroborate the observation that the elderly's complaints are quickly attended to. Katherine Gould-Martin and Ngin Choorswang (1981) provide another perspective on family care in their discussion of "patching" or restoring *peng-an,* peace and harmony. The *peng-an* of a family can be lost by the repeated or severe and lengthy illness of a family member. Thus an elderly family member in continuous ill health is not easily dismissed as just being old, for such a state of affairs affects the whole family.

Lest this picture seem too idyllic, it is important to note that the status "old" in and of itself is not sufficient to secure support and assistance. Without a social context in which the status of elder plays a meaningful role, as in a family, care, support, and respect are not necessarily accorded the elderly individual.

Although attention to health was an important part of everyday life in the age-homogeneous society of the nunnery, it was not uncritical. One member expressed concern about her physical condition at every turn. She was one of the part-time members who periodically took outside jobs as a servant to make money for the nunnery. As a trained, experienced servant she could get a good salary, but when offered a choice she repeatedly chose the lower-paying job if it was less strenuous. To the other members she justified her choices on the basis of health. They expressed little concern and considerable skepticism about the seriousness of her condition. As one member pointed out, "It's our religious duty to earn as much money as possible and to contribute it here for the good of the nunnery and the glory of the Buddha. Ah Saam shouldn't worrry so much about her health." Age alone was not sufficient to command the attention and concern of the other members for her physical problems. The demands of the specific social and in this case spiritual context help to structure a diagnosis that does not always point in the direction of support for the status and well-being of the elderly individual.

Chinese Perceptions of Old Age

Within the indigenous Chinese health-care system that we have examined, old age is not an explanation or excuse for withholding treatment. With the provocative and important exception of the elderly women who declined medical care because "in old age all the diseases come out," the elderly themselves initiate treatment at home, and if they are dissatisfied they seek further treatment for the deficits of advancing years as well as for potentially serious chronic and acute conditions. In their pursuit of health rather than treatment for disease the nuns sought to maintain a standard of well-being that precluded any but the most obvious and necessary acquiesence to physical decline. For the rest, they endeavored to reverse, prevent, or impede ill health and to maintain themselves in the best condition possible. To this end they were assisted by a medical system that understood their health problems as specific and therefore treatable. They were not dismissed or denied treatment because of the vexing etiological ambiguity of their complaints. Nor were they diminished in this attempt by cultural prejudice reflected in the medical system's blockage of access to resources of time, expertise, technology, understanding, and compassion. This pursuit of health was further sanctioned and supported by the family, whose expectations concerning old age and, as we shall see, death allowed for compassion and care unfettered by fear and denial.

Death

The differences between the Chinese and Western medical systems are not limited to the treatment of the elderly. By establishing a narrow definition of what it considers medically treatable, Western medicine declines to treat numerous problems that may accompany other stages of the life cycle, such as infancy and adolescence. Again Chinese medicine presents a contrasting approach. Chinese practitioners' willingness to treat and the limitations on treatment in the Western system are reversed at one crucial point within the life cycle—its end, death.

During my fieldwork one of the residents of the nunnery had a stroke. She was 86 and already partially incapacitated. The stroke left her paralyzed. A bed was made for her in the lightest, airiest room in the nunnery, the ancestor tablet room. This room was chosen partly for ease in caring for her and partly for the convenience of her soul should it choose to depart. But it did not depart, at least not immediately. The old nuns engaged in her care could not stay awake all night with her and still meet their demanding schedule of prayers and subsistence activity. A meeting was called of all available members and concerned friends. Some people wanted to send her to the Western hospital on the island. Others—those who lived in nearby nunneries and in the city—disagreed. They argued that she was near death, and all the hospital could do was to prevent her from dying and prolong her suffering. Anyway, one nun pointed out, she had been a vegetarian all her life; they would force her to eat meat and she would die polluted. Finally it was decided that all concerned would contribute money and that they would hire a younger nun to do the night nursing.

One can compare this paralyzed nun to the incapacitated, incontinent nursing-home resident who has been ignored by the medical profession for years, yet when he or she starts to die the most sophisticated and expensive medical technology is called into play and heroic efforts are made to save a life. Death is not a natural occurrence, but one to be treated "aggressively."

With greater or lesser degrees of awareness, Western medicine is waging a war not against disease but against death. For many highly trained specialists, prolonging life by even a few days through "aggressive" interventions is viewed as a victory over death. This orientation contributes to the antipathy physicians feel toward the elderly. From the physicians' perspective, old age is the ultimate incurable disease. There can be no hope of remission. The sheer weight of this fact and its contrariness to the goals of modern medicine accounts for much of the avoidance of elderly patients and the reluctance to treat those with whom the physician is presented.

In the Chinese system great efforts are made to treat the suffering of preterminal individuals. Their pain as well as their psychological and social stress and that of their families receives sympathetic concern and serious treatment. But once an individual is clearly and imminently dying, medical efforts cease and the individual is allowed to die. There was a special nunnery near my field site. Attached to this nunnery was a dying house. Monastery and nunnery residents on the point of death were carried there and placed on mats. Given only water, attended by the nuns, they died.

Conclusion

Biological aging is experienced as an individual matures. Whether the physiological effects of this process are interpreted as disease or as growing old is in part determined by culture and in part by the individual's social, psychological, and physical status. In both the Chinese and American contexts the distinction between old age and disease within one's own body was relatively clear, with some important exceptions. The distinction was notably less clear from the perspective of family and physician in American culture and considerably less ambiguous in the Chinese case.

In the United States the biological and cultural meaning of old age provide fertile space for the interpretation and concretization of cultural ambivalence toward the natural, physical dependence of old age as well as its intimate proximity to death and of professional conflict evoked by an inability to cure. In the Chinese case, personal and professional ambivalence toward aging and dependent individuals do not find expression through medical metaphors. Although the level and force of intervention within the two medical systems is markedly different, the Chinese system does not resort to a biological justification for the denial of treatment.

To understand the process of diagnosis from a cross-cultural perspective it is necessary to analyze the medical science of a culture as well as the social logic by which the label of illness is applied. The system of medical science within a culture—its rules of evidence, standards of health and illness, process of diagnosis, and methods of treatment—set the parameters within which medical judgments are made. No matter how rigorous the methodology is, the judgments made within these parameters are influenced by the immediate subjectivity of the patient, healer, and family and the social and cultural values associated with a particular illness label and the sick role in general. This gray area provides rich material for the cross-cultural examination of medical system dynamics.

Old age as a widely recognized social as well as biological fact can provide case studies in the cross-cultural comparison of medical systems. Such case studies can produce material for the analysis of the spaces where technology and science, reason and method, art and skill combine with cultural and social and personal logic in interpreting and treating the changes associated with the process of aging.

REFERENCES

Achenbaum, Andrew
 1978   Old Age in A New Land: The American Experience since 1790. Baltimore: Johns Hopkins University Press.
Ahern, Emily
 1975a   Sacred and secular medicine in a Taiwan village: A study of cosmological disorders. *In* Medicine in Chinese Culture: Comparative Studies of Health Care in Chinese and Other Societies, ed. Arthur Kleinman, Peter Kunstader, E. Russel Alexander, and James L. Gale. Publication no. 75-653. Washington, D.C.: National Institutes of Health, Department of Health, Education, and Welfare.
 1975b   Chinese-style and Western-style doctors in northern Taiwan. *In* Medicine in Chinese Culture: Comparative Studies of Health Care in Chinese and Other Societies, ed. Arthur Kleinman, Peter Kunstader, E. Russel Alexander, and James L. Gale. Publication no. 75-653. Washington, D.C.: National Institutes of Health, Department of Health, Education, and Welfare.
Anderson, Eugene N. and Maja L. Anderson
 1977   Modern China: The South. *In* Food in Chinese Culture: Anthropological and Historical Perspectives, ed. K. C. Chang. New Haven: Yale University Press.
Arluke, Arnold, and John Peterson
 1981   Accidental medicalization of old age and its social implications. *In* Dimensions: Aging, Culture, and Health, ed. Christine L. Fry, pp. 271–85. New York: Praeger.
Beauvoir, Simone de
 1964   Mort très douce. Paris: Soleil.
Beeson, Paul B.
 1979   Training doctors to care for old people. Annals of Internal Medicine 90(20):262.
Birenbaum, A., M. Aronsen and S. Suffer
 1979   Teaching medical students to appreciate the special problems of the elderly. Gerontologist 19(6):575.
Blacking, John, ed.
 1977   The Anthropology of the Body. New York: Academic Press.
Bowers, J., ed.
 1974   Medicine and Society in China. New York: Josiah Macy, Jr., Foundation.

Campbel, J. D.
1975 Attribution of illness: Another double standard. Journal of Health and Social Behavior 16:114–26.
Chang, K. C., ed.
1977 Food in Chinese Culture: Anthropological and Historical Perspectives. New Haven: Yale University Press.
Childress, J.
1971 Who shall live when not all can live? Soundings 53:339–55.
Clark, Margaret
1972 An anthropological approach to aging. *In* Aging and Modernization, ed. Donald Cowgill and Lowell Holmes. New York: Appleton-Century-Crofts.
1973 Contribution of cultural anthropology to the study of the aged. *In* Culture, Illness, and Health: Essays on Human Adaptation, ed. Laura Nadar and T. Maretzhi, pp. 78–88. Washington, D.C.: American Anthropology Association.
Clark, Margaret, and Barbara Anderson
1967 Culture and Aging. San Francisco: Jossey-Bass.
Croizier, Ralph
1975 Medicines and modernization in China: An historical overview. *In* Medicine in Chinese Culture: Comparative Studies of Health Care in Chinese and Other Societies, ed. Arthur Kleinman, Peter Kunstader, E. Russel Alexander, and James L. Gale Publication no. 75-653. Washington, D.C.: National Institutes of Health, Department of Health, Education, and Welfare.
Davis-Friedman, Deborah
1979 Old people and their families in the People's Republic of China. Ph.D. dissertation; Boston University.
Engle, G. L.
1977 The need for a new medical model: A challenge for biomedicine. Science 196:129–36.
Fries, James
1980 Aging, natural death, and the compression of morbidity. New England Journal of Medicine 303:130–35.
Gould-Martin, Katherine
1975 Medical systems in a Taiwan village: Ong-Ia-Kong, the plague god, as a modern physician. *In* Medicine in Chinese Cultures: Comparative Studies of Health Care in Chinese and Other Societies, ed. Arthur Kleinman, Peter Kunstader, E. Russel Alexander, and James L. Gale. Publication no. 75-653. Washington, D.C.: National Institutes of Health, Department of Health, Education, and Welfare.
Gould-Martin, Katherine, and Ngin Choorswang
1981 Chinese Americans. *In* Ethnicity and Medical Care, ed. Alan Harwood, pp. 231–74. Cambridge: Harvard University Press.

Harrell, Stevan
1981 Old age in China. *In* Other Ways of Growing Old, ed. Pamela Amoss and Stevan Harrell. Stanford: Stanford University Press.
Harris, Louis, and Associates
1976 The Myth and Reality of Aging in America. Washington, D.C.: National Council on Aging.
Hayflick, Leonard
1977 The cellular basis for biological aging. *In* Handbook of the Biology of Aging, ed. L. E. Finche and Hayflick. New York: Van Nostrand Reinhold.
Hickey, Tom
1980 Health and Aging. Monterey, Calif.: Brooks/Cole.
Hickey, Tom, and William Rakowski
1980 Older patients and their families: Negotiating the psychosocial context of gathering health information. Paper presented to the 33rd Annual Meeting of the Gerontological Society, San Diego.
Hsu, Vera, and Francis L. K. Hsu
1977 Modern China: North. *In* Food in Chinese Culture: Anthropological and Historical Perspectives, ed. K. C. Chang. New Haven: Yale University Press.
Ikels, Charlotte
1979 Urbanization and modernization: The impact on aging in Hong Kong. Ph.D. dissertation, University of Hawaii.
Institute of Medicine
1978 Aging and Medical Education. Washington, D.C.: National Academy of Science.
Kleinbach, George U.
1974 Social structure and the education of health personnel. International Journal of Health Services 4:297.
Kleinman, Arthur
1980 Patients and Healers in the Context of Culture. Berkeley: University of California Press.
Kutner, Nancy
1978 Medical student orientation toward the chronically ill. Journal of Medical Education 53:111–18.
Lucas, A. Elissen
1980 Changing medical models in China: Organizational options or obstacles. China Quarterly 83:461–90.
Mabry, John M.
1964 Lay concepts of etiology. Journal of Chronic Diseases 17:371–86.
McKeown, T.
1965 Medicine in Modern Society. London: George Allen & Unwin.
Manton, Kenneth G.
1982 Changing concepts of morbidity and mortality in the elderly population. Milbank Memorial Fund Quarterly 60:183–244.

Mechanic, David
  1962 The concept of illness behavior. Journal of Chronic Disease 15:189–94.
  1972 Social-psychological factors affecting the presentation of bodily complaints. New England Journal of Medicine 286:1132–39.
Metchnikoff, I. I.
  1906 The Nature of Man. New York: Putman.
Pernick, Martin
  1979 A calculus of suffering: Pain anaesthesia and utilitarian professionalism in nineteenth-century American medicine. Ph.D. dissertation, Columbia University.
Porkert, Manfred
  1975 The dilemma of present-day interpretations of Chinese medicine. *In* Medicine in Chinese Culture: Comparative Studies of Health Care in Chinese and Other Societies, ed. Arthur Klcinman, Peter Kunstader, E. Russel Alexander, and James L. Gale. Publication no. 75-653. Washington, D.C.: National Institutes of Health, Department of Health, Education, and Welfare.
Roebuck, Janet
  1979 The history of old age. Journal of Social History 12:416–29.
Sankar, Andrea
  1978 The evolution of the sisterhood in traditional Chinese society: From village girls' houses to chai t'angs in Hong Kong. Ph.D. dissertation, University of Michigan.
  1981 Conquest of solitude: Single people and aging in traditional China. *In* Dimensions: Aging, Culture, and Health, ed. Christine L. Fry. New York: Praeger.
Shanas, Ethel, Peter Townsend, Dorothy Wedderburn, Hennig Friis, Poul Milhø, and Jan Stehouwer
  1968 The psychology of health. *In* Middle Age and Aging, ed. Bernice L. Neugarten. Chicago: University of Chicago Press.
Stearns, Peter
  1976 Old Age in European Society. New York: Holmes & Muir.
Thomas, William C.
  1981 The expectation gap and the stereotype of the stereotype: Images of old people. Gerontologist 21(4):402–8.
Topley, Marjorie
  1970 Chinese traditional ideas and the treatment of disease. Man 5:421–37.
  1975 Chinese and Western medicine in Hong Kong: Some social and cultural determinants of variation, interaction, and change. *In* Medicine in Chinese Cultures: Comparative Studies of Health Care in Chinese and Other Societies, ed. Arthur Kleinman, Peter Kunstader, E. Russel Alexander, and James L. Gale. Publication no. 75-653. Washington, D.C.: National Institutes of Health, Department of Health, Education, and Welfare.

1976   Chinese traditional etiology and methods of cure in Hong Kong. *In* Asian Medical Systems, ed. Charles Leslie. Berkeley: University of California Press.

Verbrugge, Lois
1983   Longer life but worsening health? Trends in health and mortality of middle-aged and older persons. Paper presented at the meetings of the Population Association of America, Pittsburgh, April.

Walford, Roy L.
1969   The Immunological Theory of Aging. Baltimore: Williams & Williams.

Whyte, Martin King, and William L. Parish
1978   Village and Family in Contemporary China. Chicago: University of Chicago Press.

11

Chronology, Category, and Ritual

Ákos Östör

Age renders itself to social scientists in the West with such force and seeming objectivity that we assign it an almost universal linearity, seen in terms of stages of development, and an unvarying reality across cultures. These assumed universals and objectivity have obscured significant comparative questions: Are there similar patterns of age and aging in all societies? Is the life course divisible into beginning, middle, and end everywhere? Are the differences merely variations on predetermined, measurable distances from place to place and time to time? That people everywhere are born, mature, and then die merely begs the question: What is age, who is aging, how do men and women get old, how are we to understand these categories and processes? We attach meanings to all these terms and for that reason alone they are realities. Categories are not God-given certainties that can be invoked to illustrate specific cases. Such terms as age, life course, birth, maturity, decline, stage, grade,

This essay is part of a larger project, started at the National Humanities Center in 1980–81, concerning time as category and value in different societies. I thank David Brent, Michael Lofaro, and the editors for comments on a previous version. I have also discussed some of the arguments advanced here in seminars and lectures at the University of North Carolina, Chapel Hill, at Princeton University, and at Clemson University, and at the meetings of the American Association for the Advancement of Science in San Francisco, 1980.

seniority, and cycle are something, do something, and mean something, and we may group them, if at all, only by establishing, interpreting, and comparing them in different contexts.

These questions are inseparable from the problems of understanding time in different societies. In many societies we have to consider cyclical, plural, reversible, nonlinear, and nonmeasurable notions of time. The supposedly universal understanding thus becomes a particular indigenous folk model, that obtaining in the advanced industrial societies of the West. Age, like time, totemism, and kinship, is based on an illusion, an assumed and uninterpreted universal. It is true enough as a general expectation, but false as a skeleton to which cultures bring the varying appearances of flesh. Should the measurement of time—whatever *that* is—matter, and not the categories and the links among religion, economy, kinship, and marriage as they are culturally understood? We may get somewhere by just "counting" and "reckoning" time, and by observing the similarities and differences that emerge from such quantification, but beyond these often limited and limiting secular trends we still need to know what is meant by age and time (measurement is not enough), economy (production and distribution are not enough), politics (authority is not enough). We are left with cultural differences and the legitimate quest of interpreting them. The alternatives are not between a positive science and cultural solipsism: in commanding the tension between general and particular lies the possible contribution of a comparative anthropological science. At its very best anthropology considers the universal and the particular—moving back and forth, stressing the universality of being human but realizing that only in particular forms, men and women living in particular societies, is this experience embodied for all of us (see Dumont 1978). What follows from this observation is a promise, not the unfailing practice of anthropologists, a way of seeing ourselves as well as other societies in perspective, not just as a methodological or even a moral lesson but as constitutive of our awareness of our own society and of other societies.

Even in Euro-American societies the division of age and stage is not immutable and permanent: during the Middle Ages and as recently as the late nineteenth century the human life span was divided and interpreted differently from the way it is today. More recently the subdivision of phases at the youthful end of the life span has multiplied and the notions of passage, course, cycle, crisis themselves have changed. These changes are intimately linked to the transformation of religion, market, and politics in the eighteenth and nineteenth centuries. What happened to age and time cannot be understood without some attention to these other changes, nor can we ignore comparative data from other societies, since without the alternatives provided by Asia and Africa we cannot recognize the integration and separation of religion, economics, and politics in the West through the rise of capital-intensive production, the impact of industrialization, ideological transformations, and the like.

Time, Age, and Ritual

The meaning of ritual cannot simply be postulated as attaching to various ages and stages in society. First we must know who are the children, youth, adults, and elderly. What reorientations have taken place in society through the notions of time in different contexts and periods? How are the stages of life separated? Are the various groups and categories separated by symbols and rituals? How are we to understand fragmentation of time and ritual in relation to age and work? What are these stages, ages, and rituals, this separation and fragmentation? The cultural, symbolic studies that would provide the answers have not been done to any significant extent, so I have to make an implicit and at times evocative argument. Yet we can do more than speculate: we can outline the broad contexts and changes with which we would have to link the questions of person, age, ritual, and society.

Rather than speak of age in abstract, universal terms, it may be more helpful to think of persons in and through time in particular societies. All societies recognize persons as sentient beings, but not in the same way, in the same cycles, passing through the same stages. As with religion, kinship, and economy, so we have trouble with typologies of age.

Age is especially a problem in the West, where the very notion places the old in a liminal position: structurally outside social bounds, superfluous and expendable. The aged become a social problem because they are not in the producing economy (note the parallels with minorities, the unemployed, and welfare recipients). They are ignored until they are organized as political pressure groups, consumers of goods and services. Even in this case they have greater difficulties in gaining access to services because of the scarcity and fragmentation of time in American society. As time becomes fragmented and individuals become increasingly autonomous, the elderly become mere charges. Note the terms "care," "nursing," and "delivery," emphasizing incompetence, dependence, and infirmity, pointing to mere decrepitude, which is seen quite separately in other societies as only one of the several possible things that may happen to elders. Note also that decrepitude may be recognized universally yet age and power may also be linked differently. In India *bura* is not merely old but ripe, wise, and powerful. Furthermore, *gurujan* (elders) are respected as partakers in divinity and sacredness, quite apart from the problems of infirmity, senility, decline.

Age is inevitably linked to time and society, and thus to ideology. In the West this means linear time and capital-intensive production in democratic societies. Open-ended, cumulative, measured time emphasizes change. In other societies there is hardly anything approximating this concept: cyclical, plural, nonmeasured, nonfragmented time is not time in the same sense. Yet in both kinds of societies, we cannot consider the question without discussing other domains of social behavior, since symbolism links age, time, ritual, production, and authority. Hence we would expect that the transformation of age and time occurs in parallel with changes in these other domains. Old folks, senior citizens, the aged in America constitute a separate category and a special problem. Functional equivalents of the "aged" in other societies do not yield hypotheses about genealogical position and gerontocracy, since categories, actions, and social relations have to be constituted first, and cannot be assumed or intuited. The concomitant questions of power, control, dominance, production, and ritual also have to be examined throughout the society, not just in preestablished segments. Such a constructivist approach depends on comparison and on the (ideological) interpretation of behavior.

The basic argument of this essay is that the anthropological problem of age cannot be comprehended in the absence of a comparative cultural study of societies. For "age" this should mean, first, a recognition of the differences between advanced industrial and other societies; second, a pursuit of the changes that have occurred in advanced industrial societies in the light of these differences; and third, consideration of the changes that are transforming African and Asian societies today partly as a result of the impact of advanced industrial societies. We start with an initial comparison with other societies, and then explore changes in the past of Euro-American societies. We would expect a different division, understanding, and experience of age in America, in parallel with other changes in economy, polity, family, and religion. The American example may alert us to changes we can expect in the linking of cultural domains in industrializing societies, while the experience of the rapidly transforming societies may make us aware of the potential for change in America.

Age and Time in Anthropological Research

Anthropological studies of age, time, kinship, and family do not give the unvarnished facts about other cultures, since, as a rule, they are trying to make sense of differences in terms comprehensible to *us*. The classic study of the Nuer, for example, is an account of a singular relation between time and social structure. E. E. Evans-Pritchard (1940) notes that in ecological cycles of transhumance and cultivation, dry and wet seasons follow each other with parallel shifts in locality, habitat, and group organization; villages shift to cattle camps, and repeated short cycles of activity become, in fact, long-term regularities. Long-range, repeated patterns are central to kin and marriage relations, lineage and tribe formation, and the progression of age sets. Social segments are related and distinguished by "structural" time; the fission and fusion of lineages follow ancestors back about five generations, but beyond that, time is telescoped into another five generations, reaching, at that point, mythic origins. Linked to these cycles of ecology, lineage, and space as an aspect of "structural time" is the age-grade system, in which persons progress through a fixed cycle from birth to death, with passages of transition marked by ceremonial activities.

From one point of view age and time among the Nuer are inexorably fixed, structured so that different units (human beings grouped in different segments) pass through immutable grades, the structure being permanent, the people ephemeral. Rather than accepting this mechanical image, we may note that here time serves persons, through whom all grades and structures pass, safely removed from the accumulation of surprises, amenable to repetition and foretelling, people-oriented and serving human ends.

Evans-Pritchard's problem is that he is speaking not about Nuer time and age at all, but about *his* view of *their* social structure. The latter appears as a specific categorization of some kind of space-time universal in social life, where individuals pass through segments such as lineages, age grades, marriage, and cycles as well as seasons of cultivation and herding. Thus a Nuer concept of time becomes illusory because it is the segmentary social structure that is immutable and through which proceed an endless succession of individuals. An even more extreme mechanical example is to be found in Raymond Firth's study of the Tikopia (1957), where society is likened to a huge machine that bends and shapes individuals to its will.[1] Ideologies of industrial society intrude here, since time need not be exclusively a linear measuring stick of marked, discrete entities. Several unnoticed things are going on in the Nuer example: changes and relations among persons are marked in various ways and the social being of persons is constituted through different "times" that should be referred *to each other*, rather than to rough and ready scientific and universal equivalents such as measured time, kinship, economics, and religion.

In a more direct confrontation of relative age and kinship, Rodney Needham's pioneering study (1974) attempted to deal with time and genealogy. In scoring telling points against the notion of "kinship," however, Needham assumes age to have a given chronological meaning, with only relationship terminologies qualifying for category status. The further step of recognizing age as a cultural category is not taken, and time remains a linear, divisible, universal category.

The different aspects of ecology, kinship, politics, and age are integrated in our next example through the use of indigenous notions of person and time. In his now classic study of Bali, Clifford Geertz (1973) provides an example of how persons, cycles of time, and behavior are symbolic structures in the hands (and minds) of those who live them, providing both the integration and discontinuity (as a subdominant theme) so characteristic of nonindustrial societies. The Balinese have many ways of categorizing persons, establishing a finite set far short of the numerical possibilities. People may be named according to birth order, kinship relation, occupation, age, prestige, marriage alliance, and statuses in many different ways.

The repeating cycles of lunar/solar and task-oriented calendars do not tell what time it is; rather they tell the kind of time experienced in relation to ceremonial and other activites. The effect is to rob time of its cumulative, developmental, and transformative aspects: in Geertz's felicitous phrase, "to detemporalize time." So, too, persons are deindividualized in the sense of the Western individual as a repository of rights and responsibilities.[2]

1. I owe this insight to T. N. Madan.
2. "Persons" in this society are different from the Western construct of the "individual" (see Dumont 1980 and below).

Time thus becomes a series of forever recurrent cycles linking family, person, production, ideology, and ritual without being aggregated into steady progress, rise and fall, without a driving force such as the commodity market fueling the next phase of expansion or contraction. Geertz cautions, however, that these symbolic structures are not perfectly integrated, and their opposites may exist as contrary potentials with powerful implications for the future. A shift in any one aspect of these linked domains may yield fundamental changes in these societies. Social integration and discontinuity may both be affected; hence several possibilities are given in any society, not a single predictable and predetermined outcome.

It is exactly in the links between the symbolic structures and in the links among the various cycles of person and time that the increase in production and the expansion of the commodity market creates its msot wide-ranging effects. Let us take a specific instance of how these symbolic structures may change and how they may be related to the problem of age. While there is no direct access to the differences among and the changes going on within societies, we can outline the links between cultural domains against which these changes have to be viewed.

In India the extremes coexist. On the one hand we find capital-intensive production, a commodity market, a governmental and administrative structure inherited from the British. On the other hand, we see an enduring Indian social structure that can be understood in terms of the basic, underlying cultural principles of purity and pollution. The separation or hierarchy of groups into high and low, the division of labor from priest to untouchable sweeper, and the endogamy of groups in marriage guard the boundaries of purity. Dumont (1980) characterized this society as hierarchical, one in which the basic relationships of its units are those between encompassing and encompassed elements.

Here status and power are, relationally, separated in the link between priest and king (the former being superior), with rule, kingship, bazaar production and exchange, kinship, and marriage articulating in distinct social and regional wholes in hierarchical terms. The opposition of purity and pollution, a religious principle, is linked to notions of sacred order (*dharma*), ceremonial action (in relation to rituals of sacrifice) yielding a hierarchical whole that is sanctified by the gods and cosmic regularities.[3] Religious ideology rather than economics is dominant in this society, yet

3. Religious in the sense of the ideology of caste hierarchy.

there is no perfect fit among these symbolic structures: opposing and contrary themes exist in Islamic, Buddhist, and colonial British ideologies along with the emergent commodity market relations and other aspects of British dominance: educational, judicial, and administrative principles and systems. In the precolonial situation the bazaar existed in a hierarchical articulation with kinship and rule in terms subject to a sacred order and a sacrificial ethos.

The major question in India is the local rise and impact of commodity production and markets based on exchange value and profit which begin to differentiate the economy from other domains. This process cuts across discrete face-to-face societies that are unified only by cultural principles, and at one stroke alters the articulation of indigenous domains in a hierarchical society. The first significant changes are in the division of labor and in the autonomous, entrepreneurial activity of the market, which "liberate" the new domain from the domination of *dharma* and other cultural principles.

How, then, does the commodity market articulate with or contradict "holistic" or "hierarchical" Indian societies?[4] The regional bazaar in Bengal still articulates the production of some foodstuffs, aspects of redistribution, festivals and rituals, principles of purity and power, caste-kinship-family relations, ecological cycles, long-range trade, exchange with nonprofit bias, face-to-face social relations, need and use orientation, and handicraft production. The bazaar also symbolizes and uses an integrated, nondifferentiated stream of time, parallel to ritual, ecology, family, history, rebellion, and other indigenous constructions of reality. Hierarchy still characterizes the bazaar: the principle of *śakti* (divine female power) still infuses all action. *Śakti* appears in the kinship-marriage-caste relations that participate in the bazaar, and is also linked, in the ideology, to bazaar principles of ability/power (*khamata*) and thought/time/knowledge (*bhab*). Respect is still placed above calculation, credit is not approved as gain at someone else's expense, and time-stocks-credit-capital are still relatively undifferentiated. Temporal cycles are still unified to an extent, capable of being intuitively grasped by the participating actor.

---

4. In answering this question we have to look beyond one-dimensional studies of a single field: economy or religion or kinship and caste or polity. My own work on indigenous construction of history, rebellion, ritual, kinship, and bazaar in Bengal allows the linking of several domains apprehended ideologically and interpreted in terms of cultural categories (Östör 1980, 1983; Östör et al., eds., 1982).

Yet this integrated bazaar rhythm does not articulate with markets of commodities and finances, planning and development, central and regional politics, and administration. Rebellions, regional challenges to authority, communal conflict, and other contradictions emerge precisely because of the failing articulation of hierarchy (sacred order) with the overweening domains of market economy, and central government and administration that embody different principles. With the rise of the market and its ancillary institutions and concomitant practices, the economy becomes differentiated, and embraces and cuts across regional hierarchies that articulate societal domains in terms of an ideology of the sacred. This new commodity market draws into itself activities of other domains more centrally than any polity did before, yielding something different from hierarchy, yet also not the same as industrial society. Thus change in any of the symbolic structures discussed above signals basic change in Indian society. Although exchange market values are not anchored in the same principles, and although they dominate the bazaar, they do not replace the latter because time is still "enchanted" by ritual, festival, and ceremony.[5] Domains of living are still integrated while being dominated by the market economy, which tends to differentiate the economy from kinship and religion.

Time and Age in the Industrialization of Western Societies

In European and American societies similar changes may have been going on for centuries. Yet I know of no attempts to link the articulation of domains with cultural categories of time and age. In order to understand age in our own societies, it is not enough to invoke generation, social time, life crisis, and the like, favorite though unexamined categories of social sicence today. What has been the effect of economic and other changes on the links between person and time in the advanced industrial societies? Again we have no direct answers in the face of wide gaps in the literature. Nevertheless, the form of an approach can be outlined. Market, time, person, work, and ideology are integrally linked throughout the emergence of the capital-intensive economy.

In fourteenth-century Europe workers "struggled for the mastery of their own labor time" (Le Goff 1980), especially for setting lesiure time

---

5. Max Weber called attention to the disenchantment of the world through the rationalizing process.

aside from their working hours. This situation seems familiar yet surprising: the twentieth century thought itself unique in having to cope with the fragmentation of time. Yet the process of this breaking up has been long and incomplete. Alongside time we may expect similar things to happen with age, although our documentation in that regard is very meager. Still the work of Peter Laslett and his associates, Lawrence Stone, and others suggests that twentieth-century kinship and family systems, the position of elders, and divisions of the life span are also not a recent consequence of industrialization and capital-intensive production. A discussion of time, however, may reflect age better than family structure, genealogy, and the like, since it brings home to us the qualitative, cultural nature of the process.

In the fourteenth century, work bells already signified a regulated time in opposition to the time of events and the sacred time of festivals. Thus was born the measurable time of everyday life. Concurrently the church challenged merchants in a field crucial to emerging mercantile capitalism: credit. For the church, interest amounted to selling time, something that belongs to God alone. Time, however, is the core of a merchant's life: storage of stock, anticipation of sale, trading networks, knowledge of market and production, all are timebound, costing money. At stake were the very conditions of production: the employment of a monetary sphere required adequate measurement of time. From A.D. 1300 to 1650 the shift in time sense continued to affect labor discipline and the working people's "inward apprehension of time" (Thompson 1967); clock time contrasts with more "natural" rhythms throughout the period. Task-oriented agrarian pursuits are more humanly comprehensible than timed labor, and work and life are not sharply separated.

Yet an attention to time measurement depends on the need to synchronize labor, and this need does not become systematic till the appearance of large-scale machine-powered industry. Through the eighteenth century the pattern is one of intense bouts of labor followed by periods of idleness. At the same time it was not all "preindustrial" either: "in the transition to industrialism the stress falls upon the whole culture," including systems of power, relations of property, and religion (Thompson 1967:80).

America was, even in the 1830s, an agricultural society, characterized by a craft-based production, a mercantile system of trade, and a pattern of time still associated with the seasons and "natural" agrarian rhythms. Yet Alexis de Tocqueville saw several peculiarly American problems, most tellingly the contrast between "aristocratic" and "democratic" societies. "Amongst aristocratic nations, as families remain for centuries in the same condition, often in the same spot, all generations become as it were contemporaneous. A man almost always knows his forefathers, and respects them: he thinks he already sees his remote descendants, and he loves them. . . . Amongst democratic nations new families are constantly falling away, and all that remain change their condition; the woof of time is every instant broken, and the track of generations effaced" (Tocqueville 1954:104, 105). Social bonds are weak and so are individuals, necessitating many kinds of human association. Aristocratic societies have strong bonds under a few powerful men and no associations are needed: everyone knows and is in his place. In democratic societies the succession between generations is cut, each being condemned unto itself. Practical as against theoretical "sciences" predominate; everyone is in motion and there is a marked distaste for "meditation."

Tocqueville perceived a link between a kind of economy, polity, and ideology, even though full industrialization and the commodity economy were yet to come. This very period is now used by historians to heighten the contrast between the craft-based phase of production in the early nineteenth century and the factories of the latter part of the century. Well into the twentieth century the remaking of work habits and the needs of the machine provoked recurrent tensions. Herbert Gutman (1973) noted the conflict, unique to America, between different groups new to the machine and a rapidly changing society. The few factory workers of the early nineteenth century were bearers of a village culture. Social structure was transformed in the second half of the century, and an advanced industrial society came into being by the 1920s. Immigrants brought with them ways of work and values not associated with the industrial ethos. The question was not only of industrializing a whole culture, but of introducing new generations of factory workers to the same processes over and over.

In the Amoskoeg of 1853, mill operatives protested the cutting down of an elm tree because it was a "connecting link between past and present"; in autumn especially it was a reminder of "our mortality." The great economic changes of the late nineteenth century did not destroy the culture of previous times and places. Immigrants manage to hang onto their family, ethnic, and class ties. Communities of workers are bound together by festivals, rituals, intellectual traditions, mythic beliefs, and a structure of feeling. Workers also have their benevolent societies, holidays, sports, recreation, churches, trade unions, politicians, and reformers.

There is a parallel transformation of the work ethic and the concepts of time and play. The Puritan ethic fades out of work early, and as the rewards of industrialization bring the problem of leisure time to some, work becomes slavery for many. Yet the work ethic affirms success as a way out of the increasing encroachment on the worker's independence. For the middle classes the self-discipline of work becomes the creative spontaneity of play. For the workers the ethic erodes under the failure of rewards, and from the 1880s on irregular work patterns, increased mobility, and slowdowns are the response to the factory faith. The result is a split between rhetoric and reality: while workers affirm the dignity and value of labor, they see rewards and work opportunities decrease and practical alienation increase (see Rodgers 1978).

What are we to make of the rapid changes that occur in societies undergoing industrialization? What survives, what changes, how, and why? In a more complex vein: what are the processes and meanings of transformation, articulation, and/or contradiction? How is age affected in the process?

Suggestive though inconclusive evidence comes from the studies of Tamara Hareven and her associates of "family time" in nineteenth-century New England and of the New Hampshire factory town of Amoskoeg (Hareven, ed., 1978, Hareven and Langenbach, 1978). Harking back to the high point of industrialization, Amoskoeg workers later recall their experience with pride, as if they were talking about the earlier craft, farm, and mercantile age. There may be nostalgia in these memories, yet the valuations remain constant: availability and reward of work, good versus bad workers, pride in labor and accomplishment of hand and body, some sympathetic supervisors and some fair treatment from managers—despite widespread labor unrest during the period. Significantly, the Amoskoeg of the 1920s is favorably contrasted with the Depression era in terms of work continuity, a cycle of work-home linkages, and even the dignity of labor. The assessment of the Amoskoeg workers' experience is very different from "working for capitalism" (Pfeffer 1979), stressing what E. P. Thompson calls a more "natural rhythm," but it harks back not to the fourteenth century but to the high tide of industrialism. As we noted, there is a quality of nostalgia here, yet the work/leisure opposition is not sharp (because there is no time for leisure). Maybe women workers form a little-known culture of their own, but they also stress the value of labor and its products, of what work secures for home, independence, companionship, respect, and community.

Hareven's "family time" counters the "tyranny of the clock," a rhythm different from that of work discipline, in which celebration marks the points of entry into the stages of life, continuous and less subject to change than we would expect. These studies, however, reap some confusion from a contrast between some sort of "objective" time and the slower, more integrated patterns of family time. The latter is not related to other domains of life; its contents merely stand out. Despite this failing, the studies grope toward a constitution of otherness in nineteenth-century America. Even if Hareven's "historical" time is too single-minded a contrast to act as an outside measure of difference, at least recognition of the survival of family time is in harmony with the cultural emphasis of Thompson's, Gutman's, and Rodgers' studies.

There is a problem with all these studies: although aware of differences among societies, they reflect back into Western history as against comparative, universal, and nonwestern histories. The long-term consideration of Europe is welcome and draws out a cyclical view (stimulated by anthropological studies) beyond the short term and the unique event. At the same time historians resist the notion of structure (as proposed by Lévi-Strauss) while utilizing the mode of structural continuity in their analyses. Historians have much to learn from anthropologists, but not by the uncritical transplanting of multivocal concepts. Anthropologists, for their part, have to stop objectifying the historian's time, as if the latter's accounts were the one sure island of certainty in the face of complex links among symbols, values, practices, and social experience.

Other questions remain. If the fourteenth-century crisis involves a "new time" and yet the old rhythms continue—to the extent of causing riots in the twentieth century—then how are we to understand the opposition of fragmented time versus a flowing cyclical rhythm? And how, in Asia and Africa, an emerging time disenchanted of sacred ritual activity? And in A.D. 1335 workers of Amiens protesting night work, and in the 1970s Murray Melbin (1978) discovering the night as a frontier?

We can now pose a fundamental problem: if the "tyranny of the clock" has been in process for at least 600 years, then what of the destruction and erosion it has wrought? What have been the effects, changes, and continuities? How could the social fabric regenerate itself? Have there been qualitative differences among the various times? Where have the alternatives, even if only dreams of a qualitatively different time, come from? What is the source and structure of a continued striving for cyclical, holistic integration of person and time?

Old Age in America

It is against these processes in Europe and America that we have to view the emergence of the aged as a problem and a category in American society. Retirement, leisure time, and the unfulfilled work ethic are linked to each other, although with effects that vary with the segment of the population. Senior citizens may have the time for leisure though not the productive value that creates its rewards. Nevertheless, I put the question again: What of time and age in American society today, after the seemingly destructive and certainly major fragmentation wrought by the past 200 years?

In studying the symbolic life of Americans, Lloyd Warner (1959) showed us the confirming values of the past, age, and aristocracy that existed, albeit in tension, with democratic values in a small-town society (Newburyport, Massachusetts).

The procession celebrating the 300th anniversary of the town was the culmination of year-long preparations. The festivities oscillated around two symbols, the Permanent City and the Moving Frontier: the expanding world horizon and the declining home city within it, the value of progress and its doubting, covert contradiction. The city is the permanent New England civilization, while the frontier moves on. The permanence is detached from the past and becomes a set of movable symbols. In tones recalling Tocqueville, Warner says, ''. . . each generation is partly liberated from the thralldom and absolute authority of the preceding generation. . . . These sacred or secular objective symbols of the past or present, free from the control of their creators and their contexts of origin, as they move may radically change their meanings and the manner of their acceptance; the sacred word may become secular, or the secular marks of economic and political agreement of the Charter become semi-sacred'' (1959:214–15). The city stands for time eternal, while present time has gone elsewhere. Clock time is applied to the regulation of social time. Human values are attributed to social time; thus the life cycle, social status, and the activities of the self are measured by clock time.

The partly sacred rituals of association exhibit a dual tendency in American society: one toward the increasing formation of individuals into autonomous units, the other the unification of segmenting units into overall symbol systems. The cults of the dead relate the living to the sacred, providing communal representations of the ways persons fit into the secular world of the living and the spiritual world of the dead. The funeral "removes the *time*-bound individual from control by the forward direction of human time" (Warner 1959:281).

The purely sacred symbols of Christian values exhibit an opposition between Catholics and Protestants. The masculinity of Protestant worship eliminated the cult of the Virgin Mary. If Mary stood for a symbolic moral approval of the species, then Protestantism was a movement against the value placed on species life by the traditional church. The revival of the cult reestablishes the focus on species life: women as procreative partners, bearing and caring for children. Hence Mother's Day and other celebrations of the family in Protestant churches of the 1950s. Puritanism was authoritarian, male-dominated, with a religious symbolism from which female elements were banished. This cutting of ties to family through the mother may have helped to autonomize and free the individual, but it also helped to separate monads from their species being.

Sacred sexuality transforms the species life and the values/beliefs of a society. Sexuality, procreation, and marriage are central to Christian symbolism. The sacred year, following the life cycle of Jesus, is infused with the ultimate values and beliefs of the moral order and acts out a story about the symbolic significance of human existence. This sacred time transforms both "social time" and "technological [objective] time" into the powerful symbols of a god-man's life span. The different "times" are thereby bound to the significant crises of human individual experience. Technological time thus yields to the crises of birth, life, and death. Ordinary existence, secular mortality, sequence of past events and future projection disappear into the liturgical stillness of the present (Warner 1959:399–400).[6]

6. We may note in criticism that it was a mistake to single out "objective" time as an outside measuring stick to which everything can be referred as impartial arbiter. This kind of time is also a symbolic construct, mediated through Western ideologies. In India, for example, planetary motions are linked to a cycle of time with quite different effects. The same confusion marks Warner's linking of objective reality with chronological time in American history, something that can be discovered incontrovertibly and absolutely. Thus "scientific" objectivity is also ideological in that it gives a value as well as concept/category context to time, becoming one among the kinds of time in advanced industrial societies. *We* give "objective" time its character and value, and apply its standards to other domains of life. Lloyd Warner (1959) realizes this when he suggests that the sacred year reconciles social and scientific time, thus transforming time values for the community of the faithful.

Different kinds of time continue to be categorized, experienced, valued, and symbolized in American societies to this day: ecological and seasonal cycles; clock time; scientific time (with its variations from microseconds to light-years);[7] fragmented work time and leisure or free time; historical cycles; social time; a telescoped secular ritual time of the past; associational and political time; and finally the eternal, unchanging cycle and moment of sacred time.

Age, time, and ritual are linked to the question of the individual in American society. Here Dumont's (1980) distinction of person and individual helps to clarify the problem. The individual as an autonomous unit allows the abstraction of the aged from the rest of society. The elderly are cut off from economic and political (i.e., productive) roles and the person is split up into role performances—a circumstance that is quite impossible and meaningless in an integrated, holistic society, where the whole person acts in integrally linked social domains. What is the culture of the aged in America in relation to class, region, work? Especially work, since in fact the work ethic is contradicted in the widespread recognition of the declining possibility for most workers to attain the rewards available for the few. Further questions relate to the secularization and the lack of enchantment in the lives of the old. The time of the elderly is not enchanted by ritual and myth that is shared by the whole society. The individual, as Tocqueville stated, is condemned unto himself alone. Mere age becomes a marker of status, separation, role, bereft of value and wisdom. The link between generations is cut and the past no longer informs the present.

In the United States atomized time and fragmented domains separate work and home, contributing to the measurement and categorization of age. Schneider's (1980) work suggests that the old could have particular significance in the home, family, and kin domain, yet this domain is in a dominated, subordinated position in the society. In comparison, precisely these aspects of social relations are left to the surviving precapitalist formations in Africa and Asia, and the emerging domains of economy and polity cannot cope with integration, holism, and hierarchy (see Bourdieu's suggestive work [1979]). Thus, in America, "homes" for the aged try to reconstitute the family-kin domain, but in a separate way, detached from the rest of society. The reconstitution of the elderly in America as a society with its own rituals (à la Myerhoff 1978) would run into problems

---

7. This particularly felicitious coupling I owe to Charles Ryan.

because in African and Asian examples the whole society passes through cycles, grades, and rituals, and the whole society experiences production, polity, and the sacred. At least the parts act in relation to the whole or to an understanding and experience of the whole. The elderly off by themselves with their esoteric and feeble rites, without disturbing the rest of society, may be just what the latter wants, but such an arrangement would be inconceivable in the societies of a particular time in Africa and Asia, from which the examples of integrative, holistic ritual are derived. These lessons cannot be transplanted directly, since the articulation of domains in the two kinds of society differs; persons are differently positioned in time, ritual, and other domains, and domains themselves are differently oriented to the whole society. Ritual, symbol, and myth are not a mere reflection of a social and/or economic base. Society must also be constituted (partly through ritual) in terms of category and ideology. Going further, ritual may be constitutive of time, age, and person; hence symbolic and cultural approaches acquire a new significance in the comparative understanding of societies. Though many are prepared today to claim that ritual constitutes reality, few actually demonstrate just how it does so. More often than not the problem devolves into a mere minimalist claim: ritual as police, expressing and resolving social conflict and tension.

The problem with ritual is that in other parts of the world rites are acted out still, in many cases, in integrated social contexts, with everyone participating in the same universe. The separate world of the old in the United States is in a dominated, isolated position, even if reinvented through ritual, and remains detached, with the significance of symbolic action unrelated to the rest of society. In part this is the reason for the lack of ritual in the later phases of the American life course. Though crises are much emphasized, divorce, death, illness, and mourning are not ritualized in America, except in hastening a communal amnesia, a denial of the possibility that ritual constitutes *those* realities, or to put it differently, rituals are meant to deny and isolate, not to constitute and transcend.[8]

Conclusion

Because they ignore the cultural nature of domains and the articulation of structural and processual features, anthropological and sociological

8. An oft-voiced American complaint is that it would be easier to cope with loss, anxiety, bereavement, and separation if these experiences were more deeply embedded in ritual.

studies of age and aging reproduce a linear progression of time in other societies, past and present. Here I can do no more than call attention to category, domain, person, structure, and process. The disciplinary problems surrounding the question of age will not be resolved till comparative cultural and historical studies of the kind outlined here are carried out in advanced industrial as well as other societies. Studies of the elderly in America are particularly marked by unexamined assumptions regarding generation, measurable time, and linear chronology. "Life cycle" is a misnomer, since in fact no cycles are studied. Concepts are arranged into recurrent types, but do persons circulate through these typologies? Do groups go through the life cycle? Who returns where? "Life crisis" also proceeds from Euro-American assumptions and highlights universal stages of birth, maturity, and death, begging the questions of time and cultural meaning in different societies. "Generation" is too imprecise to refer to a group and, as Laslett has argued (1979), it subsumes a whole host of unexamined questions. Notions of cycle, crisis, and course reaffirm the older notions of age and stage typologies. Even more sophisticated and recent anthropological studies select the "old" for special attention across societies, noting but not discussing the differences in the cultural understanding of age.

Symptomatically, the Frieds' recent book on transitions is about neither age nor ritual, and certainly not about time (Fried and Fried 1981). It is about the four stages of life, as a universal given, with lots of cultural variations within each set. Stages themselves are at the center; different societies may make more or less of each. Transitions are marked in some ways. The connection between stage and ritual is tenuous. What are rituals about *beyond* some kind of marking? This is a difficult problem for current anthropology, since if ritual is constitutive of something (as many assert), then it must be more than a marker of passages (whose and for whom?). Few studies actually show just how ritual constitutes reality. The concept of the person is significant in this regard, since in India, for example, rituals complete persons and to a significant extent form an integral part of kinship/caste domain (Östör et al. 1982).

Outside anthropology the prejudice is that the life span is objective chronology with biological invariants of beginning, middle, and end that cultures divide up in their own ways. Many contributors to the volume edited by Robert Binstock and Ethel Shanas (1976) share this assumption ("social age," as the saying goes). The implication is a one-to-one correspondence between social system and the objective measuring stick of time, neither of which is discussed culturally. Most sociological and gerontological studies take time to be given and have a completely unproblematic view of it. Time-trend and time-base studies are chronological but forge links to "social generations."

Recent work, although including some promising new departures, still assumes a chronological and generational base for age. A series of edited works with a commendable cultural rather than sociological focus demonstrate clearly the advances made and the distances left to travel. The volumes edited by Barbara Myerhoff and Andrei Simic (1978), Christine Fry (1980, 1981), and Pamela Amoss and Stevan Harrell (1981) should provide the grounds for a brief assessment of the situation today.

On the whole these contributions stop short of a holistic, comparative cultural approach. Overly concerned with individual life histories and strategies and the contrast between culture and society (ideal and reality), they do not constitute the culture, do not link person to group and ideology, and do not sustain a systematic comparison between societies. Why the concentration on individual elderly? Why the neglect of indigenous categories? How are indivuduals linked to groups and in what terms is this linkage accomplished? Is there a theory for charting the individual's path through relationships within the total cultural context? Behind these drawbacks lie assumptions about analysis, theory, science, comparison, society, and meaning that account for the failure to regard time, person, historical change, and underlying differences among societies as crucial to an anthropology of age.

There are other problems with views of individual strategy and manipulation of culture. Both Myerhoff (1978) and Sally Falk Moore (1978) stress individual variations in aging and invoke "culture" as a monolithic background against individual strategies. Culture is to be used and varied according to this view, yet we are not shown what this culture is; in other words, a holistic cultural analysis is missing. We are given dyadic interactions of individuals and relations between individuals and culture. But these linkages are not accounted for. Nor are we given a theory of change that would affect the cultural constitution of person, time, and relationship in crucial ways. Furthermore, the actual reality of individual social arenas is opposed to the vague backdrop of culture, a softer reality to be manipulated by individuals. The life-history method, although an indispensable tool, can end up abstracting the individual out of the ideology and the whole society. It also begs the cultural construction of the person in different societies, as if the individual of industrial society were a universal construct. The received wisdom of cross-cultural comparison is in fact noncultural. The dialectical interplay of different societies and ideologies (the investigator's and the informant's), contextualized in history and locality, tends to get lost, and the problematic nature of constructing analytical and interpretive categories under these circumstances is hardly recognized. Much as we must admire recent striving to bring anthropology into the study of aging, the achievement so far is just a beginning. Myerhoff's sensitive and pioneering work (1978) succeeds in establishing that the elderly in America do not simply fade away but create vibrant communities complete with ritual and symbolic dimensions. The next step is to show how the communities of the elderly are related to the totality of American society. What are the ideologies of various groups in relation to each other and to what is "American"? Discussions and studies of values, symbols, histories, and regional and social variants are yet to be carried out. In addition to the elderly we need a focus on other persons, time, and the whole society. Margaret Clark, for example, ties the situation of the elderly directly to American values without giving us a symbolic and cultural study of American society. Often when values crop up they are merely invoked, presumably conjured up from the native status of the anthropologist.

Here I have not been able to realize the program I have outlined. For that the different aspects of aging held separately in disciplinary specialties of cultural, social, and economic history, anthropology and sociology, gerontology and the like would have to be brought together. Yet the outline and the promise are clear enough, as the discussion of the American case shows. The emergence of an industrial society, the continuity of preindustrial patterns of time, the growth of individualism, and the significance of history, ritual, and sacred time cannot be ignored when "aging" is discussed. Ritual and time in turn refer to the concept of person, a construct completely ignored in current studies. Yet the indication of connections is unmistakable. Work, time, person, and society are linked together in systematic cultural terms. The work ethic, capital-intensive production, sacred and nonsacred ritual, and notions of the past and of the individual converge in constituting persons in the life span, with varous categories and divisions. Particularly striking is the possibility that capitalism, Protestantism, and changing work patterns created retirement and its attendant problems. Work and age are culturally understood in American society, and production is a key value and has something to do with the separation of the elderly. The aged may have time in America but not the ability to convert time into power and afflu-ence. In this sense the situation is the opposite of Marshall Sahlins' (1972) original affluent society.

Furthermore, while time is scarce for those who produce, and therefore time means money as well as power, various categories of persons are situated in this process in very different ways. Continued work, incompe-tence (at least for production), retirement, and the separation of the old are significant links, but so are the possible ties among workers' struggles for time, ritual, and personhood in the face of rapidly diminishing re-wards and changes in ethics and leisure time. Thus workers may be in the same position vis-à-vis the whole society as are the elderly. This parallel may seem fanciful yet it is telling: just as we know little about the culture of the aged, so we know hardly anything about workers' culture through time. The indications I have given of agrarian rhythms surviving into the industrial era, the continuing relation between time and the work ethic, the separations of age and the significance of ritual (especially as regards individualism) are the starting point for a holistic anthropological study of age. The survival of nonfragmented time, of personhood (rather than statuses and roles), of values of the past, of sacred ritual time are insep-arable from the study of age. Gerontology in this sense is industrial society's folk model of aging, conducted entirely from within a particular ideology without regard for the kinds of consideration developed above.

The final piece in the puzzle is contributed by comparison. Asian and African examples should alert us to different constructions of time and person, different cultural definitions through ritual and belief. We have to journey to other societies to realize that subdominant alternative patterns of age and time survive in our society and that industrial production and capital markets did not do away with holistic symbol and meaning. Com-parison is also necessary to understand the impact of advanced industrial societies on the rest of the world. To what extent do the hierarchical aspects survive in Asian and African societies? What of the future in the whole range of societies? What elements of structure and continuity may link up to produce what kinds of changes under what sorts of conditions?

To return to our initial theme, there is nothing wrong with either universalism or relativism as such, but neither is satisfactory alone; each has to be constructed in view of the other. To begin the making of comparisons, we have to approximate assumed universals but we cannot assume we have done away with the problem by turning around and reaffirming the same approximations, often nothing more than our Euro-

American folkmodels, as proofs of universal categories. These models cannot be the much-sought universals, since we started out with them in the first place. In the same manner, translatability does not "prove" the universality of concepts, since translation itself is a symbolic mediation; the process and kind of translation arrived at are the points at issue. Even in physics different worlds have different certainties (or approximations of certainties), and universals themselves are symbolic constructs.

Age and time in an anthropological sense are not universal and objective conditions with the same meanings throughout history. They are categories and values in social relations. As categories they refer to culturally shaped indigenous concepts, determined and established through local, historical, fundamentally social experience. Such constructs order and are ordered by social relations. As such, anthropological time, age, and generation create and respond to the links among economy, kinship, religion, politics, and ideology, while these domains themselves vary from society to society but not in the same predictable way everywhere, every time. On the contrary, domains are variously constructed through history and locality, without immediate, universal meanings that leap to mind ready for comparison. Relationships and categories of age and time have to be established and interpreted to distill their comparative meanings and the promise of their application across societies. Some regularities must be observed, some classification has to be set up. But if we are to learn the lessons of comparison and recognize tendencies with implications for the future, we have to go beyond analysis and interpret ideologies in relation to practices.

REFERENCES

Amoss, Pamela T., and Stevan Harrell
  1981   Other Ways of Growing Old. Stanford: Stanford University Press.
Binstock, Robert H., and Ethel Shanas, eds.
  1976   Handbook of Aging and the Social Sciences. New York: Van Nostrand
         Reinhold.
Bourdieu, Pierre
  1979   Algeria 1960. Cambridge: Cambridge University Press.
Dumont, Louis
  1978   La communauté anthroplogique et l'idéologie. L'Homme 18:83–110.
  1980   Homo Hierarchicus: An Essay on the Caste System and Its Implications. Chicago: University of Chicago Press.

Evans-Pritchard, E. E.
1940   The Nuer: A Description of the Modes of Livelihood and Political Institutions of a Nilotic People. Oxford: Clarendon Press.
Firth, Raymond
1957   We, the Tikopia: A Sociological Study of Kinship in Primitive Polynesia. Boston: Beacon Press.
Frazer, J. T.
1966   The Voices of Time. New York: George Braziller.
Fried, Martha N., and Morton H. Fried
1981   Transitions. New York: Penguin Books.
Fry, Christine L., ed.
1980   Aging in Culture and Society. New York: Praeger.
1981   Dimensions: Aging, Culture, and Health. New York: Praeger.
Geertz, Clifford
1973   Person, time, and conduct in Bali. *In* Geertz, The Interpretation of Cultures. New York: Basic Books.
Gutman, Herbert C.
1973   Work, culture, and society in industrializing America, 1815–1919. American History Review 78:531–88.
Hareven, Tamara K., ed.
1978   Transitions: The Family and the Life Course in Historical Perspective. New York: Academic Press.
Laslett, Peter
1979   The conversation between generations. *In* Philosophy, Politics, and Society, ed. Peter Laslett and J. Friskin. Oxford: Blackwell.
Le Goff, Jacques
1980   Time, Work, and Culture in the Middle Ages. Chicago: University of Chicago Press.
Melbin, Murray
1978   Night as Frontier. American Sociological Review 43:3–22.
Moore, Sally Falk
1978   Old age in a life-term social arena: Some Chagga of Kilimanjaro in 1974. *In* Life's Career—Aging, ed. Barbara Myerhoff and Andrei Simic. Beverly Hills, Calif.: Sage.
Myerhoff, Barbara
1978   Number Our Days. New York: Dutton.
Myerhoff, Barbara, and Andrei Simic, eds.
1978   Life's Career: Aging. Beverly Hills, Calif.: Sage.
Needham, Rodney
1974   Age, category, and descent. *In* Remarks and Inventions, ed. Needham. London: Tavistock.
Östör, Ákos
1980   The Play of the Gods: Locality, Ideology, Structure, and Time in the Festivals of a Bengal Town. Chicago: University of Chicago Press.

1983   Deities, Ritualists, Merchants, and Revolutionaries: Towards the Anthropology of a Bengal Town. New Delhi: Sage.
Östör, Ákos, Lina Fruzzetti, and Steve Barnett, eds.
1982   Concepts of Person: Kinship, Caste, and Marriage in India. Cambridge: Harvard University Press.
Pfeffer, Richard M.
1979   Working for Capitalism. New York: Columbia University Press.
Rodgers, Daniel T.
1978   The Work Ethic in Industrial America, 1850–1920. Chicago: University of Chicago Press.
Sahlins, Marshall
1972   Stone Age Economics. Chicago: Aldine.
Schneider, D. M.
1980   American Kinship. 2d ed. Chicago: University of Chicago Press.
Thompson, E. P.
1967   Time, work-discipline, and industrial capitalism. Past and Present, no. 28, pp. 56–97.
Tocqueville, Alexis de.
1954   Democracy in America, vol. 2. New York: Vintage.
Warner, W. Lloyd
1959   Yankee City, vol. 5: The Living and the Dead: A Study of the Symbolic Life of Americans. New Haven: Yale University Press.

12

Rites and Signs of Ripening: The Intertwining of Ritual, Time, and Growing Older

Barbara Myerhoff

The Work of Ritual

My interpretation of the special interest of ritual for the study of aging is best begun by a brief statement of my understanding of the work that ritual may accomplish. As anthropologists have agreed, ritual is prominent in all areas of uncertainty, anxiety, impotence, and disorder. By its repetitive character, it provides a message of pattern and predictability. In requiring enactments involving symbols, it bids us to participate in its messages, even enacting meanings we cannot conceive or believe; our actions lull our critical faculties, persuading us with evidence from our own physiological experience until we are convinced. In ritual, doing is believing. Ritual dramas, especially, are elaborately staged, and use presentational more than discursive symbols, so that one's senses are stimulated and one is flooded with phenomenological proof of the symbolic reality that the ritual is portraying. By dramatizing abstract, invisible conceptions, ritual makes vivid and palpable our ideas and wishes, and, as Clifford Geertz (1965:23) has observed, "the lived-in order merges with the dreamed-of order.'' Through its insistence on precise, authentic, and accurate forms, rituals suggest that their contents are beyond question, authoritative and axiomatic. By high stylization and extraordinary uses—of objects, language, dress, gestures, and the like—ritual calls attention to itself, so that we cannot fail to distinguish its contents as set apart from ordinary affairs.

Ritual inevitably carries a basic message of order, continuity, and predictability. New events are connected to preceding ones, incorporated into a stream of precedents so that they are recognized as growing out of tradition and experience. By stating enduring and underlying patterns, ritual connects past, present, and future, abrogating history and time. Ritual always links participants to one another and often beyond, to wider collectivities that may be absent, even to the ancestors and those yet unborn. Religious rituals go further still, connecting humankind to the forces of nature and the purposes of the deities, reading the form of macrocosm into the microcosm. And when rituals employ sacred symbols, they may link the celebrants to their very selves, through the stages of the life cycle, making individual history into a continuum, a single phenomenological reality.

Because rituals dramatize a message about continuity, predictability, and tradition, they are inherently connective, providing integration of several kinds: of the self with itself as it contemplates its movement through biological and historical change; of the self with the culture, by the use of familiar, often axiomatic common symbols; of the self with others, joining celebrants into an often profound community where all manner of distinctions may be transcended in all all-embracing, sacred unity that Victor Turner (1977) has called communitas.

Rites of Passage

Of the myriad forms of human ritual, it is those that mark transitions in the life cycle—rites of passage—that we might expect to yield the most valuable information concerning the interplay of aging and ritual. In his now classic study of these rituals, Arnold Van Gennep (1908) first outlined the three-part progression through which these ceremonies proceeded as they moved initiates through transitional states involving permanent transformations in status and age, first by identifying and segregating them (Phase I, separation), then by isolating and confining them to each other's company as marginal beings, on the threshold (*limen*) between categories (Phase II, liminality), finally by reincorporating them into full membership in the society (Phase III, reaggregation). In the course of these transformative rituals, the interaction of culture, humanity, and biology is most clearly observed, for these ceremonies occur most prominently at the edge of our animality, at the intersection of our creatural existence and our cultural pretensions: at birth, reproduction, and death. During rites of passage distinctions are made most clear between the fundamental categories that set humans apart and define them: young and old, male and female, living and dead. As humans, we all are born, mate, and die; but we manipulate these constancies endlessly, so that biology with all its imperatives and universals can often be only faintly distinguished beneath the templates of symbolic and ritual forms that overlap it. Here we confront one of the many paradoxes that rituals characteristically handle that we mortals belong as much to nature as to culture, that these conditions are inseparable, that we play seriously and perpetually with our joint membership in the human and animal kingdoms, now reminding ourselves, now denying the one element or the other; now transcending, now exploiting our ineradicable oneness with all other creatures, usually enjoying ourselves in the act of self-contemplation, realizing in the end that we seem to be the only creatures so much and long amused by our play with categorical distinctions and self-definitions.

Occasionally biology and culture are closely coordinated, as when a girl's marriageability is celebrated with the onset of menstruation. But often these personal physical changes are not acknowledged or are out of synchrony with cultural identities. A thirteen-year-old boy bar mitzvahed in the Jewish religion may be sexually immature though he is socially transformed into a man by this rite of passage. Menarche, one of the clearer physiological changes in the human life cycle, seems to be little acknowledged formally, though older women as a category are often accorded special privileges and considered to have special powers. But again, sociological indicators that accord privileges may or may not coincide with the physical condition of a particular woman at a particular moment.

In contemporary industrialized nations, old age as a life stage seems particularly to be dominated by social rather than physiological criteria. In such societies, the "old" retire at a specific, legal moment, chronologically rather than functionally determined. Ever after, they are sharply separated from the "useful," fully participating members of the society, for the most part without reference to individual desire or capability. Here nature and culture stand at great remove from each other. Among the Eskimo, in earlier times, the closeness of fit between function and retirement was especially striking: when people could no longer help others or support themselves, they were put out onto the ice. As long as an old woman was able to chew garments into softness, she was a valued participant. When her teeth wore down, she committed suicide voluntarily. The discrepancy between individual capacity and cultural/legal definitions of old age are sharp in Western modern societies for many well-known reasons, including the dominance of technological tasks; formal, universalistic social definitions; and the complex, specialized division of labor, with all it implies. The fact that old age is a period of growing duration in absolute terms, given everlengthening life expectation, means that more and more people are older and older. This situation makes our ill-defined conflicting attitudes and dearth of expectations and rituals surrounding and punctuating the latter part of the life cycle all the more serious. That "old age" may last for three decades, lacking even demarcations provided by clearly named phases, goals, or features, is astonishing. Within the immense category we call "the old" there are "young old" and "old old," fit and frail, strong and invalid, independent and destitute, powerful and isolated, but none of these features is regularly specified by our social and legal conceptions.

Certainly anthropologists have not rigorously studied the phases and rites, the conceptions and ceremonies that characterize the latter part of the life cycle—neither in their own societies nor in those more remote in which they have worked. Nevertheless, one gets the impression that the degree of social and ceremonial specificity surrounding old age in most societies, of all levels of technological complexity, is generally less than that accorded earlier phases in the life cycle. While this cultural vagueness often creates anomie and isolation, at the same time it offers calculating, resourceful elders in many settings occasions in which they may innovate and exploit the rolelessness, a set of fruitful possibilities. Often freed from heavy social obligations and prohibitions for the first time, the elderly may become deft manipulators and enterpreneurs, justifying stereotypes concerning their unconventionality, originality, and wisdom. The wily old man, the truly frightening powerful old witch, the curmudgeon recluse in the hills, the mysterious, unpredictable old crone are types of exploiters of cultural freedom and confusion. If culture is conceived as a cognitive map, the inconsistencies and incomplete areas are not merely the unknowns; they are also contingencies—invitations to culture making and innovation—and in this light the relative normlessness surrounding the aged and old age holds promise as well as penalties.

But the disadvantages of the lack of rituals for the latter part of life probably outweigh the advantages, for rites of passage are moments of dramatic teaching and socialization, occasions that societies construct to inculcate and clarify, to make its members most fully and deeply its own. Rites of passage in later life could go far toward teaching the elderly and their juniors the meaning of their existence, the justifications for their continued being. Such rites would surely minimize the existential uncertainty that is one of the hardest states to bear at any time of life. Rites of passage present a society's members with a paradigm for the future, for the individual and the social order. Such rites are held at moments of great anxiety and social-biological tension.

Inevitably, rites of passage arouse self-consciousness in their subjects and invite profound self-questioning, at the very moment when they are pressing their designs and interpretations on the subjects, sometimes literally inscribing symbolic codes on the bodies of initiates in the form of tatooing, scarification, and mutilation. The Dalinese who reaches maturity must undergo a tooth-filing ceremony during which the canine tooth, the mark of the beast in humanity's heritage, is smoothed, to make the smile less reminiscent of an animal's snarl. And in some African societies, according to Victor Turner (personal communication), a youth being initiated into manhood may ingest a powder made from the foreskins of previous initiates, incorporating and sustaining in his own body the vitality and power of his predecessors. James Fernandez (1980) describes an initiation ceremony in which a neophyte stares into a looking glass until the face of an ancestor appears and merges with his own. The identification between the ancestor behind the glass and the living descendant in front of it presents, literally, a picture of genealogical continuity between the living and the dead and allows the initiate to pass into a new state of being. In such instances the human body itself is a symbolic statement, presenting to the society and the individual the message that the group and its members are inseparable, that they are vehicles for each other and must coexist. The fundamental, recurrent theme that appears in so many teachings during rites of passage is reducible to that: the interdependence of the collective and the individual; the group and the separate people who are to carry its purposes forward.

Because rites of passage occur at moments of great anxiety, at naturally transitional, dramatic moments, exaggerated by the society, the subjects are considered most malleable. Yet it is during such rites, when the group most avidly presses its messages upon members, that it also invites doubt and questioning. Self-consciousness is likely to be aroused through the regular play with mirrors, masks, costumes, and novelty so often found in rites of passage. Borders are crossed; identity symbols are stripped away, familiar roles and customs suspended. These are the very conditions under which one is likely to experience the sense of radical aloneness and uniqueness, freedom and awareness, the irreversible moment of reflexive consciousness, in the middle of the group's efforts to persuade initiates of its purposes. Thus rites of passage both announce our separateness and individuality and at the same time remind us most vividly that existence apart from the group is impossible. This paradox expresses one of the basic truths of the human condition: that while all societies attempt to absorb the individual and shape him or her into a bona fide self-regulating member, they never wholly succeed. Even in the most highly integrated, small, stable tribal societies there are distinguished individuals: old or outstanding men and women whose traits and thoughts go beyond those required by their offices, roles, and circumstances.

Victor Turner (1975) has elaborated Van Gennep's early study of rites of passage, focusing on the middle phase, liminality, when the individual is in transition between known states. This phase may be a period of marginal existence that passes, or it may become a role extended through a lifetime entirely given to the principles and practice of uncertainty, exploration, innovation, rebellion, and many varieties of nonbelonging. Then we may speak of specialists in disorder: the ritual clowns, transvestites, shamans, poets, rebels, mystics, and vagabonds who move perpetually at the borders of known categories and agreements. Whether viewed as a phase in the life cycle, as a state of mind, or as a full-time role, liminality is conducive to the generation of social criticism, creativity, and play, with its built-in affinity for paradox, symbolic and social opposition, and disorder. It is not unusual to find old people who are liminal beings, living beyond the fixed and regulated categories, beyond the constraints of the superego, which can effectively warn against penalties for transgression. Such penalties have diminished bite when the future is short and uncertain. Often, the less future, the less to lose, from the point of view of the individual, and from the point of view of society; often old people are dispensable, their conduct a matter of little consequence, their controls a matter of diminished importance. It may be, then, that the often-noted but little-studied toughness, fearlessness, idiosyncrasy, and creativity among the elderly in many societies result from this combination of social irrelevance and personal autonomy. Carl Jung's term "individuation" refers to the personal evolution that may come with time and age, as older people free themselves from the conventional fetters that tightly bind younger, productive, structurally essentially members of society. Folk wisdom has it that old people "are the same as they have always been, only more so." Liminality—being socially in limbo—anomie, rolelessness, neglect, and social irrelevance may have the complex advantage of leaving old people alone, to be themselves only more so. It is with affection and nostalgia that adults regard the innate creativity of unsocialized children. But usually they are blind to the creativity of *de*socialized elders at the other end of the life cycle, people whose reemerging originality—stemming from social detachment, long experience, the urgency of a shortened future—may be as delightful, surprising, and fruitful as anything to be found among the very young. Among them are personal and social resources that have yet to be mined and appreciated.

Intolerance for "bad behavior" among the elderly is part of our blindness to their gifts. Margaret Clark (1967) has documented what we all perhaps sense: that in our society we ask above all that the elderly not make waves. We assign them roles that represent a limited range of stereotypes—serene, detached, disengaged, wise, and so on—all closely related to maintaining a manageable problem population, easily institutionalized and patronized. Traits that in middle life often lead to worldly success—aggressiveness, independence, individualism, competitiveness, initiative, future orientation, and the like—bring to the old people who manifest them the label of "maladjusted."

Ruth Benedict (1956) long ago called such reversals in expectation "discontinuity in cultural conditioning." Such discontinuity between adulthood and old age is especially severe in our society. At the same time that we lament such inconsistency, it is impossible to release the elderly from all standards of reasonable behavior. That ultimately is the most degrading position of all, with the final effect of reducing old people to nonpeople. Ronald Blythe puts this idea felicitously: "Just as the old should be convinced that, whatever happens during senescence, they will never suffer exclusion, so they should understand that age does not exempt them from being despicable." We must not allow the old to fall into purposelessness, for "this is to fall out of all real consideration. . . . To appreciate the transience of all things is one matter, to narrow the last years—and they can be numerous—down to a dreary thread is another." But it is to this dreary thread that we often confine the elderly, and then we are appalled at the self-indulgent mindlessness of old age, which Blythe calls "its most intolerable aspect." Both young and old are uninformed in the management of old age; neither knows what it may or may not ask and expect of the other. "Perhaps," says Blythe, "with full-span lives the norm, people may need to learn how to be aged as they once had to learn to be adult (Blythe 1979:22).

Rites of passage that socialize, clarify, and demarcate phases of old age exist in many societies in nascent and nonsystematic forms. In our own society, we do acknowledge some transitions: fiftieth wedding anniversaries, great-grandparenthood, special birthdays. These occasions are usually celebrated. We have no comparable rites for losses: giving up the family home, transferring property and privilege to children, completing menopause, relinquishing one's driver's license, moving into an institution, accepting a wheelchair or hearing aid, and the many large and small events that are usually thought of as failures and signposts indicating that the end is ever nearer. Even the gross forms of change, such as senescence and becoming a legal ward, are but crudely acknowledged. While these are undeniably negative and painful events, the clear public acknowledgment of them by others who accept and care about them has clarifying, healing consequences that redefine relationships and identities for all those involved. Retirements and funerals are crude markers for the stark beginning and end of old age; in between there is a universe of differentiation that remains a cultural wasteland for each to calculate and navigate alone, without the aid of ritual, ceremony, or symbol.

There is some irony in this absence of public social rituals during later life, since a great many older people create their own private rituals with enthusiasm, even obsessiveness. Just as children fastidiously work to bring some cosmos into the chaos of their emerging world of boundless complexity, so older people are often noted to fuss obsessively with trivial items, ordering a life that is ending, using the predictability and certainty that ritual provides during times of anxiety and helplessness. When things are finally coming undone, when the last rupture is imminent, the old often set about putting their house in order. It is an activity akin to the nesting that mothers-to-be engage in late in pregnancy, a nesting that is also a cleaning, sorting, classifying preparation for a drastic change. Among the very old, often it is memories and mementos that are sorted and integrated, a last look at what has been, combined with moving objects about, discarding and arranging papers and things: a final imposition of one's human purpose on the last random, untidy event of all.

In sum, it seems that the life sequences are segmented in all societies, with varying fineness. The life cycle is recognized in large part through ritual. The earlier stages in general are more highly defined, and adolescence in particular is abundantly celebrated and acknowledged. Later, at the end of life, mortuary rituals are often quite rich, as Richard Huntington and Peter Metcalf (1979) demonstrate, but between the rites that mark the beginnings of social-sexual maturity—puberty and marriage—and those that mark the end, distinctions are less rich and rituals more sparse. Lately some attention has been given to the dearth of literature on the adult life cycle in our society. Gail Sheehy (1974) and Roger L. Gould (1978) have written in some detail on the necessity for conceptualizing the phases of maturity in terms of predictable, normal adult crises. Bernice Neugarten (1980) has suggested some refinements in our approach to the phases of adult life, emphasizing the crudeness of our view of aging. She suggests that at the very least we make a distinction between the young-old and the old-old. The former have much to offer society, and our task as a group is to find ways they may make a meaningful contribution, though they may be occupationally retired. The old-old are frail and in need of care. The problems they present are entirely different.

Helpful as such theories are in suggesting a less simplistic approach to the life cycle, none of them draws our attention to ritual. The authors provide some guidance in making clear the characteristics of each age and, implicitly, the nature and meaning of a change from one to another. But they do not help us to identify *ceremonies* that define and accentuate the changes. But then, psychologists should perhaps not be expected to cast their studies in the form of rituals, which are, ultimately, social matters, even though they are enacted individually. It seems more appropriate to look to anthropologists for insights as to how ceremony and ritual might be usefully considered as part of the life cycle; but even anthropologists do not agree on the importance of rites of passage. Martha and Morton Fried (1980) cast doubt on the utility of these rites. They examine four critical transitions—birth, puberty, marriage, and death—in cultures deliberately selected to provide variation in geographical distribution and technological and social complexity. All the societies they examine celebrate some transition points in the life cycle, and all place a

symbolic template over the facts of biology, treating it as socially manip-
ulable. It is often thought, they note, that societies without profound
rituals, particularly adolescent rites, are asking for trouble. But in their
survey they find no association between the absence of ritual and the
presence of social problems, as indicated by high rates of delinquency or
suicide. They remark (1980:268): "It is possible, then, for cultures to
survive with relatively small attention to ritual and also with extraordinarily rich preoccupation with ritual, including life transition ceremonies. We cannot say for sure that a culture cannot exist unless it has a
bare minimum of such rituals. But we have no record of societies up to
the present that have existed without ritual, hence if such existed they did
not survive." They therefore assume that rituals play some adaptive role
in the process of cultural evolution. They claim that human—that is,
cultural—life came into existence considerably in advance of the first
clear evidence of ritual. The latter is dated by the Frieds at roughly
40,000 B.C., in the flower-strewn remains of Neanderthals who used
flowers to acknowledge and celebrate death. Since culture is now regarded as definitely manifested by the appearance of tools, two million
years ago, it may be that rites of passage have existed for only two
percent of the history of culture—a relatively recent, hence optional
development, as things go (1980:269–70). Rites of passage may be functionally adaptive at the social level but probably are not necessary for the
survival of individuals, the Frieds conclude.

But can we be so certain that individuals and social evolution are as
separable as the Frieds maintain? Surely the ability of individuals to cope
with increasing complexity, conflict, and isolation contributes to the evolution of society. Human beings are the carriers of culture, and they may
transmit their culture more or less successfully, in confusion and disarray
or with a sense of coherence and well-being. The well-being of the units
of a society, the living people, surely cannot be so sharply severed from
the success of the society, even in terms of mere survival and evolution.
Emile Durkheim's classic study *Suicide* (1952) long ago indicated that
social anomie may be expressed by the individual in the form of suicide.
Rites of passage certainly do not *cause* social intergration; rather they
may be expected to reflect and enhance it.

Rituals as Cultural Performance

As far as we can tell, one of the characteristics that is limited to
humanity is its capacity, even drive, for reflexive knowledge. Another

distinctly and exclusively human feature is the capacity of many creatures to live well into old age, far beyond what is required for the perpetuation of the species in the course of evolutionary survival. These two tendencies become confounded and combine to exaggerate the human fascination with its own condition, the self's desire for understanding of its being, for old age is regularly associated with growing consciousness of self, interest in reflexive knowledge, and philosophical/escatological reflection. We have concrete evidence of this tendency in literate cultures and the suggestion of it in nonliterate ones, where elders may be freed from mundane labors associated with making a living (involuntarily freed through loss of physical function or, where materials and funds are abundant, freed as a privilege); then they are absolved from conventional prohibitions, tasks, and roles. Prestige, time, freedom, and sheer life experience are fodder for reflectiveness. In his theory concerning the social-psychological developmental tasks that must be accomplished through the course of the life cycle, Erik Erikson (1977) designates old age as a time for integration, during which the meaning of the entire cycle of life is affirmed. Old people create a sense of immortality "not only for the leaders and the elites but also for every participant" in a society by "tying life cycle and institutions into a meaningful whole (Erikson 1977:112). Erikson cites William Blake, who points to elders' natural affinity for the task of integrating and understanding:

> The Child's Toys and the Old Man's Reasons
> Are the Fruits of the Two Seasons.

(Erikson is one of the few writers who suggests that senescence and senility may be a genuine, though not inevitable, stage in the life course. He attributes "unavoidable attitudes of despair and disgust" [1977:112] to that stage in life but does not make clear whether he means that these are attitudes *toward* the senile by society or attitudes held by the senile about themselves—an important distinction.)

It is safe to say that in societies of all kinds, the old experience an inevitable heightening of awareness by virtue of the anticipation of the nearness of death. Rousseau is said to have remarked, "I only began to live when I looked upon myself as dead." Of course cultures may encourage or discourage such inquiries into our nature, at any time of the life cycle, but as I have maintained throughout this essay, the hold society has over the life (especially the inner life) of elders, who have less to lose with each passing day, diminishes with the mere passage of time. As I remarked, Victor Turner interprets liminality as giving rise to questions and doubts, to rebellious conceptions and engagements with the social order. Elders are liminals par excellence, often associated with the power, awe, or dread of the already dead, and with the natural forces that seem so close to reclaiming them. They have the penalties and privileges of being "the other," not entirely "us."

But the relation of ritual to reflexive knowledge is always complex. On one hand, rituals, especially rites of passage, invite questions, playing as they often do with fixed conceptions that carry us far beyond our rational imaginings, daring us, it sometimes seems, to see through their patent artifices to our own existential imaginings and wishes. Because of their very predictability, rituals provide the safeguards within which we may risk ultimate enterprises and ideas. Because by definition we know the outcome of a ritual in advance, within it we find the courage to perform our most far-reaching symbolic and mythic formulations. We provide ourselves with a view of reality, reshaping relationships between subject and reality, reorganizing the Self and its experience at the same time, to paraphrase Sherry Ortner (1978). This reorganization creates a subjective psychological state that restructures meanings, changes consciousness, and even solves certain problems. In this view ritual is far more than merely expressive or communicative. It can be an active agent of change, of society, by altering the consciousness of its members. Ritual allows us to perform our thoughts, inhabit the invisible worlds of our imaginings, and experience them as real in the structures that we create for them. In the subjective mood that ritual creates, the moral order is seen from a new perspective. Conformity or questioning may result.

On the other hand, there are those who emphasize the purely persuasive aspect of ritual. With its insistent repetitive driving quality, it may still rather than arouse reflection. Its strict coordination and formality may refuse entry to individual questions. Geertz, for example, stresses the "busyness" of ritual as likely to discourage thoughtfulness; indeed, that may be part of rituals' basic task. In discussing a Balinese funeral, he remarks, "Funeral ceremonies consist largely of a host of detailed little busy work routines, and whatever concern with first and last things death may stimulate is well submerged in a bustling ritualism" (Geertz 1973; 183). A funeral ceremony, he suggests, stifles one's view of mortality and distracts one from seeing oneself and one's destiny in the corpse.

But surely after a funeral or cremation one does not think about the corpse, or even one's own death, in the same way, with the usual daytime, direct, orderly consciousness that characterizes mundane life. On another, deeper, less rational level, we *do* understand something about death in general and our own death is particular by participating in rituals involving a corpse. Symbolic experiences—whether in dreams, poetry, myth, the arts, trance—hold their own kind of information, eluding words but nonetheless significant and real. Ritual deals with unconscious knowledge, and its work and teachings cannot be adequately assessed only in terms of what people may tell us about their impact and purpose.

Certain circumstances in addition to mere chronological aging and the approach of death may generate the self-consciousness and self-knowledge that are dealt with by ritual. Situations that promote severe invisibility among the elderly seem to call for symbolic and ritual elaboration. Immigrant populations, for example, sharply and permanently cut off from their natal country, populations that expect total ideological or biological extinction, groups that have lost natural progeny who can carry forward their traditions and stories, people and collectivities that have no natural heirs or witnesses to validate their individual claims to have lived a worthy life: these are some of the situations that create a sharp need for the elderly to dramatize and ritually display their own version of themselves and their histories.

The group with which I have worked for the past decade provides a vivid example here (Myerhoff 1980). Self-documentation is among the most passionate concerns of these elderly people, for onto them has fallen the task of indicating what their earlier lives were, and what their worth and places were. These people, now in their eighties and nineties, are immigrants from Eastern Europe, now living on their own in a Southern California urban community, often in severe economic and physical straits. The focus of their social and cultural life is a senior citizens' day center where they have been meeting now for nearly three decades, creating an alternative world based on their earlier shared sacred language, history, and culture. That their natal culture, the Yiddish world of Eastern Europe, was definitely and abruptly destroyed by the Holocaust, that their children have become assimilated Americans, geographically and culturally removed, that the rest of society has turned away from them, left them on their own, means they have had to become their own witnesses to their own stories. The transmission of tradition is in their hands, and their failure is nearly certain. The separation from ordinary stable rhythms of a known and familiar past and future is almost complete. Though most are culturally Jewish, they are secular. For them there is no assurance that God or man will remember their names. Death means not only personal but cultural extinction. Wherever they could, and by whatever means possible, these individuals have improvised and performed a lively, syncretic culture, made up of a common childhood past combined with their values and experiences of adulthood and old age. Using any means at hand, they bring themselves to light through ritual and ceremony, to portray and proclaim the meaning of their lives and experiences.

Old people are said to be naturally drawn to review their lives, and Jews are reputed to be addicted to talk of this nature, "talking as if their lives depended upon it, but with no 'as if.'" That is how folklorist Barbara Kirshenblatt-Gimblett put it (personal communication). These old Jews are virtuoso talkers, exegetes, arguers, and dialecticians, and many reasons for this articulateness may be suggested. The historical facts of their history since the Dispersion from the Hold Land have exacerbated their passion for self-scrutiny, for so much time spent among hostile outsiders in so many differing countries requires explanation. The Holocaust further intensified their awareness of their distinctiveness and urgently called for explanation. These people did not experience the Holocaust at firsthand; they left the Old World before so many of their peers, family, and companions who remained behind were destroyed. They did not directly experience the most important event of their generation, perhaps of the century; yet they did, for just as those who are victims of atrocity petition the gods to know why they are afflicted, those who escape by accident demand to know why they have *not* been taken. "Why me?" becomes "Why not me?" and the ones who survive seem universally to detest no intrinsic justice in their escape, usually believing that it was always the best who perished, the least deserving who did not. Much has been written on the subject of "survivor's guilt." Robert Jay Lifton, speaking about survivors of Hiroshima as well as Jews who survived Hitler, suggests that those who remain after mass destruction of their fellows become "seekers after justice," devoting themselves to careful examination of their own lives and of history, trying to find evidence of something aside from chaos to account for their sufferings (Lifton 1967:526). An explanation is sought, some indication is required of a moral and sane accountable universe. Disaster once named and conceptualized becomes bearable when, as Einstein observed, one can at the very least manage to believe in the modest assumption that God is not playing dice with the universe (cited in Geertz 1965:15). Such scrutiny is extraordinarily painful; but as one of the old people I worked with put it, "Why do we torture ourselves with such memories? The one who studies history loses an eye. The one who does not loses two eyes."

Surviving and survivor's guilt, then, can serve as transformative agents, taking the base materials of ordinary existence and disaster and working the alchemical miracle upon them until they result in consciousness. The consequence is a development of the capacity to lead an examined life. Through this consciousness, the elders are able to focus their remaining moments, enliven and enrich every detail of daily life, in the light of what has been extinguished and lost. "If we lose ourselves now, if we give up our traditions, if we become like everyone else, then we finish ourselves off. We do Hitler's work for him," said one of the women. They owe living fully to those who are gone. And they often feel a bittersweet triumph at having persisted despite so many and such exaggerated attempts to do away with them. Outliving historical enemies (Hitler was the last in a series, after all) is a personal accomplishment in which they take pride.

Memory, Re-membering, and Reminiscence

Memory is a continuum, ranging from vague, dim shadows to the brightest, most vivid totality of an original experience. It may offer opportunity not merely to recall the past but to relive it, in all its primary freshness, unaltered by intervening changes and reflections. Such magical Proustian moments are pinpoints of the greatest intensity, when a sense of the past as never truly lost is experienced. The diffuseness of life is then transcended, the sense of duration overcome, and all of one's self and one's memories are felt to be universally valid. Simultaneity replaces sequence and a sense of oneness with one's past is achieved. Often such moments involve childhood memories, and then one experiences the self as it was originally, and knows beyond doubt that one is still the same person as the child who yet dwells within a time-altered body. Integration through memory with earlier states of being surely provides the sense of continuity and completeness that may be counted as an essential developmental task of old age.

Freud (1965) has suggested that the completion of the mourning process requires that those left behind develop a new reality that no longer includes what has been lost. But it must also be said that full recovery from mourning may restore what has been lost, maintaining it through incorporation in the present. Full recollection and retention may be as vital to recovery and well-being as the forfeiture of memories.

The term "re-membering" is hyphenated to distinguish it from ordinary recollection. Re-membering is the reaggregation of one's members, the figures who properly belong to one's life story, one's own prior selves, the significant others without which the story cannot be completed. Re-membering, then, is a purposive, significant unification, different from the passive, continuous, fragmentary flickerings of images and feelings that accompany other activities in the normal flow of consciousness. The focused unification provided by re-membering is requisite to sense and order. Through it a life is given shape that extends back in the past and forward into the future, a simplified, edited tale in which completeness may be sacrificed for moral and aesthetic purposes. Then history approaches art, myth, and ritual. Perhaps this is why Mnemosyne, the goddess of memory, is the mother of the Muses. Without re-membering we lose our history and ourselves

Ritual is a form by means of which culture presents itself to itself. It creates a setting in which desire and interpretation may *appear*, to participants and to an audience. It allows old people in particular to present claims regarding their vanished past and proof of their continuing existence and honor. It provides public occasions for re-membering. In my work I have identified a form of these events as definitional ceremonies: ritualized performances that provide arenas for garnering honor and prestige, for enacting and displaying one's own interpretation of oneself, against the play of accident, chaos, and negative interpretations that may be offered up by history and outsiders. On these occasions, existence and worth are dramatized, and by being performed and seen are (to some extent and for some time) believed. Ritual as an inherently persuasive and rhetorical form accomplishes this task of convincing and reassuring participants and (with luck) witnesses about its claims. The importance of ritual as a persuasive form is highlighted among the elderly by their heightened need for physical verification and sensory proof of their ongoing vitality when evidence of the senses may have grown dim, and when sharp distinctions between dreaming and waking may have become blurred. Then participation in a ritual gives one the sensory experience of continuing existence and vitality, of being still in life.

Often performance and reminiscence blend in ritualized reminiscence and storytelling. That reminiscence is an appropriate and healthy activity for the elderly was suggested several years ago by Robert Butler (1968). The search through one's life for enduring patterns, sense, and coherence, for a recognition of the self over time, is striking in old age, as I have said. Often such reminiscences are formalized and publicly made. Often cultural templates are provided by myths, employed to give a story shape and clarity. A life is read retrospectively and scrutinized for those definitive moments that provided connectedness to the present and to the collective, even sacred symbols of the culture. Then storytelling becomes myth, and one comes to see oneself as embodying an ancient hero or ancestor. In one life story I collected, a modest tailor who was an outsider in his group, perpetually at odds with the other members, identified with the prophet Jeremiah, the gadfly whose task it was to stand apart and criticize, to keep his people morally alive.

Time, Ritual, and Age

For some old people, the search through their past is not linear; precedent is eschewed in favor of epiphanies that seem to contain the distilled truth of an entire life, unforgettable experiences of being utterly alive or moments of clairty when time stops. T. S. Eliot refers to "the still point at the center," when one's life is most fully known. Then no longer need we fear having "the experience but missing the meaning." (1958:133). At these moments "we learn from all our exploring where we started and know the place for the first time" (Eliot 1958:145).

With various models and purposes, the old point the way to the search through life experience from the perspective of the present, sorting and rearranging the past for the understanding that is required before it is too late. Painful moments as much as joy transform mere experience into meaning, and then all becomes bearable. Wilhem Dilthey puts it this way: "Because both our fortunes and our own natures cause us pain, so they force us to come to terms with them through understanding. The past mysteriously invites us to know the closely-woven meaning of its moments." This is the foundation for the historical vision that can give "a second life to the bloodless shades of the past," as he puts it (cited in Rickman 1979:215).

These pinpoints of intensity and understanding that crystallize a lifetime of experience may be thought of as a vertical rather than a horizontal integration. The latter stresses continuity, recurrent patterning, a linear, unidirectional view of time as flowing by without interruption, a steady stream from which the individual selects and joins certain similar themes, recognizes unifying elements that finally provide linkage despite underlying and random variation. In this view, a life is evaluated and known in a cumulative fashion, adding up to what can be called a life career. The vertical approach stresses a timeless transcendent recognition that does not involve change. Quite the opposite, it escapes change, focuses on total illumination of the enduring elements of a life that do not pass away. These illuminations have been given various names: epiphany, moments of being, revelation, satori, qualitative time, transcendence. They approach the religious experience by escaping life's repetitiveness and evanesence. Indeed, these moments may never recur, yet they may give a whole life its focus and justification. A fine example is to be found in the concluding song in Gustav Mahler's *Leid von der Erde,* "Ewig," in which life's final mystery is revealed as a person faces death, an almost wordless moment, soaring beyond time, at once joyful and grave: "Everywhere and always a blue glimmer on the horizon: Forever, forever, forever . . ." This song differs from the earlier ones in which Mahler contemplates his personal death, realizes his part in the repetitive dimension of the human and natural cycle of death and rebirth. Then he sings of "my peaceful heart, awaiting its hour . . . the beloved earth everywhere flowers and is green again." (The English translations by Deryck Cooke are from the jacket notes of the London recording.) "Ewig" is about immortality, the impersonal eternity that the individual may glimpse at last; the earlier song is about individual death, the renewal of life, processes within which one is included—the great temporal progression with change at its very heart.

Haim Hazan (1982) has described theories of aging as based on alternative, contrasting approaches to time. In one view, change, progress, advancement, mobility, and achievement dominate our attitudes toward time. The elderly are at a basic disadvantage in a society that approaches in this way, but some compensation is possible through an emphasis on the cumulative, processual aspects of life. Time is linear and the fundamental orientation to change gives a teleological cast to it. Ultimately, the old lose; it is only a matter of losing well or badly, quickly or slowly. An alternative view is what Hazan calls autoletic; here time is cyclically perceived, as a mythical, total, noncumulative system (Hazan 1982; see also Hazan 1980). Here we are dealing not with teleology or completion, but with eternity. Sacred autobiographers, mystics, and poets have long recognized these moments.

Being at one with all things of the world, nonrepetitively, is the vision of life outside of the self, outside process, nature, and change (see Gray 1981). In Western cultures this is a privileged experience, and it is the blessed individual who escapes time even for a moment to realize him- or herself as mysteriously eternal, or as part of the eternal. But of course in many cultures such a theory of time is generally shared, and then everyone, not merely the elite and elect, may know time as cyclical, non-teleological, and noncumulative. Stephen Lansing (1980), for example, describes the experience of time in Bali and its consequences for the concept of aging in his discussion of a fundamentally Buddhist world-view. According to him, Balinese calendars show a world view in which the processes of growth and decay proceed at different rates for all things, at all times, in part because there are no seasonal changes in Bali, whose tropical rain forests are located so near to the equator. All living things are thus regarded as existing in their own growth cycle, different for a person or a flower or a rock. These cycles mesh in this human manifest world, "the Middle World," to create the lives of mortals. Age is no impediment here, indeed, it is irrelevant, and most Balinese do not know how "old" they are. Death is not an ending but "a movement out of the Middle World into some space . . . in the Balinese Heaven. . . . The very old and very young are closest to the unseen worlds and hence to a state of purity and detachment from this world" (Lansing 1980:35). In such a system the concept of absolute age, indeed the concept of "lifetime," is nearly meaningless. An individual moves through a life cycle of statuses from newborn to elder village head to ancestor spirit and back to child many times. To be an old Australian aborigine living in the Dream time; to be an aging Taoist monk who believes that the Tao is forever and though the body ceases it cannot be destroyed, to be a Christian or Jew dating life, time, and mortality from the time of the Fall, awaiting the end of days, when time stops forever—these are among the innumerable cultural conceptions of time that profoundly influence the experience of aging.

There are of course countless important subtler variations within Western Judeo-Christian linear time conceptions that invite examination, particularly as they impinge on the experience of aging. Hazan (1980); for example, describes a group of old people who have collectively created a social world outside of time, in which accomplishments and failures of earlier periods in the life cycle are viewed as irrelevant. Among the people he studied, "change is arrested and progress and planning are eliminated; and yet people find themselves doing meaningful, purposeful things within a well-defined, structured social arena. Theirs is a change-proof environment that is not stagnant, aimless or anomic," derived from the incongruities and ambiguities commonly considered unavoidable and inexorable, he notes (1980:183). They see time as neither cyclical nor linear, but as literally and figuratively inconsequential. There are, then, many kinds of time in many cultures. Time as expendable resource; as an endlessly renewing flow; as merely a reflection of the physical or social universe; as irrelevant—these are some of many ideas of the utmost importance in our efforts to interpret the meaning of the human life course, and of old age and death especially. This is an imperative and largely neglected subject that must be taken into account if we hope to understand the experience of age in any society or setting.

Any discussion of ritual is, finally, a discussion of time and continuity; when a ritual deals with death or birth, the themes of time and continuity are thrown into sharp relief. Ritual alters our ordinary sense of time, repudiating meaningless change and discontinuity by emphasizing regularity, precedent, and order. Paradoxically, it uses repetition to deny the empty repetitiveness of unremarked, unattended human and social experience. From repetition ritual finds or makes patterns, and these patterns are scrutinized for hints of eternal designs. In ritual, all forms of change are interpreted by being linked with the past and incorporated in a larger framework, where inevitable variations are equated with grander, tidier totalities. When traditional elements are inserted into the present, the past is read as prefiguring what is happening in the here and now, and by implication the future is seen as foreshadowed in all that has gone before. Religious rituals are more sweeping than secular ones in this elongation of time and reiteration of continuity. The latter usually confine themselves to remembered human history, whereas the former transform history into myths, stories with no beginning and no end. Then time is obliterated and continuity is total.

To do their work, rituals must disrupt our ordinary sense of time and displace our awareness of events coming into being and disappearing in discrete, precise, discontinuous segments. That experience of continuous episodes is part of our everyday sense of time, from which societies must coordinate collective activities. It is largely external to the individual in origins and referents, and does not take into account private responses, stimulation, states of mind, or motivation. Public chronological time is anathema to the mood of ritual, which has its own time. Rituals attempt to sweep us away from the everyday time sense, and from the public, objective instrumental frame of mind that is associated with it. By merely absorbing us sufficiently, ritual, like art, lets us "lose ourselves" and step out of our usual conscious, critical mentality. When successful, ritual replaces discontinuous, chronological, collective time with the experience of flowing duration, paced according to personal significance. Sometimes this experience is so powerful that we are altogether freed from a sense of time and an awareness of self. This we may call ritual time, and it must be present to some degree to mount the mood of conviction concerning the messages contained in a ritual.

But ritual is still a social event, and it is necessary that within it individuals' temporal experiences be coordinated. They must be delicately synchronized, without obliterating the individual's sense of an intense personal experience. Ordinary time is suspended and a new time instituted, geared to the event taking place, shared by those participating, integrating the private experience into a collective one. These moments of intensely shared experience have been called by Martin Buber (1961) *Zwischenmenschlicheit.* They are often the euphoric, religious experiences that, paradoxically, occur when the self stands outside itself—ecstasy.

Much exploration remains to be done concerning physiological correlates and causes associated with ritual's manipulation of time and emotional states. An important work in this area has made a tantalizing beginning, taking up the study of ritual from a physiological or more precisely "biogenetic structural" point of view (D'Aquili et al. eds., 1979). Barbara Lex (1979) points out that a change in neurophysiological functioning is the goal of rites of passage; this view might well be extended to all rituals. Lex indicates several circumstances in which rituals or ritualized conduct can alter neurophysiological states; she mentions the efficacy of the systematic practice and modification of such "expressive movements" as posture, gesture, speech, and singing, noting that in certain situations "feedback from proprioreceptors, as in singing and dancing, seems to evoke new patterns of affective response to the hypothalamus, limbic system and neocortex" (Lex 1979:117–51). She mentions as well the tendency for rituals to shift consciousness to the right cerebral hemisphere of the brain, associated with perceptions of unity and holism.

In rituals "individuals, eager or reluctant, are integrated into a group, not only by the sharing of pleasurable emotions through participation in formalized, repetitive, precisely performed interaction forms, but also by a mode of thought that reinforces feelings of solidarity" (1979:143–44).

Among the salient features of all ritual are the performative, sensory dimensions, clearly important for their physiological, neural, central involvements. The action aspect of ritual is what enables a participant to retrieve earlier states of being. Actors know and use this capacity in what they call "body memory," according to Richard Schechner (personal communication), who points out that the Stanislavskian teaching methods use this device regularly. The actor in training is encouraged to recall an appropriate moment in his or her past and the feelings that accompanied it, which will be annealed onto the character being portrayed in the present. The actor does not merely recall this memory cognitively; he or she proceeds to enact it, recognizing that the body movements will return some of the original feelings associated with them. Feelings are to follow, not precede, the gesture.

In my own fieldwork among the elderly, I was particularly struck by the frequency with which certain actions recalled the past. Songs, ritual storytelling, dancing, and gestures were recurrent occasions when time was transcended. One of the elderly women with whom I was working explained this experience most precisely, referring to the significance of a prayer accompanied by certain ritual gestures. "When I make the movements, circling the Sabbath candles, calling their holiness to me, covering my eyes, then I feel my mother's hands on my smooth cheeks." Often on such occasions the elderly looked transformed. Their posture, energy, movements, facial expressions lightened, quickened, expressed freedom, and took on what can only be called an air of youthfulness. Then their songs, dances, and the like were not *about* anything else; though symbolic forms, they were not secondary experiences or interpretations, but original experiences, immediate and satisfying in themselves, *sui generis*. The past returned along with the ritual circumstance in which they had first been experienced, bringing unaltered fragments of prior time. Marcel Proust was fascinated by this process. His work examines how the past may sometimes be recaptured with all its original force, unmodified by intervening events. This reexperiencing may occur when the conscious mind, with its interpretations and associations, is bypassed. Experiences of past time come back unaltered, often as spontaneous responses to sense stimuli; as Adam Mendilow (1952) describes this process, it occurs when the chemistry of thought is untouched by intervening events and the passage of time. These numinous moments carry with them their original, pristine associations and feelings. This is timelessness and the past is made into the present. It is "a hermetical magic, sealed outside of time, suspending the sense of duration, allowing all of life to be experienced as a single moment. . . . These are pin-points of great intensity, concentrations of universal awareness, antithetical to the diffuseness of life" (Mendilow 1952:137). Then the self is experienced as eternally valid; simultaneity replaces sequence.

Conceivably, any kind of ritual has the capacity to retrieve a fragment of past life. Rituals associated with and originating in childhood are more likely to do so, and they carry opportunities to provide personal and historical continuity. Two characteristics of these ritual are salient here: first, their intensely physiological associations, and second, their great power and immediacy, coming as they do from the individual's first emotional social experiences. They arise in a context of nurturance and dependence, evoking the familiar domestic domain, preceding language and conceptualization. In a modern world of pluralistic cultures, first experiences of nurturance set in the context of domestic life are often associated with ethnic origins, bound up with first foods, touch, language, song, folkways, and the like, carried and connoted by rituals and symbols learned in that context. In my study of a community of elderly Eastern European Jews in Los Angeles (Myerhoff 1980) I have called such rites "domestic religion," emphasizing their personal context and the sacrality endowed by their embeddedness in local tradition. Ethnic rituals are often redolent with the most profoundly emotional associations, and are often the means for carrying one back to earlier times and selves. Consider the statement made by an elderly man, reminiscing about his first experience with mortuary ritual: "Whenever I say kaddish [the Jewish prayer for the dead], I chant and sway, and it all comes back to me. I remember how it was when my father, may he rest in peace, would wrap me around in his big prayer shawl. All that comes back to me, like I was back in that shawl, where nothing bad could ever happen."

Ultimately we are interested in ritual because it tells us something about the human condition, the mythic condition, and our private lives all at once. It demonstrates the connection between the human being and humanity. It does more than tell an eternal tale; it sheds light on our own condition. Rituals do not change the hard realities of aging. But if people lived by hard realities only, there would be no need for rituals and symbolic forms. The power of ritual is to change our experience of the world and its worth. It may make the oblivion of an individual life a little less certain, presenting a life as belonging not only to the individual who lived it but to the world, to progeny, to witnesses who are heirs to embodied traditions. Ritual allows the elderly to find and enact linkages between their shared beliefs and values and specific historical events. Particularities are subsumed and equated with grander themes, exemplifying ultimate concerns. Then the elderly may be regarded as exemplars, fulfilling themselves and embodying their traditons at the same time.

REFERENCES

Benedict, Ruth
    1956   Continuities and discontinuities in cultural conditioning. *In* Personality in Nature, Society, and Culture, ed. Clyde Kluckhohn et al., pp. 522–31. New York: Knopf.
Blythe, Ronald
    1979   The View in Winter: Reflections on Old Age. New York: Penguin.
Buber, Martin
    1961   I and Thou. Trans. R. G. Smith, Edinburgh: Clark.
Rutler, Robert N.
    1968   The life review: An Interpretation of reminiscence in the aged. In Middle Age and Aging, ed. Bernice L. Neugarten, pp. 486–96. Chicago: Chicago University Press.
Clark, Margaret
    1967   The anthropology of aging. Gerontologist 7:55–64.
D'Aquili, Eugene G., Charles D. Laughlin, Jr., and John McManus, eds.
    1979   The Spectrum of Ritual: A Biogenetic Structural Analysis. New York: Columbia University Press.
Durkheim, Emile
    1952   Suicide. Trans. John A. Spaulding and George Simpson. London: Routledge & Kegan Paul.
Eliot, T. S.
    1958   The Complete Poems and Plays, 1909–1950. New York: Harcourt, Brace.
Erikson, Erik
    1977   Toys and Reasons: Stages in the Ritualization of Experience. New York: Norton.
Fernandez, James
    1980   Reflections on looking into mirrors. Semiotica 30:27–39.

Freud, Sigmund
1965   Death, Grief, and Mourning. New York: Doubleday.
Fried, Martha N., and Morton H. Fried
1980   Transitions: Four Rituals in Eight Cultures. New York: Norton.
Geertz, Clifford
1965   Religion as a cultural system. In Anthropological Approaches to the
       Study of Religion, ed. M. Banton, pp. 1–46. New York: Praeger.
1973   "Internal conversion" in contemporary Bali. *In* Geertz, The In-
       terpretation of Cultures, pp. 170–89. New York: Basic Books.
Gould, Roger L.
1978   Transformation: Growth and Change in Adult Life. Louisville,:
       Touchstone.
Gray, Rockwell
1981   Time present and time past: The ground of autobiography. Soundings
       64:52–74.
Hazan, Haim
1980   The Limbo People: A Study of the Constitution of the Time Universe
       among the Aged. London: Routledge & Kegan Paul.
1982   Aging—from course to cycle: Temporal transformations in old age.
       Unpublished manuscript.
Huntington, Richard, and Peter Metcalf
1979   Celebrations of Death: The Anthropology of Mortuary Ritual. Cam-
       bridge: Cambridge University Press.
Jung, C. G.
1959   The Archetypes of the Collective Unconscious. Vol. 9, pt. 1 of The
       Collected Works of C. G. Jung. Princeton: Princeton University Press.
Lansing, J. Stephen
1980   Circles of time. Parabola 5(1):34–37. Special issue.
Lex, Barbara W.
1979   The Neurobiology of Ritual Trance. *In* The Spectrum of Ritual: A
       Biogenetic Structual Analysis, ed. Eugene G. D'Aquili et al., pp.
       117–51. New York: Columbia University Press.
Lifton, Robert Jay
1967   Death in Life: Survivors of Hiroshima. New York: Simon & Schuster.
Mendilow, Adam A.
1952   Time and Experience. London: Peter Nevill.
Myerhoff, Barbara
1980   Number Our Days. New York: Simon & Schuster.
1982   Life history among the elderly: Performance, visibility, and re-mem-
       bering. In A Crack in the Mirror: Reflexive Perspectives in Anthropol-
       ogy, ed. Jay Ruby, pp. 99–120. Philadelphia: University of Pennsyl-
       vania Press.

Neugarten, Bernice L.
1980   Acting one's age: New rules for old. Psychology Today (April).
Ortner, Sherry B.
1978   Sherpas through Their Rituals. Cambridge: Cambridge University Press.
Rickman, H. P.
1979   Wilhelm Dilthey, Selected Writings. Cambridge: Cambridge University Press.
Sheehy, Gail
1974   Passages: Predictable Crises of Adult Life. New York: Dutton.
Turner, Victor
1975   Dramas, Fields, and Metaphors: Symbolic Action in Human Society. Ithaca: Cornell University Press.
1977   The Ritual Process: Structure and Anti-Structure. Ithaca: Cornell University Press.
Van Gennep, Arnold
1908   The Rites of Passage. Trans. M. B.Vizedon and G. L. Caffee. Chicago: University of Chicago Press.

Contributors

CYNTHIA M. BEALL, a biological anthropologist at Case Western Reserve University, received her doctorate in 1976 from Pennsylvania State University. She has conducted fieldwork in the Peruvian Andes and the Nepalese Himalayas. She has recently edited a special issue of *Social Science and Medicine* (1982).

RONALD COHEN, a political anthropologist who has worked extensively in Africa, currently teaches at the University of Florida. Among his books are *The Kanuri of Bornu* (1967) and various co-edited volumes, including *Handbook of Method in Cultural Anthropology* (with Raoul Naroll, 1970) and *Origins of the State* (with Elman Service, 1978).

PHYLLIS DOLHINOW is a biological anthropologist at the University of California, Berkeley, specializing in primate studies. Her fieldwork includes studies of nonhuman primates in India, East Africa, South Africa, and Southeast Asia, with special emphasis on Indian langurs and rhesus monkeys. Since the early 1970s she has been studying the behavior of langurs in colony. Her publications include several edited volumes and numerous articles on primate behavor and development.

PENELOPE ECKERT received her Ph.D. in linguistics from Columbia University in 1978. Her initial work in sociolinguistics was based on field study of a dying dialect of Gascon, spoken in a small peasant community in the French Pyrenees. In 1979 she began to study the role of adolescent social categories in linguistic change with fieldwork in suburban high schools in the United States, and she is currently examining the spread of linguistic change through the adolescent population of the Detroit suburban area. She recently completed a monograph on adolescent social categories titled "Adolescent Social Class."

NANCY FONER is an associate professor of anthropology at the State University of New York, Purchase. She graduated from Brandeis University and received her Ph.D. from the University of Chicago. She has done fieldwork in rural Jamaica (1968–69) and among Jamaican migrants in London (1973) and New York (1982). Her publications include *Status and Power in Rural Jamaica: A Study of Educational and Political Change* (1973), *Jamaica Farewell: Jamaican Migrants in London* (1978), and *Ages in Conflict: A Cross-Cultural Perspective on Inequality between Old and Young* (1984).

MEYER FORTES, William Wyse Professor of Social Anthropology, emeritus, at the University of Cambridge, has been one of the most influential figures in modern social anthropology. Following studies with Bronislaw Malinowski and Charles Seligman after receiving his doctorate in psychology from London, Fortes began his fieldwork in West Africa. His publications include *African Political Systems (co-edited with E. E. Evans-Pritchard, 1940), The Dynamics of Clanship among the Tallensi* (1945), *The Web of Kinship among the Tallensi* (1949), and *Kinship and the Social Order* (1969). Meyer Fortes died in 1983, shortly after completing his chapter for this volume.

RHODA HALPERIN received her Ph.D. in anthropology from Brandeis University. She is associate professor of anthropology and assistant clinical professor of family medicine, University of Cincinnati. She has edited and authored books and articles in economic anthropology, the political economy of peasants, and medical behavioral science, including *Peasant Livelihood: Studies in Economic Anthropology and Cultural Ecology,* which she co-edited with James Dow (1977).

EUGENE A. HAMMEL is a social anthropologist at the University of California, with interests in demography, analytic methodology, and computer use. He has done fieldwork in Peru, Mexico, Yugoslavia, and Greece, much of it focused on the effects of industrialization on kinship and household systems. His recent work has dealt with the historical demography of the Balkans and the use of computer micro-simulation to build models of demographic and social structure.

JENNIE KEITH received her Ph.D. in anthropology from North-western University in 1968. She is Professor of Anthropology at Swarthmore College. She has done fieldwork in France and in the United States on age groups and age differentiation. Major publications include *Old People, New Lives: Community Creation in a Retirement Residence* (1977) and *Old People as People: Social and Cultural Influences on Aging and Old Age* (1982). She is codirector (with Christine Fry) of Project A.G.E. at Swarthmore, a cross-cultural study of community factors that affect well-being in old age.

DAVID I. KERTZER is a social anthropologist at Bowdoin College who has worked primarily in Italy. His interests include age, historical demography, and the interrelationship of politics and religion. Among his other books are *Comrades and Christians* (1980), *Family Life in Central Italy* (1984), and, coedited with Michael Kenny, *Urban Life in Mediterranean Europe* (1983).

DAVID MAYBURY-LEWIS, a social anthropologist at Harvard University, has conducted extensive research among the Gê peoples of Central Brazil. He has been especially interested in kinship and anthropological theory, and has been active in attempts to protect indigenous peoples and cultures in South America and elsewhere. His books include *Akwe-Shavante Society* (1967), *The Savage and the Innocent* (1967), and an edited volume, *Dialectical Societies* (1979).

BARBARA MYERHOFF received her Ph.D. in anthropology from the University of California, Los Angeles, in 1968. She is professor of anthropology at the University of Southern California. She has done research in Latin America and in the United States on ritual, myth, ethnicity, and old age. Her major publications include *The Peyote Hunt* (1976), *Life's Career: Aging* (1978, with Andrei Simic), and *Number Our Days* (1980), the basis of an award-winning film and of a play.

ÁKOS ÖSTÖR, who studied history at Melbourne University and anthropology at the University of Chicago, has conducted fieldwork in India and Sudan. He is author of *The Play of the Gods* (1980), *Europeans and Islanders in the Western Pacific 1520–1840*, and *Deities, Ritualists, Merchants, and Revolutionaries* (1983); coauthor (with Lina Fruzzetti) of *Kinship and Ritual in Bengal* (1983); and coeditor (with

Lina Fruzzetti and Steve Barnett) of *Concept of Person: Kinship, Caste, and Marriage in India* (1982). He has taught at the University of Minnesota, Khartoum University, Harvard University, and Bowdoin College.

ANDREA SANKAR received her Ph.D. in anthropology from the University of Michigan. She conducted fieldwork in 1975–76 in Hong Kong and in 1980–81 in San Francisco. In 1979–81 she was a fellow at the Medical Anthropology Program, University of California, San Francisco. Currently she is a postdoctoral fellow of the National Institute on Aging at the Institute of Gerontology, University of Michigan. She has published various articles on aging and health in Hong Kong and the United States.

Index

Library of Congress Cataloging in Publication Data
Main entry under title:

Age and anthropological theory.

   Includes index.
   1. Aged—Addresses, essays, lectures. 2. Aging—
Addresses, essays, lectures. 3. Anthropology—Philosophy—Addresses, essays, lectures. I. Kertzer, David I.,
1948–   . II. Keith, Jennie.
GN485.A33 1984   305.2′6   83-21060
ISBN 0-8014-1567-5